W0225745

# New Developments in Antirheumatic Therapy

INFLAMMATION AND DRUG THERAPY SERIES
VOLUME III

# New Developments in Antirheumatic Therapy

Edited by

**KD Rainsford**
Department of Biomedical Sciences
McMaster University Faculty of Health
Sciences
Hamilton, Ontario
Canada

**GP Velo**
Institute of Pharmacology
University of Verona
Italy

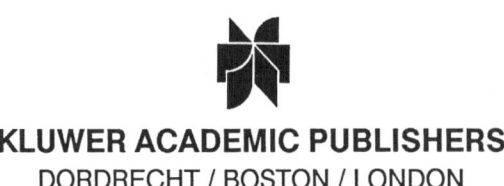

**KLUWER ACADEMIC PUBLISHERS**
DORDRECHT / BOSTON / LONDON

**Distributors**

*For the United States and Canada:* Kluwer Academic Publishers,
PO Box 358, Accord Station, Hingham, MA 02018-0358, USA
*For all other countries*: Kluwer Academic Publishers Group,
Distribution Center, PO Box 322, 3300 AH Dordrecht, The
Netherlands

**British Library Cataloguing in Publication Data**

New developments in antirheumatic therapy.
  1. Man. Joints. Arthritis & rheumatic diseases.
Therapy
  I. Rainsford, K.D. (Kim D.), *1941–* II. Velo, G.P. (Giampaolo)
*1943–* III. Series
  616.7'206

ISBN-13: 978-94-010-7056-0       e-ISBN-13: 978-94-009-1253-3

DOI: 10.1007/978-94-009-1253-3

**Copyright**

Published in the United Kingdom by Kluwer Academic Publishers,
PO Box 55, Lancaster, UK.

Kluwer Academic Publishers BV incorporates the publishing
programmes of D. Reidel, Martinus Nijhoff, Dr W. Junk and
MTP Press.

# Contents

# Preface

At present we may be at the cross-roads in the therapeutic approaches we have for the treatment of the 100 or more rheumatic conditions. This is because we now recognise that although some advances have been made with the development of a large range of non-steroidal and steroidal drugs during the past two decades or so, we now recognise that many, if not all, of these have rather limited effects on many of the disease processes which underlie the manifestations of the various rheumatic states. Advances in molecular biology in the past 5–10 years have enabled these tools to be applied extensively for developing further our understanding of the rheumatic disease processes. In some cases these molecular tools (e.g. γ-interferon, interleukin-2, T-cell antibodies) have been directly employed as therapies themselves. While the outcome from trials with such agents in rheumatoid arthritis in particular has not been as would have been hoped, these results as with cyclosporin A and low-dose methotrexate in the therapy of rheumatoid arthritis have given us important indications for the approach employing what are generally described as "immunomodulators" to control this disease. But this may not be the same type of approach which is desirable for all types of rheumatic conditions. Indeed, even the way which the present range of drugs and other therapies are applied may not be the most effective and safe means of treating different types of arthritic conditions.

Thus, it was considered that the time is appropriate to review what we understand about the current range of therapies; what basic developments are occurring in the search for the newer, more specific and more effective agents; and what progress has been made in the understanding of the disease processes which can give clues or leads for future therapeutic approaches. While it may be considered that the coverage of some areas may be limited because of the size limitations necessary for such a book, it should be pointed out that further consideration is being given in some newly emerging approaches in the fields of, for example, neuro-inflammation, the broader range of cytokines other than interleukin-1, and the non-articular rheumatic conditions in companion volumes which are currently in preparation.

Special thanks are given to the valued efforts of the contributors, Dr Peter Clarke (Publishing Director, Kluwer Academic Publishers) and Mrs Veronica Rainsford-Koechli for her help in proof-reading the manuscripts.

*K D Rainsford*
*Hamilton, Ontario, Canada*
*February 1989*

# List of Contributors

**M.E.J. BILLINGHAM**
Lilly Research Centre
Eli Lilly and Co.
Windlesham, Surrey GU20 6PH
UK

**M.L. BLIVEN**
Department of Immunology and
Infectious Diseases
Pfizer Central Research
Groton, CT 06340
USA

**J. CHANG**
Immunopharmacology Subdivision
Wyeth-Ayerst Research Inc.
CN 8000
Princeton, NY 08543-8000
USA

**A. CONFORTI**
Istituto di Farmacologia
Università di Verona
Policlinico Borgo Roma
37134 Verona
Italy

**A.J. COYLE**
Department of Pharmacology
King's College
University of London
Chelsea Campus, Manresa Road
London SW3
UK

**C.W. DENKO**
Departments of Rheumatology and
Medicine
Case Western Reserve University
Cleveland, OH 44106
USA

**D.R. HAYNES**
Department of Pathology
University of Adelaide
GPO Box 498
South Australia 5001
Australia

**B.L. HAZLEMAN**
Rheumatology Research Unit
Addenbrooke's Hospital
Hills Road
Cambridge CB2 2QQ
UK

**A.S.HEIMAN**
Center for Anti-inflammatory Research
College of Pharmacy
Florida A&M University
Tallahasee, FL 32307
USA

**I.M. HUNNEYBALL**
The Boots Company plc
Nottingham NG2 3AA
UK

**H.J. LEE**
Center for Anti-inflammatory Research
College of Pharmacy
Florida A&M University
Tallahasee, FL 32307
USA

**L.A. MARSHALL**
Immunopharmacology Subdivision
Wyeth-Ayerst Research Inc.
CN 8000
Princeton, NY 08543-8000
USA

**E.D. MOYER**
KabiVitrum Inc
1311 Harbor Bay Parkway
Alameda, CA94501
USA

**P. NASH**
Rheumatology Research Unit
Addenbrooke's Hospital
Hills Road
Cambridge CB2 2QQ
UK

**I.G. OTTERNESS**
Department of Immunology and
Infectious Diseases
Pfizer Central Research
Groton, CT 06340
USA

**C.P. PAGE**
Department of Pharmacology
King's College
University of London
Chelsea Campus, Manresa Road
London SW3
UK

**A.L. PARKE**
Department of Biochemistry
University of Surrey
Guildford GU2 5XH
Surrey
UK

**D.V. PARKE**
Department of Biochemistry
University of Surrey
Guildford
Surrey GU2 5XH
UK

**M.C. POWANDA**
Letterman Army Institute of Research
Presidio
San Francisco, CA 94129
USA

**K.D. RAINSFORD**
Department of Biomedical Sciences
McMaster University Faculty of Health
Sciences
Hamilton, Ontario
Canada L8N 3Z5

**A.M. SYMONS**
Department of Biochemistry
University of Surrey
Guildford
Surrey GU2 5XH
UK

**I.B. TARAPOREWALA**
Center for Anti-inflammatory Research
College of Pharmacy
Florida A&M University
Tallahasee, FL 32307
USA

**F.M. VERONESE**
Dipartimento di Scienze Farmaceutiche
Centro di Chimica del Farmaco e dei
Prodotti Biologicamente Attivi del CNR
Università di Padova
Padova
Italy

**G.P. VELO**
Istituto di Farmacologia
Università di Verona
Policlinico Borgo Roma
37134 Verona
Italy

**M.W. WHITEHOSE**
Department of Pathology
University of Adelaide
GPO Box 498
South Australia 5001
Australia

# 1
# Recent developments in antirheumatic therapy

**P. Nash and B.L. Hazleman**
Rheumatology Research Unit
Addenbrooke's Hospital
Hills Road, Cambridge CB2 2QQ

## I. INTRODUCTION

This chapter will discuss recent developments in anti-rheumatic therapy and serve as an introduction to later chapters in which a variety of novel therapeutic approaches will be discussed in more detail, including topics from newer avenues of immunomodulation to alternative methods of drug delivery.

In any discussion of the therapy of rheumatic disease the important role of the physical therapies, i.e. physiotherapy and occupational therapy, in patient management, should not be underemphasized. However, this review will deal specifically with pharmacological, immunotherapeutic and radio-therapeutic approaches to therapy and concentrate on those developments that have occurred in established as well as experimental areas of treatment. Wherever possible the results of human clinical trials will be described and experiences detailed to indicate the efficacy of the new developments and trends in current clinical practice.

## II. NON-STEROIDAL ANTI-INFLAMMATORY DRUGS (NSAIDs)

Some of the newer NSAIDs under evaluation seek 'disease modifying' activity in addition to their anti-inflammatory action whilst striving to improve the adverse effect profile common in classical agents in this group. Those with longer plasma half-lives and 'slow release' preparations are becoming popular in attempts to improve patient compliance. Response or lack of it to one agent does not predict response to another. Tailoring drug efficacy, e.g. by the choice of drug and titrating the dosage is therapeutically worthwhile. Interpatient variation in response to NSAIDs has been discussed at length

*New Developments in Antirheumatic Therapy.* Rainsford, KD and Velo, GP (eds),
Inflammation and Drug Therapy Series, Volume III.

recently[1]. Actions and side effects of these agents which are currently being examined will be discussed.

## III. CARTILAGE PROTECTION

Coke, in 1967, first raised the issue of the possible detrimental effect of long-term NSAID usage upon articular cartilage[2]. A number of reports followed suggesting a causal role for these agents, particularly the salicylates and indomethacin, in accelerating destructive arthropathy, particularly that affecting both femoral and acetabular components of the hip joint ('analgesic hip'). This is characterized radiographically by marked bone attrition, paucity of osteophytes, frequent protrusio acetabuli, and disproportionate retention of joint space[3-5]. These studies, predominantly retrospective, and more recent work supported by *in vitro* studies using cartilage explants or isolated chrondrocytes from animal species, have in the main, shown a dose-dependent suppression of sulphated glycosaminoglycan synthesis[6-8], reduced fracture healing[9], and inhibition of bone remodelling[10]. Other work suggests that some NSAIDs have affects totally independent of their ability to inhibit prostaglandin synthesis. For example, some authors have shown that NSAIDs can inhibit superoxide anion production from polymorphs and macrophages, reduce the production of free oxygen radicals important in the destructive arthritic process, and that chondrocyte subcellular ultrastructure can be altered by NSAIDs[11-12]. Of clinical relevance is the demonstration that these effects are not universal to all of these agents suggesting, theoretically an advantage of some agents over others.

**Table 1** Effects of NSAIDs on proteoglycan synthesis[14]

| Suppression | Enhancement |
| --- | --- |
| fenoprofen | benoxaprofen |
| flufenamic acid | diclofenac |
| ibuprofen | piroxicam |
| indomethacin | sulindac |
| isoxicam | tiaprofenic acid |
| phenylbutazone | |
| salicylates | |
| tolmetin | |

**Polymorph superoxide radical production**

| Inhibition | | No effect |
| --- | --- | --- |
| piroxicam | diclofenac | aspirin |
| chloroquine | naproxen | ibuprofen |
| azapropazone | sulindac | flurbiprofen |

In a reappraisal of the 'analgesic hip', Doherty et al.[13] showed that NSAIDs could not be incriminated in the development of this form of arthropathy in their patients. They also found a striking resemblance to apatite-associated destructive arthritis in their subjects with evidence that a crystal related disease process was occurring in other joints. Nevertheless, evidence continues to accumulate that various NSAIDs adversely affect the metabolism of cartilage. Table 1 outlines the effects of a variety of NSAIDs on cartilage metabolism but caution needs to be exercised in directly extrapolating from in vitro studies and those from animal models to man. Further work is required before prescribing recommendations can be made.

## IV.  MUCOSAL GASTROPROTECTION AND RELATED GASTROINTESTINAL ISSUES

Gastrointestinal adverse effects of NSAIDs remain the biggest drawback to their usage. Renal effects, including deterioration in creatinine clearance, hyperkalaemia and interstitial nephritis are well recognized and these effects have been reviewed recently[15]. Similarly, recent reviews[16] detail less common side-effects of therapy with these drugs. The gastrointestinal tract of patients with rheumatic diseases is receiving increasing attention. The relationship between peptic ulcer disease (PUD) and NSAID therapy is complicated. Thus, endoscopic studies of patients under treatment have been hampered by a lack of adequate control subjects. This is particularly relevant in diseases that produce chronic stress and pain both of which may contribute to a higher incidence of PUD in this patient population regardless of therapy.

Patients with rheumatoid arthritis (RA) have a three to four times higher incidence of PUD than the general population. Malone et al. showed a high incidence of upper GI ulcers and lesions. In RA this was 15%, whereas in osteoarthritis it was 18%. Similar PUD rates were evident in patients with RA and osteoarthritis when the history of the intake of drugs, smoking and alcohol consumption was taken into account. A common factor, which was probably the NSAID therapy, was considered responsible[17]. Acute haemorrhage from peptic ulceration and perforated peptic ulcer, particularly in females over 65 years, has been significantly related to NSAID usage[18-20]. Armstrong and Blower[21], reviewed 235 consecutive patients with a life-threatening complication of PUD who either died or were admitted to hospital for surgery. They found 60% of patients were taking a NSAID and in 58.2% of these the first sign of PUD was a life-threatening complication. Nearly 80% of all ulcer related deaths occurred in patients taking anti-inflammatory medications. Similar findings have been reported by other workers[22-23].

Given this background, clinicians have looked at two major areas of therapeutic intervention.

1.    $H_2$-blockers are widely used for PUD and trials looking at their prophylactic use with NSAID are underway. In one study Davies *et al.*[24] maintained NSAID therapy for their patients with endoscopically proven PUD, and placed one group on placebo treatment and the other on cimetidine. At 6 weeks, ulcers had healed without significant difference in both placebo (60%) and cimetidine treated groups (69%). The inferences from this and other similar studies are:

      (a)    peptic ulceration can occur and resolve in patients on NSAID therapy unsuspected by the patient and treating physician; and

      (b)    reduction in gastric acid alone in the presence of continued NSAID usage does not appear to influence repair of the mucosal lesion.

2.    Mucosal 'cytoprotection' and the role of prostaglandins (PG) in maintaining gastro-duodenal mucosal integrity are currently receiving much attention. Gastroprotection is a more satisfactory term despite the former having wide usage. The E and I type prostaglandins can afford mucosal protection[25] by:

      (a)    'strengthening' the gastric mucosal barrier with a reduction in hydrogen ion back-diffusion;

      (b)    stimulating gastric and duodenal mucous and bicarbonate secretion;

      (c)    a role in controlling gastric mucosal blood flow; and

      (d)    stimulating the regeneration of superficial mucosa from mucosal basal cells.

There is conflicting data concerning levels of PGs in the gastric mucosa of patients with gastric ulceration. Both high and low levels have been found, but a PG deficiency state has been more convincingly shown in duodenal ulceration. It has been well demonstrated that endogenous gastric $PGE_2$ and 6-keto $PGF_1$ synthesis are almost totally inhibited by chronic NSAID therapy[26]. Subsequently, double-blind controlled trials of three PG analogues, misoprostol, enprostil and arbaprostil have been performed and their effectiveness in healing gastric and duodenal ulcers demonstrated. However, it appears that the doses required for ulcer healing are those required for antisecretory activity rather than the lower cytoprotective effects. These doses required for cytoprotective effects have been shown to prevent gastric mucosal damage and decrease gastrointestinal blood loss. However, large-scale placebo-controlled trials are needed to determine if gastro-duodenal damage caused by NSAIDs can be prevented. In addition, these studies need to determine whether or not NSAID anti-inflammatory efficacy is impaired by the concurrent administration of PGs and their analogues being used for mucosal gastroprotection.

4

Other issues gaining attention recently include the increasing evidence that NSAID ingestion may affect small and large intestinal mucosal integrity and function in man. Studies have shown small bowel and colonic perforations and/or haemorrhage and the development of small bowel strictures significantly associated with NSAIDs usage. The effect has been shown to be due to increased intestinal permeability that is systemically mediated and related to potency of NSAIDs inhibition of cyclo-oxygenase. Increased permeability is followed, in animal models, by macroscopic inflammation probably representing bacterial mucosal invasion[27]. $PGE_2$ and broad spectrum antibiotics have been shown to modestly reduce this effect. Further work examining the effects of more stable, longer acting PG analogues is required.

Another issue that requires resolution is the role of *Campylobacter pyloridis* (CP) infection in PUD in patients with rheumatic diseases. This organism is found colonising the gastric antrum in 90–100% of patients with duodenal ulceration, 70% of patients with gastric ulceration, and half of the patients with non-ulcer dyspepsia[28]. When present this organism is invariably associated with histological evidence of gastritis. Further, lower relapse rates have been shown in patients with duodenal ulceration treated with tri-potassium bismuth (which eradicates CP) when compared with $H_2$-blockers (which are ineffective against CP)[29]. If CP infection can be shown to be an important aetiological agent in PUD and in patients with rheumatic diseases, independent of NSAID therapy, effective anti inflammatory drugs need not be withheld, or at least a theoretical advantage could be argued for a choice of anti-ulcer therapy having inhibitory effects on CP, e.g. tri-potassium bismuth, whilst continuing NSAID treatment.

Finally unexpected benefits from NSAID therapy have been recently demonstrated. With the exception of indomethacin, NSAID therapy may decrease the development of cataracts[30] and Inman *et al.* has found that the risk of acute myocardial infarction is 30–80% less during, as compared with after the use of NSAID therapy[31]. As these two conditions contribute significantly to the morbidity and mortality in the community these benefits, if further substantiated may be of importance.

## V.  DISEASE REMITTING ANTI-RHEUMATIC THERAPY

### (1)  Established drugs

There has been a resurgence of interest in a number of well established medications in the treatments of rheumatic disease, particularly sulphasalazine (SAS) and methotrexate (MTX). These drugs are used after an adequate trial of first-line drug therapy fails to relieve symptoms satisfactorily. As the alternative name of slow-acting would suggest, such drugs are thought to have an influence on the underlying disease process, though they do take several weeks or months to exert this effect. These drugs: (a) decrease pain,

5

morning stiffness and joint swelling; (b) effect an associated increase in grip strength and an increase in a feeling of well-being; (c) when elevated, the ESR or C-reactive protein should fall and the haemoglobin should rise; (d) should create a fall in the titre of rheumatoid factor, and the rate of bony erosion visible on radiographs may be slowed.

These drugs will reduce disease activity, but will not abolish symptoms and signs altogether. Relapse will occur if the drug is discontinued. Unfortunately, patients whose symptoms and signs have been well controlled on the drugs may relapse despite continuing their therapy. The mechanism of this late relapse is unexplained. Occasionally a beneficial effect can be regained by increasing the dose of the drug.

The toxicity of these drugs is such that regular monitoring is required. In part, inappropriate use without proper monitoring has contributed to a reputation for toxicity which is perhaps unjustified. Nevertheless less than 20% of patients will be taking one drug for more than four years. The drop out rate for toxicity or inefficacy with time is still high.

There is no clear evidence that any of these drugs influence the rate of joint damage in RA. The reason that X-ray changes have assumed such prominence in assessment is because the radiological abnormalities are thought to closely reflect the degree of joint damage. In particular emphasis is placed on erosive damage, because this is the most specific change for RA; however, cartilage loss may be equally important.

In general, active RA is more likely to be associated with marked X-ray progression than less severe disease, but in any one patient it is not possible to predict whether or not they will show continuing joint damage based on the acute-phase response. There is some evidence to suggest that patients whose disease activity is reduced by disease modifying drugs will have less X-ray progression in the second six months of therapy when therapy is continued for 12 months or more[32]. It does suggest that there is an indirect relationship between joint damage and the acute-phase response.

## (2)  Sulphasalazine

An extensive literature now documents the usefulness of SAS in RA. Situnayake et al.[33] have reviewed their experience with 317 patients treated with SAS and compared its use with D-penicillamine (163 patients) and intramuscular gold (210 patients). Table 2 lists the pertinent findings at 5 years follow-up suggesting that SAS was less efficacious than the comparable agents, but well tolerated over long periods with fewer adverse effects leading to withdrawal. Particularly noticeable was the lower incidence of serious adverse effects.

The benefits of SAS treatment for the peripheral arthritis of patients with HLA B27 associated spondyloarthropathies has been documented[34]. Recent studies suggest similar efficacy in the spondylitis of these patients. Dougados et al. studied 60 patients with active ankylosing spondylitis in a

6

double blind placebo controlled trial using 2 g/day SAS for 6 months. Efficacy was considered to be 'good' or 'very good' in 50% of the patients treated (16% withdrew because of gastrointestinal intolerance and 7% because of treatment failure). There were significant improvements reflected in functional index and reduction in the consumption of NSAID requirements. Further work is needed to look at the effects of therapy upon bowel flora, intestinal permeability and on the effect upon ankylosis.

## (3)  Methotrexate

Methotrexate in a low dose, once-per-week regimen (7.5–15 mg/week) is being increasingly used in unresponsive cases of RA, psoriatic arthritis and chronic Reiter's disease. The use and action of this drug has been reviewed at length recently[36-38]. The problem of long-term methotrexate hepatoxicity and its optimal management still requires resolution.

Table 2

| Drug | Gold (%) | D-Penicillamine (%) | SAS (%) |
|---|---|---|---|
| Treatment termination | | | |
| –   all reasons | 92.0 | 83.0 | 81.0 |
| –   inefficacy | 29.5 | 38.1 | 41.2 |
| Adverse effects (withdrawal) | | | |
| –   all | 57.0 | 41.2 | 37.0 |
| –   serious | 17.4 | 12.3 | 1.6 |

## (4)  Methylprednisolone pulse therapy

Infusion of a pulse dose of methylprednisolone have been used at the time of introduction of a disease remitting agent in patients with RA to see if this could bridge the gap between commencement of therapy and delayed response to these drugs. Pulse intravenous therapy with 1 g methylprednisolone daily for three days reduces the clinical signs of inflammation, ESR and C-reactive protein with improvement lasting 3–6 weeks[39]. Neumann et al.[40] compared pulse methylprednisolone alone, the combination of methylprednisolone and D-penicillamine, methylprednisolone and sulphsalazine, and contrasted this with D-penicillamine or SAS alone. They found that the addition of pulse methylprednisolone was well tolerated and accelerated the response to additional therapy by 6 weeks. However, Hansen et al.[41] and Bijlsma et al.[42] performed similar studies in patients with active RA. They were unable to show any benefit from intravenous pulse methylprednisolone, apart from the short-lived anti-inflammatory response previously described when they used pulse methylprednisolone with gold, D-penicillamine or azathioprine. As this form of therapy has been occasionally associated with

7

Table 3 Combination chemotherapy

| Author | Patient No. | Study type | Study duration | Regimen | Results | Comments |
|---|---|---|---|---|---|---|
| Sharp et al.[48] | 56 | Double blind placebo controlled | 2 years | D-Pen + OHCHL<br>D-Pen + placebo<br>OHCHL + placebo | No significant differences between groups | Inadequate drug doses high withdrawals for non-toxicity reasons |
| Bitter et al.[49] | 71 | Open | 5 years | (1) IMI Gold alone<br>+ Levamisole<br>+ Chloramb.<br>+ D-Pen<br>(2) D-Pen alone<br>+ Levamisole<br>+ Chloramb. | Sig. improvement Joint score not ESR (Gold comb. & D-Pen + Levamisole) Remission Gold combinations 26.6% D-Pen 12% Gold + D-Pen effective | Toxicity Gold combs / D-Pen combs. Early 6.7% / 0%. Late 13.4% / 6%. Leading to withdrawal 30.0% / 18% |
| Lewis & Hazleman et al.[50] | 70 | Open | 7 years | Azathioprine (5 mg/kg/day) + Gold IMI (50 mg) | Well tolerated No increase in malignancy | Withdrawal of azathioprine led to increased disease activity |
| Gibson et al.[51] | 72 | Single blind | 1 year | D-Pen + OCHCL and each alone | Significant improvement joint score Response same by 12 months | Toxicity and withdrawal higher in combination group |
| Bunch et al.[52] | 56 | Placebo controlled double blind | 2 years | D-Pen + OCHCL and each alone | D-Pen alone better than combination | Toxicity similar all groups |

8

**Table 3 Combination chemotherapy (continued)**

| Author | Patient No. | Study type | Study duration | Regimen | Results | Comments |
|---|---|---|---|---|---|---|
| MacKenzie et al.[53] | 20 | Open | Mean 14.7 months | Methotrexate (0.117 mg/kg/wk) mean dose Azathioprine (1.43 mg/kg/day) mean dose | Improvement 50% – morning stiffness, ESR, grip strength and joint count | Minor toxicity, previously failed gold, hydroxychloroquine, methotrexate or azathioprine alone |
| Tiliakos et al.[54] | 12 | Open | 16–25 months | Hydroxychloroquine 400 mg/day Cyclophosphamide 25 mg/day Methotrexate 5 mg/week | 50–90% improvement grip strength, joint pain/ swelling ESR | 7 patients recorticated erosions 45–60 days to onset of response plateau by 6–8 months |
| Dawes et al.[55] | 101 | Double blind | 12 months | Gold IMI 50 mg with placebo or hydroxychloroquine 450 mg/day | Rate of response accelerated in active group. Less disease activity at 12 months active group | Withdrawals from adverse effects 18 (active) 10 (placebo) |
| Taggart et al.[56] | 30 | Open | 6 months | Sulphasalazine vs sulphasalazine + D-penicillamine | Disease activity including global Score, ESR and CRP 50% SAS alone 90% SAS + D-Pen | Onset with 4–8 weeks quicker response than either SAS or D-Pen alone Combination more adverse effects – 50% withdrawals before 6 months (2 thrombocytopenia) |

9

sudden death, seizures, arrhythmias and avascular necrosis, this treatment modality has a questionable place in therapy in RA[62-64].

Pulse methylprednisolone therapy has an established role in the management of severe systemic lupus erythematosis (SLE), particularly in complicated lupus nephritis[46].

## VI. COMBINATION CHEMOTHERAPY

Studies in RA have been undertaken using combination chemotherapy regimens similar to those used for haematological malignancies. These have resulted as a consequence of dissatisfaction with individual disease-remitting drugs and the similarities between the locally invasive, destructive, predominantly lymphocytic synovial infiltration seen in chronic arthritis and the histology of malignant lymphoproliferative disorders.

In 1982, McCarty and Carrera[47] treated 17 patients with progressive erosive seropositive RA refractory to conventional therapy, with cyclophosphamide (mean daily dose 38.5 mg/day), azathioprine (mean 55 mg/day) and hydroxychloroquine (mean 220 mg/day). These low doses were chosen to minimise toxic effects. Five patients achieved complete remission, nine of seventeen partial remission and three patients did not respond. Prednisolone therapy could be reduced or ceased in a significant number of patients and healing of erosions occurred in a similar number. Progressive disease occurred in three patients.

Spurred on by these results a number of other combinations have been tried and these are tabulated in Table 3. This approach warrants further intensive investigation. It will be important in these studies to establish a number of fundamental characteristics of both T and B cell arms of the immune response. The time sequence for macrophage and T and B cell subset turnover (and their immunoglobulin and lymphokine products), analogous to the phases of the cell-cycle, require clear elucidation so that specifically active and cell-cycle targeted chemotherapy can be developed to produce remission-inducing and then maintenance regimes of treatment.

## VII. IMMUNOMODULATION

A number of novel strategies to modulate the immune system to provide specific and limited immunosuppression in those patients with intractable rheumatic disease, particularly RA and SLE, have been under intensive investigation. Advances in the delineation of defects in cell mediated immunity have led to avenues of therapeutic intervention aimed particularly at the T cell arm of the immune response, e.g. anti-T cell monoclonal antibodies. Table 4 lists some of these approaches.

**Table 4 Strategies to modulate the immune system**

---

Cyclosporin A
Immune tolerance inducers, e.g. to autoantibodies
Interferons
Intraarticular autologous activated T suppressor cells
Lymphokines, e.g. IL-2 with activated killer cells
Monoclonal Antibodies, e.g. to T cell subsets, Interleukin (IL) 2 receptors, Ia antigens
Thoracic duct drainage/lympho/plasmapheresis
Thymic hormones – nonathymulin, thymopoietin pentapeptide, thymosin-1
Total nodal irradiation

---

## VIII. CYCLOSPORIN A

This agent, which inhibits both humoral and cell mediated immunity by a specific and reversible action on T-cells (suppression of activating message so that lymphokine production, e.g. I-L2 is reduced to subnormal levels[57] has featured in several clinical trials. Table 5 outlines a number of clinical trials using cyclosporin A in RA.

Trials of cyclosporin A (CyA) in RA show that more than 3 mg/kg/day is required for efficacy whilst doses above 5 mg/kg/day (plasma troughs > 500 ng/ml) are associated with significant toxicity particularly nephrotoxicity. This toxic effect of cyclosporin A is dose dependent, exacerbated by NSAIDs and can be reduced or prevented by the administration of synthetic pros-taglandins[64]. However, Ruffel et al. have demonstrated loss of immuno-suppression along with reduced nephrotoxicity when subcutaneous prostaglandin $E_2$ was administered with cyclosporin A. They showed the mechanism to be related to impaired CyA absorption with peak plasma levels being reduced by a factor of > 3[65].

Table 6 tabulates the small published experience of the treatment of SLE patients with cyclosporin. These patients seem better able to tolerate higher doses of CyA with less nephrotoxicity, even in the presence of lupus nephritis, in comparison with treated RA patients. Patient numbers are small but the results look promising in refractory and severe disease.

## IX. TOTAL LYMPHOID IRRADIATION (TLI)

Total lymphoid irradiation has been tried in intractable RA based upon the premise that the proliferative synovitis of this disease may respond in a similar fashion to the neoplastic lymphoid infiltrate of Hodgkin's disease. Similar trials have used total lymphoid irradiation in patients suffering from SLE[71] as well as in an anecdotal report of a patient with dermato-poly-myositis[72].

The predominant chronic effect of total lymphoid irradiation on im-mune function has been shown to be the selective depletion of OKT4 (hel-per) T lymphocytes with the generation of large immature radioresistant and antigen-nonspecific suppressor cells which result in defective cellular and

Table 5 Cyclosporin A in rheumatoid arthritis

| Author | Patient No. | Study type | Study duration | Regimen | Results | Comments |
|---|---|---|---|---|---|---|
| van Rijthoven et al.[58] | 36 | Placebo controlled double blind | 6 months | 10 mg/kg/day for 2 months 7.5 mg/kg/day for 2 months 5.0 mg/kg/day for 2 months | Significant improvement-Ritchie score and joint index. No improvement ESR or titre, rheumatoid factor. Radiological progression | Significant partially irreversible increase in creatinine. All patients gastrointestinal adverse effects. 50% drop-out (half gastrointestinal) |
| Weinblatt et al.[59] | 10 | Open | 6 months | 6 mg/kg/day | Significant improvement joint pain, joint swelling and morning stiffness by 12 wks. No remission. | 40% significant renal dysfunction Follow-up study same patient using 3 mg/kg/day showed loss of efficacy with retained toxicity |
| Dougados et al.[60] | 12 | Open | 12 months | 5 mg/kg/day | Significant improvement. Clinical assessments Reduction in prednisolone No decrease ESR/Rh factor | Onset efficacy 1 month and maintained 12 months. 50% increase creatinine 50% drop-out |
| Modhok et al.[61] | 20 | | | 5 mg/kg/day | Significant improvement Joint index and ESR | Dose dependent revesible decrease of renal function |
| Forre et al.[62] | 24 | Open controlled | 6 months | 10 mg/kg/day | Significant improvement Clinical and lab. parameters (CRP, RhF) | Comparison with aza-thioprine in favour of cyclosporin |
| Yocum et al.[63] | 31 | Double blind | 6 months | 10 mg/kg/day or 1 mg/kg/day | Significant improvement. Clinical assessment high dose not low dose. | Significant nephrotoxicity. 3 withdrawals each group from adverse effects 25% low dose group drop-outs because uncontrolled disease |

12

Table 6 Cyclosporin A in SLE

| Author | Patient No. | Study type | Study duration | Regimen | Results | Comments |
|---|---|---|---|---|---|---|
| Miescher et al.[66] | 20 | Open | | 5 mg/kg/day | 17/20 improved including proteinuria | Response more favourable with steroids Reductions in titres d.s. DNA and C3d found |
| Bambauer et al.[67] | 7 | Open | 6 months | 7–15 plasma exchange + 2.5 mg/kg/day (through 200 mg/ml) | 6/7 no new attacks | 4 cystitis Able to decrease methylprednisolone dose |
| Deteix et al.[68] | 4 | Open | 8–26 months | 9 mg/kg/day | Significant improvement. Reductions d.s. DNA titres. Normalized complement | Able to reduce prednisolone |
| Halloran et al.[69] | 7 | Open | | 8 mg/kg/day | 5/7 no benefit | 4 deaths – 2 from sepsis |
| Fentgren et al.[70] | 12 | Open | 6 months | 5–10mg/kg x 5 then 5 mg/kg x 7 | 7/8 improvement with relapse if dose 3 mg/kg/day. Reduction in prednisolone requirements | 6/8 reversible nephrotoxicity and hypertension |

**Table 7 Total nodal irradiation in rheumatoid arthritis**

| Author | Patient No. | Study type | Study duration | Regimen | Results | Comments |
|---|---|---|---|---|---|---|
| Tanay et al.[74] | 32 | Open | 24 months | Total 2000 RAD | 75% improved by 1/4 20% required further immunosuppression to maintain improvement after 2 years | Peak improvements 6 months 4 deaths (include myocardial infarction) and rheumatoid lung disease with infection 13 infections. Most patients on prednisone |
| Crook et al.[75] | 6 | Open | 6 months | Total 150 cGy | Minimal effect | Well tolerated transient pancytopenias |
| Brahn et al.[76] | 12 | Open | 15–40 months | Total 3000 RAD | Improved joint score | 7 infections: 2 septic arthritic; 2 fatal; 2 cardiac deaths; 1 hypothyroid |
| Sherrer et al.[77] | 34 | Open | 32 months | Total 2000 RAD | Two thirds required subsequent treatment | 20% infective episodes + 50% zoster 4 deaths including rheumatic lung disease and myocardial infarction. Bone marrow toxicity 20% ceasing therapy |
| Nusslein et al.[78] | 11 | Open | 6–24 months | Mantle 150–200 RAD x 2–3 weeks + 2000 RAD infradiaphragm | Improvement by 6 months. Relapse by 24 months. No change ESR or titre rheumatoid factor | Amyloid with renal failure (2), cardiac arrest (1), septic arthritis (1) |
| Hanly et al. | 20 | Open | 10 months | Total 750 RAD vs Total 2000 RAD | 35% major reduction disease activity improvement peaked at 3–6 months | Efficacy of 750 RAD same as 2000 RAD |

humoral immune responses[73]. Table 7 contains a summary of experience with this treatment modality.

Review of experience with this treatment has highlighted a number of concerns, which may be summarized as follows:

(i)   Rheumatoid patients appear to be prone to serious infections throughout the period of follow-up; associated use of prednisone further complicates this issue.

(ii)  A number of deaths related to coronary artery disease and acceleration of rheumatoid lung disease suggest that coronary artery and alveolar endothelial damage may be implicated. Hodgkin's disease patients treated with total nodal irradiation have been shown to have accelerated coronary artery disease[80].

(iii) A significant proportion of patients relapse and require subsequent treatment by 2 years post therapy.

(iv)  Improvements in clinical parameters have not been accompanied by improvements in biochemical and haematological parameters as normally seen in disease-remittive therapy.

(v)   Oncological experience suggests an increased risk of malignancy following combined cytotoxic and radiotherapy[81]. A considerable percentage of intractable RA patients will receive cytotoxic therapy and follow-up to-date has been too short to exclude this potential problem with this form of therapy.

Although these studies have reported use of total dose of irradiation that have been in excess of that required to achieve an improvement, as Hanly *et al.* demonstrated when comparing 750 and 2000 RAD treatment regimes, the above concerns are sufficient to seriously question the use of this treatment modality in intractable RA.

## (1)  Interferons

Recombinant interferon-gamma has antiproliferative, antiviral and immunomodulatory activity in animal models. Low doses in RA produce a consistent increase in natural killer cell activity and HLA-DR expression. Studies by Emery *et al.* suggest that levels of interferon-gamma are raised in patients in disease remission[82]. Franchmont has also shown that in active RA peripheral blood mononuclear cells show significantly reduced interferon-gamma production[83]. Results of clinical trials in RA to date are tabulated in Table 8.

15

**Table 8 Interferon gamma in rheumatoid arthritis**

| Author | Patient No. | Study type | Study duration | Regimen | Results | Comments |
|---|---|---|---|---|---|---|
| Lemmel et al.[84] | 40 | Open Phase II | 3 weeks | Daily20 patients subcutaneous | No serious adverse 25% improvement pain and function | effects 50% non-responders 3 patients accelerated disease activity |
| Verbruggen et al.[85] | 26 | Double blind | 24 weeks | Subcutaneous 100 µg daily x 5 days then twice weekly | Significant improvement tender joint index | Minimal adverse effects favourable response in other measure not reaching statistical significance |
| Machold et al.[86] | 13 | Double blind | 16 weeks | | No significant difference active | Improvements in fibrinogen and thrombocytosis |
| Firestein et al.[87] | 12 | Open | 12–17 weeks | $1.3 \times 10^6$ units subcutaneous | 75% unchanged. Two patients 50% improvement, 1 flare leading to withdrawal | Minor adverse effects e.g. fever, rash 6 dose reductions because of fever and fatigue |
| Cannon et al.[88] | 105 | Double blind | 12 weeks | 100 µg | 11 patients disease flare (7 active group) 5 adverse effects (2 active group) | Placebo group large response mitigating significant differences |

16

## (2) Monoclonal antibodies

The potential for monoclonal antibodies to be utilized therapeutically is enormous and is as yet untapped. Approaches to therapy could include:

(a)    The use of antibodies that are cytotoxic to targeted cells, in combination with host complement or killer cells, e.g. recombinant human I-L2 with autologous lymphokine-activated killer cells have been tested in advance malignancy[89].

(b)    Conjugation of antibodies to a drug or isotope to deliver the agent specifically to targeted areas.

(c)    Antibodies that react with cell surface molecules mediating cellular proliferation.

(d)    Use of anti-idiotype antibodies to block auto-antibodies.

Some investigation along these lines has occurred in the fields of oncology and marrow transplantation[90].

In five models of autoimmune disease (experimental allergic encephalitis, myasthenia gravis, SLE-like syndrome of NZB/WF$_1$ mice, collagen arthritis and autoimmune thyroiditis) monoclonal antibodies against products of the I-a subregion of the major histocompatibility complex or against the L3/T4a molecule on helper/inducer T cells either prevent the development of clinical signs when given prior to auto-immunization) or reverse the ongoing disease[91].

Hazleman and colleagues[92] used Campath 1, a monoclonal Ab against T cells expressing I-L2 receptors in three intractable RA patients aiming for limited and specific immunosuppression that would spare resting T cells, lead to restricted cell lysis and potentially alter the immune response to allow conventional immunosuppressive agents a better chance of sustained effect. Using 25 mg Campath 1 in daily saline infusions over 10 days they were able to show symptomatic benefit lasting into the second month of follow-up but all patients subsequently relapsed. Further work is anticipated from this area of research.

## (3) Thymic hormones

Thymic hormones (e.g. thymosin-1, thymopoietin and nonathymulin) act predominantly on T cell maturation and differentiation and show a variety of biological effects. Thymopoietin has been shown to induce early T cell differentiation, including the regulation of cytotoxic lymphocyte precursor cells. Veys *et al.*[93] treated RA patients with thymopoietin pentapeptide (TP5), the pentapeptide was shown to retain the biological activity of thymopoietin. Thirty one patients were treated with placebo or TP5 (subcutaneous injections 1 mg, 10 mg or 50 mg, 3 per week) for 6 months but no statistically significant improvements were demonstrated despite important improvements

17

in individual patients and the absence of serious adverse effects. Two randomized double blind placebo-controlled trials in RA patients treated with nonathymulin (subcutaneous injections 1, 5 and 10 mg/day) found significant improvement in grip strength, Lee Index and global assessment as well as allowing a modest reduction in steroid consumption. The effect was maximal at 5 mg per day, and was associated with minimal toxicity which was interpreted as being the result of suppressor T cell stimulation, although immunological studies performed were contrary to this[94].

## (4) Other immunotherapeutic approaches

Other interesting immunotherapeutic approaches are briefly mentioned. Sutton et al. have been shown that synovial fluid T lymphocytes from active rheumatoid joints show defective suppressor T cell activity whilst the same patients' peripheral blood lymphocytes have intact function. Using a model diffusion chamber system analogous to a joint their results suggest that intra-articular injection with autologous peripheral blood lymphocytes may be of therapeutic benefit[95].

Bond and workers[96] have attempted to induce tolerance to DNA antigens in humans, in vivo, using DNA fragments bound to gamma globulins.

## XI. DISEASE REMITTING ANTI-RHEUMATIC THERAPY

A range of medications and approaches have been examined in trials in the search for new and improved agents with disease-remitting anti-rheumatic activity. Table 9 lists some of these agents. While results are preliminary, these experimental agents do not appear particularly promising. They do however, illustrate interesting directions in therapy presently under scrutiny.

**Table 9**

---

Captopril
Iron chelation
Isoprinosine
Neurotransmitter, e.g. regional intravenous guanethidine
Phenytoin
Sex hormones, e.g. nandrolone decanoate

---

## (5) Novel drugs

*Phenytoin*

Bobgrove et al. reported two patients with RA and one with psoriatic arthritis whose joint symptoms and ESR improved when phenytoin was given for concurrent epilepsy[97]. Phenytoin can inhibit collagenase[98], selectively decrease IgA and is mildly immunosuppressive[99]. Grindulis et al.[100] thus performed a pilot study of 18 patients with active RA treated with 300 mg phenytoin per day. They showed significant improvement in clinical score, articular index and visual analogue score, which persisted after 8 weeks off treatment but no improvement in laboratory markers of disease activity suggesting an anti-inflammatory effect alone. Richards et al., compared phenytoin and intramuscular gold in 60 patients and found phenytoin to have a less potent second line effect than gold but influenced laboratory indicators of disease activity more than clinical variables[101].

### Sex hormones

The majority of rheumatic diseasse have a marked female predominance. For example, SLE affects 10 females at childbearing age, for each male. However, the ratio falls to 3:1 after the age of 50 years. Sex hormone metabolism influences inflammation and autoimmunity and this factor has been examined in one recent study[102]. RA has been thought to improve in the presence of oestrogens whilst in SLE these hormones case a deterioration[103-4]. Androgen therapy in NZB/NZW murine SLE/models have been shown to afford significant improvements in both morbidity and mortality[105]. Sex hormones have been shown to affect lymphocyte subsets[106], induce specific lymphokines[107] and to induce receptors for thymocytes and CD8 T cells. Agnello et al.[108], studied seven SLE patients treated with Danazol (an impeded androgen) and found reduction in anti-d.s. DNA antibodies, increased serum complement, and some clinical improvement in mildly active disease. In another study nandrolone decanoate (50 mg intramuscularly every third week for 2 years) was given to 47 RA patients on grounds that this anabolic steroid may benefit the patients disease, muscle wasting and osteoporosis. Using a variety of assessments there was no demonstrable effect on activity of disease or bone metabolism, however improvement in chronic anaemia was seen within 6 months of therapy[109].

### Neurotransmitters

Experimental work in the rat adjuvant arthritis model has shown that chemical sympathectomy is associated with less severe joint injury in the rat[110]. Levine et al.[111] investigated regional sympathetic blockade following intravenous guanethidine infusion in 24 patients with active RA in a randomized double blind study over 14 days. They were able to show an improvement in pain measures in the treated limb which persisted up to 14 days (the blockade was expected to last 2 to 3 days). They postulated that the depletion in catecholamines in postganglionic efferent nerves was a possible mechanism of the action of guanethidine. Substance P and other neuropeptides have been implicated as neurogenic mediators of the inflammatory response[112] and therapy targeted along these lines provides an interesting approach, particularly for the future of analgesic therapy.

*Captopril*

Martin *et al.*[113], noted the similarity of molecular structure between captopril and D-penicillamine (shared thiol group-acid group). Both agents bind copper, have similar adverse effects (rash, nephrotic syndrome, dysgeusia, agranulocytosis) and are immunosuppressive as determined in models of PHA-stimulated lymphocytes *in vitro*. They performed an open study in 15 patients with active RA using 75–150 mg/day of captopril followed for 48 weeks. After 8–12 weeks they found a significant improvement in 7 patients and a moderate improvement in 3 more (articular index, grip strength, pain score, levels of C-reactive protein, IgM and in plasma viscosity). Withdrawals were due to rash gastrointestinal upset and hypotension (one patient each). It was postulated that the mechanism of action may have included blockade of inflammatory and pain mediators via interference with the kinin system.

*Iron chelation*

High levels of synovial iron have been shown to be associated with a poorer prognosis in RA[114]. Moreover iron dextran treatment can exacerbate disease, an effect mediated by the iron rather than dextran component[115]. Andrews *et al.*[116] induced mild iron deficiency in the rat adjuvant arthritis model with the iron chelator desferrioxamine. This reduced the incidence and severity of joint inflammation without altering the systemic sequelae. There was however, a reduction in soft tissue swelling and bone erosion. It was postulated that the effects were as a consequence of reduction of iron available for the promotion of hydroxyl radical formation with subsequent tissue damage, and to reduction in prostaglandin $E_2$ production.

*Isoprinosine*

Viral infection has long been postulated as an aetiological factor in the development of rheumatic disease, particularly RA. Isoprinosine is an antiviral immunostimulating drug which has been subjected to open trials in RA. Sadowska *et al.* treated 10 patients with short duration and non-erosive disease in regimes of 1.5–2.0 g/day over a 4 week period. They found significant improvement in number of painful and swollen joints, grip strength and duration of morning stiffness with reduction in rheumatoid factor titre in 40% and no change in ESR[117].

## X. DIET AND ARTHRITIS

The role of diet in the aetiology and management of patients with rheumatic disease remains controversial. A number of observations suggest that diet may have a significant role in rheumatic diseases either aetiologically or by exacerbating existing pathology. Diet may influence inflammation by mechanisms relating to:

1.    Alterations in the balance of essential fatty acids precursors of prostaglandins and leukotrienes.

2.    Food or drug related alterations in gut permeability leading to invasion of organisms, absorption of immunogenic proteins, biologically active compounds, e.g. plant flavinoids, vasoactive monoamines, immune complexes etc.

3.    Vitamin and mineral deficiencies, e.g. copper and zinc, or

4.    Alterations in gut flora, e.g. *Klebsiellae, Clostridiae* or *Proteus* species.

There exists a strong relationship between gastrointestinal disease and arthritis as evidenced by:

(a)    Gastrointestinal infection, e.g. *Yersiniae, Salmonellae, Shigellae, Klebsiellae*, and the HLA B27 associated spondyarthritides.

(b)    The arthropathy associated with inflammatory bowel disease – coeliac disease, ulcerative colitis and Crohn's disease.

(c)    Jejuno-ileal by-pass arthropathy.

(d)    Whipple's disease.

A number of attempts at therapeutic intervention by dietary manipulation have been published. Patients with classic rheumatoid arthritis partially fasted for 7 to 10 days then commenced on a lacto-vegetarian diet showed improvement after fasting followed by relapse on the diet[118]. Hicklin et al.[119] reported improvement in a third of patients with RA treated with an exclusion diet. Anecdotal case studies exist suggesting dietary manipulation improving RA patients with dairy product intolerance[120], corn intolerance[121] and milk intolerance[122].

In a 12 week prospective double-blind controlled study of 37 RA patients, Kremer et al. compared the effects of a high polyunsaturated fat diet and supplemental eicosapentaenoic acid (EPA) (1.8 g/day) with a high saturated fat diet with placebo supplement. Results at 3 months showed significant improvement in the morning stiffness and number of swollen joints. Within 8 weeks of cessation of the diet the patients had relapsed[123].

In another randomized, double-blind, placebo-controlled, crossover trial 40 RA patients continued with their normal diet and drug therapy but in addition took placebo or 2.7 g/day of EPA. A tendency for improvement was seen for a variety of activity measures but only a reduction in number of swollen joints and time to fatigue reached statistical significance when compared with placebo treated patients. However, when compared with baseline, patients treated with EPA showed significant improvement in ARA class, physician's global assessment, number of tender and swollen joints and fatigue time. The benefits lasted to 4 weeks, after cessation of the supplement, and were associated with reductions in measured neutrophil leuco-triene B4 levels[124].

A number of possible mechanisms for improvement have been suggested. The addition of EPA would produce relatively inactive 3-series prostaglandins in place of the proinflammatory 2-series PGs. In addition, EPA will compete with arachidonic acid for the cyclo-oxygenase pathway producing less inflammatory mediators and may interfere with cell membrane responsiveness as a result of the introduction of EPA instead of linoleic and arachidonic acids into the membranes of immunologically active lymphocytes and macrophages[125].

The Dong diet (diet free of additives, preservatives, alcohol, red meat, dairy products, fruit and herbs and spices) was examined in a 10 week study by Panush *et al.* but no benefit was found[126].

A trial of EPA supplementation for 12 months in 30 mild SLE patients showed no significant activity against this disease although a rebound of disease activity was seen after stopping the trial[127].

Considerable work is required to elucidate the benefits or hazards of diet in arthritis. Supplemental EPA would seem to have the effect seen with NSAIDs in respect of soft tissue swelling and pain relief but has no apparent disease modifying activity.

## XII. CONCLUSION

This chapter has highlighted a number of recent developments in anti-rheumatic therapy and described a number of avenues of treatment under intense scrutiny, partly because of dissatisfaction with established therapeutic modalities. This is illustrated by recent studies. Wolfe and Hawley[128] reviewed treatment in their 438 RA patients, and found 18.8% achieved remission (ARA criteria). This contrasts with remission in 13.6% of patients who received no remittive therapy. Median length of remission when obtained was only 10 months and only 7.8% of the observed time course of their patients was spent in remission.

Scott *et al.*[129], prospectively studied 112 consecutive RA patients over a 20 year period. They found a 35% mortality (often attributable to RA) and 19% of patients severely disabled with function deteriorating particularly in the second decade of follow-up.

These results highlight the necessity to tackle the treatment of rheumatic diseases with novel and aggressive approaches. It further emphasizes the need to consider all rheumatic patients as study or trial patients, whether it be to examine the use of novel therapies, to examine dietary manipulation, or to act as controls. Treatment of these chronic diseases provides a challenge. The following chapters will outline a number of areas of research aimed at meeting that challenge.

# REFERENCES

1. Day, R and Brooks, P (1987). Variations in response to NSAIDs. *Br J Clin Pharm*, **23**, 655-8
2. Coke, H (1967). Long term indomethacin therapy of coxarthrosis. *Ann Rheum Dis*, **26**, 346
3. Arora, J (1968). Indomethacin arthropathy of Hips. *Proc R Soc Med*, **61**, 669
4. Milner, J (1972). Osteoarthritis of the hip and indomethacin. *J Bone Joint Surg*, **54b**, 752
5. Solomon, L (1973). Drug induced arthropathy and necrosis of the femoral head. *J Bone Joint Surg*, **55b**, 246
6. McKenzie, L, Horsburgh, B and Gosh, P *et al.* (1976). Effect of anti-inflammatory drugs on sulphated glycosaminoglycan synthesis in aged human articular cartilage. *Ann Rheum Dis*, 487-97
7. Palmoski, M, Brandt, K (1979). Effect of salicylate on proteoglycan metabolism in normal canine articular cartilate *in vitro*. *Arth Rheum*, **22**, 746-54
8. Palmoski, M and Brandt, K (1983). Relationship between matrix proteoglycan content and the effects of salicylate and indomethacin on articular cartilage. *Arth Rheum*, **26**, 528-31
9. Ro, J, Sudman, E and Marton, P (1976). Effect of indomethacin on fracture healing in rats. *Acta Orthop Scand*, **47**, 588-99
10. Sudmann, E (1975). Effect of Indomethacin on bone remodelling in rabbit ear chambers. *Acta Orthop Scand*, suppl. 160, 91-115
11. Herman, J and Hess, E (1984). Non-steroidal anti-inflammatory drugs and modulation of cartilaginous changes in osteoarthritis and rheumatoid arthritis. Clinical implications. *Am J Med*, **48**, 16-25
12. Brandt, K and Palmoski, M (1984). Effects of salicylates and other non-steroidal anti-inflammatory drugs on articular cartilage. *Am J Med* **77 (1a)**, 65-9
13. Doherty, M, Holt, M, MacMillan, P *et al.* (1986). A reappraisal of "analgesic hip". *Ann Rheum Dis*, **45**, 272-6
14. Herman, J, Appel, A, Khosla, R *et al.* (1986). The *in vitro* effect of select classes of non-steroidal anti-inflammatory drugs on normal cartilage metabolism. *J Rheum*, **13**, 1014-18
15. Clive, DM and Stoff, JS (1984). Renal syndromes associated with NSAIDs. *Nw Engl J Med*, **310**, 563-72
16. O'Brien, WM and Bagley, GF (1985). Rare adverse reactions to NSAIDs. *J Rheum*, **12**, 13-20
17. Malone, D, McCormick, P, Daly, L *et al.* Peptic ulcer in rheumatoid arthritis - intrinsic or related to drug therapy.
18. Collier, D St J and Paine, JA (1985). NSAIDs and peptic ulcer perforation. *Gut*, **26**, 359-63
19. Somerville, K, Faulkner, G and Langman, M (1986). NSAIDs with bleeding peptic ulcer. *Lancet*, **1**, 462-4
20. Committee on the Safety of Medicines (1986). CSM update: NSAIDs and serious GIT adverse reactions - 2. *Br Med J*, **292**, 1190-1
21. Armstrong, C and Blower, A (1987). NSAIDs and life threatening complications of peptic ulceration. *Gut*, **28**, 527-32
22. Catford, J and Simpson, R (1986). Confidential enquiry into deaths from peptic ulcer. *Health Trends*, **18**, 37-40
23. Hunt, PS, Hansky, J and Korman, M (1979). Mortality in patients with haematemesis and melaena: a prospective study. *Br Med J*, **1**, 1238-40
24. Davies, J, Collins, AJ and Dixon, St J (1986). The influence of cimetidine on peptic ulcer in patients with arthritis taking anti-inflammatory drugs. *Br J Rheum*, **25**, 54-8

25. Sontag, S (1986). Prostaglandins and acid peptic disease. *Am J Gastro*, **81 (11)**, 1021-27

26. Rachmilewitz, D, Ligumisky, M, Fich, A *et al.* (1986). Role of endogenous gastric prostanoids in the pathogenesis and therapy of duodenal ulceration. *Gastroenterology*, **90**, 963-9

27. Bjarnson, I, So, A, Levi, A *et al.* (1984). Intestinal permeability and inflammation in rheumatoid arthritis: effects of NSAIDs. *Lancet*, **2**, 1171-74

28. Axon, AT (Editorial)(1986). Campylobacter pyloridis: what risk in gastritis and peptic ulcer. *Br Med J*, **293**, 772-3

29. McLean, AJ, Harrison, PM and Joannides-Demos, L (1984). Microbes, peptic ulcer and relapse rates with different drugs. *Lancet*, **2**, 525-630.
    Van Heyningen, R and Harding, J (1986). Do aspirin-like analgesics protect against cataracts? *Lncet*, **i**, 1111-13

31. Inman, WHW (1985). Comparative study of 5 NSAIDs. In: *Prescription Event News*, No.3. (Southampton: Hamble Valley Press)

32. Davies, P, Fowler, P and Jackson, R (1986). Prediction of progressive joint damage in patients with rheumatoid arthritis receiving gold or D-penicillamine therapy. *Ann Rheum Dis*, **45**, 945-9

33. Situnayake, R, Grindulis, K and McConkey, B (1987). Long term treatment of rheumatoid arthritis with sulphasalazine, gold or D-penicillamine: a comparison using life-table methods. *Ann Rheum Dis*, **46**, 177-83

34. Feltelius, N and Hollgren, R (1986). Sulphasalazine in ankylosing spondylitis. *Ann Rheum Dis*, **45**, 396-9

35. Dougados, M, Boumer, P and Amor B (1986). Sulphasalazine in ankylosing spondylitis: a double blind controlled study in 60 patients. *Br Med J*, **293**, 911-4

36. Kremer, J (1985). Long term methotrexate theray in rheumatoid arthritis: a review. (suppl. 12), **12**, 25-8

37. Willkens, R (1985). Short term efficacy of methotrexate in treatment of rheumatoid arthritis. *J Rheum*, (suppl. 12), **12**, 21-4

38. Bookbinder, S, Espinoza, L, Fenske, N *et al.* (1984). Methotrexate: its use in the rheumatic diseases. *Clin Exp Rheum*, **2:2**, 185-95

39. Williams, I, Baylis, EM and Shipley, ME (1982). A double blind placebo controlled trial of methylprednisolone pulse therapy in active rheumatic diseases. *Lancet*, **2**, 237-40

40. Newman, V, Hopkins, R and Dixon, J (1985). Combination therapy with pulse methylprednisolone in rheumatoid arthritis. *Ann Rheum Dis*, **44**, 747-51

41. Hansen, T, Dickmeiss, E, Henning, J *et al.* (1987). Combination of methylprednisolone pulse treatment and remission inducing drugs in rheumatoid arthritis. *Ann Rheum Dis*, **46**, 290-95

42. Bijlsma, J, Schenk, Y, Ramselaar, A *et al.* (1986). Methylprednisolone pulse therapy in conjunction with azathioprine in rheumatoid arthritis. *Clin Rheum*, **5:4**, 499-504

43. Suchman, A, Condenii, A and Leddy, J (1983). Seizure after pulse therapy with methylprednisolone. *Arth Rheum*, **26**, 117

44. Moses, RE, McCormick, A and Nickey, W (1981). Fatal arrhythmia after pulse methylprednisolone therapy. *Ann Intern Med*, **95**, 782

45. Williams, I, Warren, D and Smith, R (1983). High dose prednisolone. *Lancet*, **1**, 593-4

46. Lupus Nephritis (1987). NIH Conference. *Ann Int Med*, **206**, 79-94

47. McCarty, D and Carrera, G (1982). Intractable rheumatoid arthritis. *J Am Med Assoc*, **248** (14), 1718-23

48. Sharp *et al.* (in press)

49. Bitter, T (1984). Combined disease-modifying chemotherapy for intractable rheumatoid arthritis. *Clin Rheum Dis*, **10**, 427-8

50. Lewis, P, Hazleman, B, Bulgen, D *et al*. Clinical and immunological study of high dose azathioprine combined with gold therapy. In: Gordon, J and Hazleman, B (eds), *Rheumatoid Arthritis, Cellular Pathology and Pharmacology*, 280. (Amsterdam, Holland)

51. Gibson, T, Emery, P, Armstrong, R *et al*. (1986). Combined chloroquine and D-penicillamine in rheumatoid arthritis - better or worse? (Abs.) *Br J Rheum*, **25**, 114-5

52. Bunch, T, O'Duffy, J, Tompkins, R and O'Fallon, W (1984). Controlled trial of hydroxychloroquine and D-penicillamine singly and in combination in the treatment of rheumatoid arthritis. *Arth Rheum*, **27**, 267-74

53. Mackenzie *et al*. In press

54. Tiliakos, N *et al*. (1986). Low dose cytotoxic drug combination therapy in intractable rheumatoid arthritis (abst). *Arth and Rheum*, **29**, 4

55. Dawes, PT, Tunn, E, Fowler, P *et al*. Combined gold and hydroxychloroquine in rheumatoid arthritis. *Br J Rheum*, suppl

56. Taggart, A, Hill, J, Astbury, C *et al*. Sulphasalazine alone or in combination with D-penicillamine in rheumatoid arthritis. *Br J Rheum*, **26**, 32-6

57. Borel, J and Gunn, H (1986). Cyclosporin A as a new approach to therapy of autoimmune diseases. *Ann NY Acad Sci*, **475**, 307-20

58. Van Ritjthoven, A, Dijkmans, B and Goei, H (1986). Cyclosporin A treatment in rheumatoid arthritis: A multicentre placebo-controlled double-blind study. *Ann Rheum Dis*, **45**, 726-31

59. Weinblatt, M, Coblyn, J and Fraser, P (1987). Cyclosporin A treatment of refractory rheumatoid arthritis. *Arth Rheum*, **30** (1), 11-17

60. Dougados, M, Amor, B *et al*. (1987). Cyclosporin A in rheumatoid arthritis: Preliminary clinical results of open trial. *Arth Rheum*, **30**, 83-7

61. Madhok, R and Capell, H (1987). Cyclosporin A: A potential disease modifying drug in rheumatoid arthritis. *Arth Rheum* (Abs), C16

62. Forre, O, Bjerkhoel, F, Salvesen, C *et al*. (1987). An open controlled randomised comparison of Cyclosporin A and Azathioprine in the treatment of rheumatoid arthritis. Preliminary report. *Arth Rheum*, **30**, 88-92

63. Yocum, D, Wilder, R, Wahl, S *et al*. (1987). A double blind randomized trial of high dose (HD) and low dose (LD) Cyclosporin A in rheumatoid arthritis. *Arth Rheum* (Abst) 30, 4, S58

64. Makowka, L, Lopatin, W, Gilas, T *et al*. (1986). Prevention of Cyclosporin A nephrotoxicity by synthetic prostaglandins. *Clin Neph*, **25** (Suppl), S89-94

65. Ruffel, B, Donatsch, P, Hiestand, P and Mihatsch, M (1986). Prostaglandin E$_2$ reduces nephrotoxicity and immunosuppression of Cyclosporin A in rats. *Clin Neph*, **25** (Suppl), S95-9

66. Miescher, P and Miescher, A (1985). Combined Cyclosporin A - steroid treatment of systemic lupus erythematosis. In: Schindler (ed), *Cyclosporin A in Autoimmune Diseases*, pp. 337-45. (Berlin: Springer Verlag)

67. Bambauer, R, Jutgler, G, Pees, H *et al*. (1985). Cyclosporin A and therapeutic plasma exchange in steroid resistant SLE. In: Schindler (ed), *Cyclosporin A in Autoimmune Diseases*, 346-55. (Berlin: Springer Verlag)

68. Deteix, P, Lefrancois, N, Laville, M *et al*. (1985). Open therapeutic trial of Cyclosporin A in SLE - preliminary results in 4 patients. In: Schindler (ed), *Cyclosporin A in Autoimmune Diseases*, pp. 361-5. (Berlin: Springer Verlag)

69. Halloran, P, Cole, E, Boohinan, A *et al*. (1985). Possible beneficial effects of Cyclosporin A in some cases of severe SLE. In: Schindler (ed), *Cyclosporin A in Autoimmune Diseases*, pp. 356-64. (Berlin: Springer Verlag)

70. Fentgren, G, Oussin, S, Chatenoud, L *et al*. (1985). The effects of Cyclosporin A in 12 patients with severe systemic lupus erythematosis. In: Schindler (ed), *Cyclosporin A in Autoimmune Diseases*, pp. 366-72. (Berlin: Springer Verlag)

71.    Ben-Chetrit, E, Gross, D, Braverman, A *et al*. (1986). Total lymphoid irradiation in refractory SLE. *Ann Intern Med*, **105**, 58-60
72.    Morgan, S, Bernstein, R and Hughes, G (1985). Intractable polymyositis: prolonged remission induced by total body irradiation. *J R Soc Med*, **78**, 496-7
73.    Slavin, S (1987). Total lymphoid irradiation. *Immunol Today*, **8**, 88-92
74.    Field, E, Hoppe, R, Tanay, A *et al*. (1987). Long term follow up of rheumatoid arthritis patients treated with total lymphoid irradiation. *Arth Rheum*, **30**, 1-9
75.    Crook, P, Lucraft, H, Evans, R *et al*. (1986). Lack of effect of total body irradiation in rheumatoid arthritis. *Brit J Rheum*, **25**, 384-7
76.    Brahm, E, Strober, S, Hoppe, R, Bloch, D, Strober, S *et al*. (1983). Sustained improvement of intractable rheumatoid arthritis after total lymph irad. *Arth Rheum*, **26**, 937-46
77.    Sherrer, Y, Block, D, Strober, S *et al*. (1987). Comparative toxicity of total lymphoid irradiation and immunosuppressive drug treatment in patients with intractable rheumatoid arthritis. *J Rheum*, **14**, 46-51
78.    Nusslein, H, Herbert, M, Manger, B *et al*. (1985). Total lymphoid irradiation in patients with refractory rheumatoid arthritis. *Arth Rheum*, **28**, 1205-10
79.    Hanly, J, Hassan, J, Mornaity, M *et al*. (1986). Cyclosprin A in intractable rheumatoid arthritis. *Arth Rheum*, **29**, 16-25
80.    Simon, EB, Ling, J, Mendizabel, R *et al*. (1986). Radiation-induced coronary heart disease. *Am J Med*, **81**, 183-4
81.    Tester, W, Kinsella, T, Waller, B *et al*. (1984). Second malignant neoplasms complicating Hodgkin's disease: the National Cancer Institute experience. *J Clin Oncol*, **2**, 762-9
82.    Emery, P and Hertzog, P (1987). Evidence of increased interferon production in patients with rheumatoid arthritis in remission. *Clin Exp Rheum*, Suppl. 2 (Abst)
83.    Franchimont, P (1987). Tumor necrosis factor (alpha), interferon (alpha) and interleukin 2 production by peripheral blood mononuclear cells from subjects with active and inactive rheumatoid arthritis. *Clin Exp Rheum*, **5**, Suppl. 2 (Abst)
84.    Lemmel, E, Francke, M, Grus, W *et al*. Recombinant human interferon gamma in the treatment of rheumatoid arthritis: a multicentre phase 2 trial. *Arth Rheum*, **29**, 4, Suppl., (Abst)
85.    Verbruggen, G, Veys, E and Mielants, H (1987). Recombinant interferon gamma in rheumatoid arthritis. A double blind study comparing immuneron with placebo. *Clin Exp Rheum* (Abst), F167, 5/S 2
86.    Machold, K, Flener, R and Smolen, J (1987). Double blind placebo controlled crossover study of human recombinant gamma-interferon therapy in rheumatoid arthritis - preliminary results. *Clin Exp Rheum*, F168, 5/S 2
87.    Firestein, G, Weisman, M and Zvaifler, N (1987). Parenteral interferon gamma in rheumatoid arthritis: effect on disease activity and peripheral blood monocytes. *Arth Rheum* (Abst), E13, 30, Suppl. 4
88.    Cannon, G, Schindler, J and Emkey, R (1987). Double blind trial of recombinant interferon gamma in rheumatoid arthritis. *Arth Rheum* (Abstr), 49, 30, Suppl. 4
89.    Belldegrum, A, Webb, D, Austin, H *et al*. (1987). Immunotherapy for advanced cancer. *Ann Inter Med*, **106**, 817-22
90.    Fahey, J, Sarna, G, Gale, R *et al*. (1987). Immunointerventions in disease. UCLA Conference. *Ann Int Med*, **106**, 257-74
91.    Steinman, L, Waldor, M and Zanwil, S (1986). Therapy of autoimmune diseases with antibody to immune response gene products or to T cell surface markers. *Ann NY Acad Sci*, **475**, 274-83
92.    Hazleman, B *et al*. Intravenous anti-T cell monoclonal antibodies (Campath) in the treatment of rheumatoid arthritis. In press

93.  Veys, E, Mielants, H, Verbruggen, G *et al*. (1984). Thymopoietin pentapeptide in the treatment of rheumatoid arthritis. A compilation of several short and long term clinical studies. *J Rheum*, **11**, 462-6

94.  Amor, B, Dougados, M, Mery, C *et al*. (1987). Non-athymulin in rheumatoid arthritis: 2 double blind placebo controlled trials. *Ann Rheum Dis*, **46**, 549-54

95.  Sultan, A, Jawad, A, Berry, H *et al*. (1986). Immunotherapy in rheumatoid arthritis by T suppressor lymphocytes: experimental model *in vitro*. *Clin Rheum*, **5**, 450-8

96.  Bond, H, Bastian, D and Cooper, B (1986). A possible new therapy of systemic lupus erythematosis. *Ann NY Acad Sci*, **475**, 296-305

97.  Bobgrove, AM (1983). Possible beneficial effects of phenytoin for rheumatoid arthritis. *Arth Rheum*, **26**, 118-9

98.  Eisenberg, M, Williams, JF, Stevens, L *et al*. (1974). Mammalian collagenase and peptidase estimation in normal skin and in skin of patients suffering from epidermolysis bullosa. *J Int Res Comm*, **2**, 1732

99.  Sorrel, T and Forbes, I (1975). Depression of immune competence by phenytoin and carbamezapine. *Clin Exp Immunol*, **20**, 273-85

100. Grindulis, K, Nichol, F and Oldham, R (1986). Phenytoin in rheumatoid arthritis. *J Rheum*, **13:6**, 1035-9

101  Richards, I, Fraser, S and Hunter, J (1987). Comparison of phenytoin and gold as second line drugs in rheumatoid arthritis. *Ann Rheum Dis*, **46**, 667-9

102. Talel, N, Ahmed, A and Dauphinee, M (1986). Normal approaches to immunotherapy of auto immune disease. *Ann NY Acad Sci*, **475**, 320-7

103. Chapel, T and Burug, R (1971). Oral contraceptives and exacerbation of SLE. *Am J Obstet Gynaecol*, **110**, 366-9

104. Jungers, P, Dougados, M, Pelissier, C *et al*. (1982). Influence of oral contraceptive therapy on the activity of SLE. *Arth Rheum*, **25**, 618-23

105. Roubinian, J, Talal, N, Greenspan, J *et al*. (1979). Delayed androgen treatment prolongs survival in murine lupus. *J Clin Invest*, **63**, 902-11

106. Ansar Ahmed, S, Dauphinee, M and Talal, N (1986). Effects of sex hormones on autoantibody producing B cells bearing Ly-1 antigen (abstract). *Arth Rheum* (suppl), **29**, 34

107. Ansar Ahmed, S, Penhale, W and Talal, N (1985). Sex hormones, immune and autoimmune responses: mechanisms of sex hormone action. *Am J Pathol*, **121**, 531-59

108. Agnello, V, Pariser, K and Gell, F (1983). Preliminary observations on Danazol therapy of systemic lupus erythematosis: effects on DNA antibodies, thrombocytopaenia and complement. *J Rheum*, **10**, 682

109. Bird, H, Burkinshaw, L, Pearson, D *et al*. (1987). A controlled trial of nandrolone decanoate in the treatment of rheumatoid arthritis in postmenopausal women. *Ann Rheum Dis*, **46**, 237-43

110. Levine, J, Clark, R, Helins, C *et al*. (1984). Interneuronal substance P contributing to severity of experimental arthritis. *Science*, **226**, 547-9

111. Levine, J, Fye, K, Heller, P *et al*. (1986). Clinical response to regional IV guanethidine in patients with rheumatoid arthritis. *J Rheum*, **13**, 1040-3

112. Iversen, L (1985). Editorial - the possible role of neuropeptides in the pathophysiology of rheumatoid arthritis. *J Rheum*, **12**, 3

113. Martin, M, McKenna, F, Bird, H *et al*. (1984). Captopril: A new treatment for rheumatoid arthritis. *Lancet*, **1** (a83910), 1325-8

114. Blake, D, Gallagher, P, Potter, A *et al*. (1984). The effect of synovial iron on the progression of rheumatic disease. *Arth Rheum*, **27**, 495-501

115. Blake, D, Lunec, J, Ahern, M *et al*. (1985). Effect of IV iron dextron on rheumatoid synovitis. *Ann Rheum Dis*, **44**, 183-8

116. Andrews, F, Morris, C, Kondratowicz, G *et al*. (1987). Effect of iron chelation on inflammatory joint disease. *Ann Rheum Dis*, **46**, 327-33

117.    Sadowska-Wrolblewska, M, Wroblewska, J, Przybylska, J *et al*. (1987). Isopinosine in the treatment of early rheumatoid arthritis. *Clin Exp Rheum* (abstract), **5** Supppl. 2, 54

118.    Skoldstram, L, Larsson, L, Lindstrom, F *et al*. (1979). Effects of fasting and lactovegetarian diet on rheumatoid arthritis. *Scand J Rheum*, **8**, 249--235

119.    Hicklin, J, Mcewen, L, Morgan, J *et al*. (1980). The effect of diet in rheumatoid arthritis. *Clin Allergy*, **10**, 463-7

120.    Parke, A and Hughes, G (1981). Rheumatoid arthritis and food: A case study. *Br Med J*, **282**, 2027-9

121.    Williams, R (1981). Rheumatoid arthritis and food: A case study. *Br Med J*, **283**, 563

122.    Panush, R, Stroud, R and Webster, E. Food - induced (allergic) arthritis. *Arth Rheum*, **29**, 220-5

123.    Kremer, J, Michaelek, A, Lininger, L *et al*. (1985). Effects of manipulation of dietary fatty acids on clinical manifestations of rheumatoid arthritis. *Lancet*, **2**, 184-7

124.    Kremer, J, Jubiz, W and Michalek, M (1987). Fish-oil fatty acid supplementation in active rheumatoid arthritis. *Ann Intern Med*, **106**, 497-503

125.    Lee, T, Hoover, R and Williams, J (1985). Effect of dietary enrichment with eicosapentanoeic and decosahexanoeic acids on *in vitro* neutrophil and monocyte leukotriene generation and neutrophil function. *N Engl J Med*, **312**, 1217-24

126.    Panush, R, Carter, R, Katz, P *et al*. (1983). Diet therapy for rheumatoid arthritis. *Arth Rheum*, **26**, 462-71

127.    Moore, G, Yarboro, C, Sebring, N *et al*. (1987). Eicosapentanoieic acid in the treatment of systemic lupus erythematosis. *Arth Rheum*, **30** Abstr., 138

128.    Wolfe, F and Hawley, D (1985). Remission in rheumatoid arthritis. *J Rheum*, **12**, 245-52

129.    Scott, D, Symmons, D and Coulton, B (1987). Long term outcome of treating rheumatoid arthritis: results after 20 years. *Lancet*, **2**, 1108-11

# 2
# Osteoarthritis: a metabolic disorder

**C W Denko**
Associate Clinical Professor
Rheumatology/Medicine
Case Western Reserve University
Cleveland, Ohio 44106

## DEFINITION

Osteoarthritis (OA) is a common systemic disorder characterized in humankind by painful, stiff, swollen joints that show cartilage loss and bony overgrowth of radiographic examination. X-rays show joint space narrowing, bony eburnation, osteophytes and bony spurs. The joint with OA is usually bony hard with irregular knobby contours and somewhat limited in motion. Cartilage loss and osteophyte formation are usually detected simultaneously but either may precede the other. The presence of these characteristic radiographic changes in the joints without clinical symptons is considered physiologic degeneration and does not warrant the diagnosis of OA which is a disorder characterized by both signs and symptoms.

## PATHOLOGIC CHANGES

Earliest changes in OA start in the articular cartilage, showing a focal loss of metachromasia with swelling of cartilage matrix. Collagen fibrils are altered, developing surface irregularities and fibrillation, with progressive denudation to underlying bony cortex. New bone formation takes place in two separate locations in relation to the joint surface, at the margins of the articular process and immediately adjacent. Inflammatory reactions are common, especially in primary generalized OA[1].

## CLASSIFICATION

In the absence of known antecedent metabolic disorders and in the absence of trauma, OA is considered primary OA. Primary OA may take several forms. It can localize in one joint or a set of joints such as spine or knees. When three or more joints are affected, OA is considered generalized OA.

*New Developments in Antirheumatic Therapy.* Rainsford, KD and Velo, GP (eds), Inflammation and Drug Therapy Series, Volume III.

A form of OA involving the terminal interphalangeal joints is termed Heberden's nodes which may occur in families involving mother to daughter transmission. A less common form of primary OA is the hip disorder, malum coxae senilis. Secondary OA encompasses all forms associated with other disorders including gout, rheumatoid arthritis, ochronosis, and heritable articular diseases.

## BIOCHEMICAL CHANGES

Although popular concepts regard OA as the end result of use and abuse and trauma acting on joints with individual genetic, metabolic, and developmental characteristics, this is only part of the pathogenesis in specific subsets of OA. When OA emerges, declaring itself by joint pain and characteristic anatomic radiographic patterns, alternations occur in serum proteins compatible with changes found in patients with generalized inflammatory disorders[2]. These perturbations in acute phase proteins are protective and follow two patterns. The first type is increased synthesis, by the liver, of acute phase reactants. Each acute phase reactant (ceruloplasmin, acid glycoprotein, and antitrypsin) reduces inflammation[3-5]. The second pattern is decreased synthesis, by the liver, of carrier proteins (transferrin and albumin) which are pro-inflammatory (Table 1)[6].

Table 1 Acute phase reactants[*] in serum of patients with osteoarthritis (OA)

| Group | (n) | Age | T[*] (mg/dl) | Cp[*] (mg/dl) | Alb[*] (mg/dl) | AGP[*] (mg/dl) | AT[*] (mg/dl) |
|-------|-----|-----|------|------|------|------|------|
| Women | | | | | | | |
| OA | 107 | 65 | $266 \pm 67$ | $49 \pm 18$ | $4104 \pm 634$ | $146 \pm 86$ | $291 \pm 107$ |
| N | 41 | 51 | $280 \pm 56$ | $43 \pm 11$ | $4100 \pm 608$ | $105 \pm 36$ | $267 \pm 61$ |
| P | | | n.s. | 0.02 | n.s. | 0.01 | 0.05 |
| Men | | | | | | | |
| OA | 39 | 65 | $242 \pm 49$ | $40 \pm 12$ | $4288 \pm 881$ | $143 \pm 64$ | $273 \pm 84$ |
| N | 32 | 58 | $265 \pm 41$ | $36 \pm 8$ | $4418 \pm 669$ | $110 \pm 31$ | $241 \pm 60$ |
| P | | | 0.02 | 0.07 | n.s. | 0.01 | 0.04 |

[*]Acute phase reactants: T = transferrin; Cp = ceruloplasmin; Alb = albumin; AGP = acid glycoprotein; AT = antitrypsin.

In addition to these inflammation-related actions by which the liver responds by altering serum proteins, there is the response of neuronal tissue and other cells making up joint structures in altering neuropeptide levels. Perturbations in peptide levels occur in the serum of the patients with OA. As with acute phase proteins, one group of peptides is anti-inflammatory while the other group is pro-inflammatory. Beta-endorphin, a 31-amino acid compound, is reduced in OA and in other rheumatic disorders[7], while substance P, an 11-amino acid compound, is pro-inflammatory and is increased (Table 2). Beta-endorphin exerts its anti-inflammatory action by modifica-

30

tion of the pro-inflammogenic effects of prostaglandins[8]. On the other hand, substance P exerts its pro-inflammatory action by stimulating the release of pro-inflammatory prostaglandins from synoviocytes[9].

**Table 2** Substance P (SubP) serum levels in patients with osteoarthritis (OA), in patients with rheumatoid arthritis (RA) and in normal controls

| Group | (n) | SubP (pg/ml) | P |
|-------|-----|--------------|---|
| RA | 21 | 69 ± 41 | 0 |
| Control | 37 | 25 ± 16 | – |
| OA | 12 | 46 ± 26 | 0.003 |

## NEW HYPOTHESIS

I suggest a multifactorial pathogenesis for OA that includes interactions of regulatory neuropeptides deranged significantly by liver dysfunction, thereby influencing complex processes in bone and cartilage metabolism. Since many steps are required for normal bone and cartilage function, OA may develop due to one or more biochemical aberrations.

When controlled, inflammation is a desirable process in containing noxious stimuli and instituting healing. Uncontrolled inflammation with its protean manifestations drives the patient to seek relief of the pain, redness, heat and swelling before loss of function occurs. Inflammation is the net result of pro- and anti-inflammatory stimuli. It may progress slowly to partial or complete loss of function, and cartilage is then destroyed. The products of cartilage degeneration promote inflammation. Malemud and co-workers have demonstrated that as cartilage progresses from normal configuration to the lesions of OA, the main change in cartilage is *quantitative*, not qualitative. The ability of cartilage to synthesize proteoglycans and related components of cartilage is not sufficient to keep up with the consuming demands of the illness. Cartilage diminishes in bulk without biochemical alteration. Analysis of discolored and fibrillated cartilage from defined areas of human femoral heads with OA showed no unique histopathologic changes[10]. As cartilage diminishes, however, bone grows and osteophytes proliferate. In this active phase of OA several neuropeptide levels change, some influencing inflammation, others influencing growth in cartilage and bone, down-regulating cartilage metabolism and up-regulating bone metabolism. The growth-promoting peptides include insulin, insulin-like growth factor-1 (IGF-1), and growth hormone (GH)[11].

An important underlying cause for altered levels of these neuropeptides is impaired hepatic function. IGF-1 is the main stimulant of cartilage metabolism while insulin stimulates bone[12]. Excess GH inhibits cartilage metabolism [13,14]. The liver in OA does not process GH adequately, forming too little beneficial IGF-1 and leaving too much toxic GH in the arena. Concomitantly, the liver does not clear the system of insulin adequately, leaving higher levels to stimulate bony growth. The stage is set for down-regulating cartilage metabolism and up-regulating bone metabolism. A constant outside stimulus is not needed. The initial inciting lesion or lesions remain unknown. The changes in neurohormone levels may attain levels high enough to modify anatomic structures.

Waine and co-workers[15] reported a relation between OA and diabetes mellitus suggesting a possible role for insulin in this constellation. Rheumatologists find obesity, hypertension (HTN), diabetes mellitus, and OA to occur commonly in various combinations. Other investigators propose insulin resistance of cellular membranes as a prominent feature in explaining obesity and HTN[16,17]. Similarly, I feel that derangement of membrane receptors for growth-promoting peptides such as insulin and GH plays a significant role in the etiology of OA.

Table 3 Growth promoting peptides - insulin-like growth factor (IGF-1), insulin growth hormone (GH) - in normotensive patients with osteoarthritis (OA) and in normotensive controls

| Group | (n) | Av. age | Glucose (mg/ml) | IGF-1 (nM/L) | Insulin (U/ml) | GH Hg/ml) | Ht (cm) | Wt (kg) |
|---|---|---|---|---|---|---|---|---|
| *Female – white* | | | | | | | | |
| Control | 11 | 68 | 90 | 14.6 ± 2 | 5.2 ± 2 | 1.1 ± 0.4 | 160 | 59 |
| OA | 7 | 71 | 90 | 9.0 ± 3 | 9.9 ± 1 | 2.1 ± 1.3 | 163 | 60 |
| P | – | – | – | < 0.02 | < 0.001 | 0.1–0.05 | – | – |
| *Male – white* | | | | | | | | |
| Control | 10 | 67 | 86 | 16 ± 2 | 6.6 ± 2 | 0.76 ± 0.2 | 173 | 73 |
| OA | 7 | 68 | 98 | 11 ± 4 | 10.7 ± 2 | 0.76 ± 0.3 | 176 | 79 |
| P | | | | < 0.01 | < 0.01 | – | | |
| *Female – black* | | | | | | | | |
| Control | 8 | 58 | 88 | 21.5 ± 4 | 6.8 ± 3 | 0.80 ± 0.6 | 163 | 72 |
| OA | 5 | 67 | 90 | 14.9 ± 4 | 16.1 ± 10 | 0.84 ± 0.8 | 168 | 78 |
| P | – | – | – | < 0.02 | < 0.05 | – | – | – |
| OA + obese + HTN | 10 | 67 | 93 | 14.6 ± 5 | 16.8 ± 7 | 0.91 ± 0.2 | 163 | 92 |
| P | – | – | – | < 0.01 | < 0.02 | – | – | – |

The availability of standard radioimmunoassay methods (INCSTAR, Stillwater, MN) for the growth promoting peptides, insulin, GH and IGF-1, led to a search for data to test the metabolic hypothesis of OA. Volunteer patients with OA who were not insulin-impaired were studied along with suitable non-rheumatic controles matched for age, sex, and race. Only euglycemic persons who were not diabetic, obese, or hypertensive were evaluated. Concomitant assays of serum levels of growth-promoting peptides have not been previously reported. Sera from OA patients and controls were treated in similar fasion (Table 3).

32

In OA patients, both white men and white women, IGF-1 was lower and insulin was higher than in the serum of suitable matched controls. In studies of black women with OA compared to black women with OA and HTN and obesity (20% over standard tables), similar patterns were found. IGF-1 was lower and insulin was higher than in normal controls. The presence of HTN and obsesity did not alter the pattern found in patients with OA alone. GH levels tended to be higher in white women with OA than in controls but the difference did not attain statistical significance. Basal GH levels were sought, a condition difficult to achieve in unfettered individuals. GH release fluctuates under the influence of numerous stimuli, such as hypothalmic effects, physical activity, and eating (Summary, Table 4).

Alterations in glucose metabolism are reported in certain types of inflammation in association with increased release of interleukin 1 (IL-1) and with increased insulin levels in the blood[18]. The presence of normal glucose levels in OA patients with hyperinsulinemia suggests that the host undergoes a type of tissue aggression that elicits neuroendocrine metabolic changes, not changes related to the immune-derived cytokine, IL-1.

## EXPERIMENTS OF NATURE

The syndrome of acromegaly that occurs in all ages is due to chronic secretion of excess GH which leads to overgrowth of bone and soft tissues. Among the complications of acromegaly in young persons is degenerative joint disease (OA) which may be crippling[19]. Hypersecretion of GH also occurs without symptons of acromegaly as has been reported in asymptomatic young women[20]. Although disc degeneration is not OA, it is a loss of cartilage and has been found in 80% of asymptomatic women past 70[21]. This degenerative process begins during the third decade of life and has been attributed to a natural aging process. Radiographic changes characteristic of OA are relatively common in asymptomatic or non-arthritic individuals. I believe that the asymptomatic young women with excess GH secretion may become the asymptomatic older women with disc degeneration.

Impaired liver function is common in Wilson's Disease, a rare metabolic disorder of young persons attributed to excess copper deposits in tissues. Many affected adults develop arthropathy characterized as OA of the wrists, metacarpophalangeal joints, knees and spine. Although the disorder is attributed to excess copper deposition in tissues, no copper has been reported in synovial biopsies showing hyperplasia with mild inflammation[22]. Following the hypothesis herein proposed that OA is a metabolic disorder, I attribute the OA of Wilson's disease to hepatic dysfunction which results in excess insulin and deficient IGF-1. After decades of living with excess insulin and deficient IGF-1 the patient develops anatomic changes characteristic of OA.

Perhaps the up-regulation of insulin production aggravates the inflammation of OA. Insulin exerted a pro-inflammogenic effect in alloxandiabetic rats challenged by injections of dextran, carrageenin and cellulose acetate into the paw[23]. There is a complex interaction between GH and the peripheral actions of insulin. Injections of GH can produce arthritis with features of OA[24].

Finally, OA is reversible by endogenous agents as yet undefined[25,26]. Spontaneous improvement in OA occurs over many years. In those who improved, the average time of observation was eleven years in one series. However, an exogenous agent, a cartilage-bone marrow extract, produced radiographic evidence of the reversal of OA in two or three years[27].

## SUMMARY

OA is a multifactorial metabolic inflammatory disorder in which too little cartilage and too much bone are synthesized because of impaired liver function in processing GH and insulin. The hepatic dysfunction results in altered peptide levels: too little IGF-1 which is required for cartilage growth and too much insulin which accelerates bony growth and osteophyte formation (Summary, Table 4).

Table 4   Summary – significant neuropeptide effects in osteoarthritis

| Agent | β-End | Sub P | GH | Insulin | IGF-1 |
|---|---|---|---|---|---|
| A. Inflammation | ↓↓ | ↑↑ | ↑↑ | ↑ | NT |
| B. Bone Metabolism | NT | NT | ↑ | ↑ | ↑ |
| C. Cartilage Metabolism | ↑↑ | ↑ | ↓ | ↑ | ↑↑ |
| Change in OA | ↓ | ↑ | ↑? | ↑ | ↓ |
| Lit. citation | 7,8 | 8,9 | 13,19,22,24 | 1,12,23 | 11,19 |

NT = Not tested
*Effect = ↓ or ↑, definite; ↓↓ or ↑↑, pronounced
**↓ or ↑ = p<0.05, ↑? = p 0.01–0.05 (see Table 3)

## REFERENCES

1.      Howell, DS (1984). Etiopathogenesis of Osteoarthritis, Chap. 7, pp. 129-146, in Moskowitz, RW, Howell, DS, Goldberg, VM, and Mankin, HJ (eds) *Osteoarthritis, Diagnosis and Treatment*, (Philadelphia: WB Saunders).

2.      Denko, CW and Gabriel, P (1979). Serum Proteins – in Rheumatic Disorders. *J Rheumatol*, **6**, 665–672.

3.      Pitt, E and Lewis, DA (1979). Anti-inflammatory properties of alpha₁-antitrypsin. *Int J Tissue Reactions*, **1**, 21–32.

4.      Denko, CW (1979). Protective role of ceruloplasmin in inflammation. *Agents Actions*, **9**, 333–336.

5.      Denko, CW and Wanek, K (1984). Anti-inflammatory action of alpha-1-acid-glycoprotein in urate crystal inflammation. *Agents Actions*, **15**, 539–540.

6.      Denko, CW (1980). Phlogistic properties of the serum proteins, albumin and transferrin. *Inflammation*, **4**, 165–168.

7.  Denko, CW, Aponte, J, Gabriel, P and Petricevic, M (1982). Serum beta-endorphins in rheumatic disorders. *J Rheumatol*, **9**, 827–833.
8.  Denko, CW (1985). Regeneration, repair and their control by pharmacological agents. Bonta, IL, Bray, MA and Parnham, MJ, (eds) in *Regeneration and Inflammation: Handbook of Inflammation*. Vol. 5, Chapter 10. (Amsterdam: Elsevier Science Publishers).
9.  Lotz, M, Carson, D and Vaughn, JH (1987). Substance P activation of rheumatoid synoviocytes: neural pathways in pathogenesis of arthritis. *Science*, **235**, 893–895.
10. Goldberg, VM, Norby, DP, Sachs, BL, Moskowitz, RW and Malemud, CJ (1984). Correlation of Histopathology and Sulfated Proteoglycans in Human Osteoarthritic Hip Cartilage. *J Orth Res*, **1**, 302–312.
11. Van Wyk, JJ, Underwood, LE (1980). Growth hormone, somatomedins and growth failure. In Krieger, DT, and Hughes, JC (eds) *Neuroendocrinology*. Chp. 32, pp. 299-309 (Sunderland, MA: Sinauer Associates).
12. DeLuise, MA and Harker, M (1988). Insulin stimulation of $Na^+$-$K^+$ pump in clonal rat osteosarcoma cells. *Diabetes*, **37**, 33–37.
13. Smith, TWD, Duckworth, T, Bergenholtz, A, Lemperg, RK (1975). Role of growth hormone in glycosaminoglycan synthesis by articular cartilage. *Nature*, **253**, 269–271.
14. Denko, CW, Bergenstal, DM (1955). The effect of hypophysectomy and growth hormone on $S^{35}$ fixation of cartilage. *Endocrinology*, **57**, 76–86.
15. Waine, H, Nevinny, D, Rosenthal, J, Joffe, IB (1961). Association of osteoarthritis and diabetes mellitus. *Tufts Folia Med*, **7**, 13–19.
16. Ferrannini, E, Buzzigoli, G, Bonadonna, R, Giorico, MA, Oleggini, M, Graziadei, L, Pedrinelli, R, Brandi, L, Bevilacqua, S (1987). Insulin resistance in essential hypertension. *N Eng J Med*, **317**, 350–357.
17. Landsberg, L (1987). Insulin and hypertension: lessons from obesity. *N Engl J Med*, **317**, 378–379.
18. del Rey, A, Besedovsky, H (1987). Interleukin 1 affects glucose homeostasis. *Am J Physiol* **253**, R794–R798.
19. Daughaday, WH, Cryer, PE (1980). Growth hormone hypersecretion and acromegaly. In Krieger, DT and Hughes, JC (eds) *Neuroendocrinology*. Ch. 31, pp. 293-298. (Sunderland, MA: Sinauer Associates).
20. Klibanski, A, Zervas, NT, Kovacs, K and Ridgway, EC (1987). Clinically silent hypersecretion of growth hormone in patients with pituitary tumors. *J Neurosurg*, **66**, 806–811.
21. Powell, MC, Wilson, M, Szypryt, P, Symonds, EM and Worthington, BS (1986). Prevalence of lumbar disc degeneration observed by magnetic resonance in symptomless women. *Lancet*, **2**, 1366–1367.
22. Gordon, DA (1979). Arthritis associated with metabolic or endocrine disease. In Cohen, AS (ed) *Rheumatology and Immunology* pp. 298-304. (New York: Grune and Stratton).
23. Leme, JG, Hamamura, L, Migliorini, and Leite, MP (1973). Influence of diabetes upon the inflammatory response. A pharmacologic analysis. *Eur J Pharmacol*, **23**, 74–81.
24. Reinhardt, WO and Li, CH (1953). Experimental production of arthritis in rats by hypophyseal growth hormone. *Science*, **117**, 295–297.
25. Perry, GH, Smith, MJG and Whiteside, CG (1972). Spontaneous recovery of the joint space in degenerative hip disease. *Ann Rheum Dis*, **31**, 440–448.
26. Storey, GO and Landells (1971). Restoration of the femoral head after collapse in osteoarthritis. *Ann Rheum Dis*, **30**, 406–412.
27. Denko, CW (1978). Restorative chemotherapy in degenerative hip disease. *Agents Actions*, **8** (3), 268–279.

# 3

# Concepts of the mode of action and toxicity of anti-inflammatory drugs. A basis for safer and more selective therapy, and for future drug developments

**KD Rainsford**
Department of Biomedical Sciences
McMaster University Faculty of Health Sciences
1200 Main Street West
Hamilton
Ontario, Canada, L8N 3Z5

## I. INTRODUCTION

The enormous range of drugs which have recently become available for the treatment of the 100 or so different arthritic conditions present the physician with a challenge to determine if there are some of these which are more suitable than others. Inspection of Table 1 indicates that of over 100 or so non-steroidal anti-inflammatory drugs (NSAIDs) these can be graded in terms of overall potency to be roughly equivalent to one of the four 'traditional' or well-established drugs, i.e. aspirin, ibuprofen, indomethacin and phenylbutazone. It could therefore, be argued that it is pointless having many of the new NSAIDs since these may be no better than those which are well established? This challenging question receives further provocate support from several well-established tenets frequently uttered by clinicians and even experts alike that (a) NSAIDs act by inhibiting the synthesis of inflammatory prostaglandins (PGs) (b) the anti-inflammatory and analgesic efficacy of these drugs is directly related to their inhibitory effects as PG synthesis inhibitors, and (c) with some few exceptions their potency as anti-inflammatory agents is correlated with their propensity to produce side-effects especially in the gastrointestinal tract[1-3]. Even the term 'Aspirin-like'[2] as frequently and, probably inappropriately, misapplied to all NSAIDs, conjures up in the mind the notion that all NSAIDs are the same, but possibly differ in potency only. If these features constitute the basis for the actions of the NSAIDs overall then it can be logically argued why do we really need all the

*New Developments in Antirheumatic Therapy*. Rainsford, KD and Velo, GP (eds), Inflammation and Drug Therapy Series,Volume III.

drugs that we have, except for the few cases they have proven unacceptably toxic. This is a very convincing argument often espoused by the more conservative physician, some experts advising Governmental drug regulatory authorities who preside over new applications for the evaluation and licensing of NSAIDs, and even teachers of medical students or graduates. Support for this tenet comes from evidence that aspirin, the oldest of all NSAIDs, by being the cheapest is still regarded in North America among the drugs of first choice for the treatment of pain and soft tissue inflammation in arthritis and this drug is frequently given for long-term therapy of this group of conditions[3,4]. The choice among others comes from the failure of aspirin to effectively control the pain with the appearance of untoward side effects and so an element of non-compliance. Following this there is the relative influence of drug sales techniques becomes apparent for the subsequent choice of drugs[4].

Faced with these pragmatic views, the pharmaceutical industry and independent medical and scientific investigators have attempted to determine if there are real differences among the NSAIDs. For industry this has great significance because of the need to establish the market for their particular drug. Recently, some companies have sought to claim that their drugs differ from others in (a) greater gastrointestinal (GI) 'tolerability' (i.e. they produce fewer GI side-effects)[7-15], (b) by exhibiting 'renal-sparing' effects in not affecting the production of urinary PGs[16-20], and now (c) in osteoarthritis they exhibit 'chondroprotective' effects by failing to affect the synthesis of cartilage proteoglycans or by inhibiting the release of interleukin 1-like cartilage-degrading proteins[21-38]. Each of these three claims does have some measure of support but it must be said the evidence for these effects especially in arthritic patients is at the stage of being suggestive and certainly not fully proven (the jury may be considered to be still 'out'!). Some of the clinical aspects of each of these claims are discussed in the first chapter in this volume by Nash and Hazleman.

**Table 1** Non-steroidal anti-inflammatory drugs currently available or in advanced stages in clinical trials

| Generic (INN) name | Trade mark names | Manufacturer(s) | Rating of therapeutic potency and special notes on use/properties |
| --- | --- | --- | --- |
| Acemetacin (indomethacin glycolate) | Rantudil | Bayer Troponwerke: Kowa | = IND |
| Acetyl salicylic acid/aspirin | Aspirin, Ecotrin | Various (Trademark for Aspirin held by Bayer in certain European countries) | |
| Alminoprofen | Minalfen, Minalfene | Bouchara | = PBZ |
| Amorfazone | | Morishita | |

38

Table 1 continued

| Generic (INN) name | Trade mark names | Manufacturer(s) | Rating of therapeutic poteny and special notes on use/properties |
|---|---|---|---|
| Antrafenine | Stakane | Synthelabo | |
| Azapropazone | Rheumox | Siegfried: AH Robins: Robapharm | = PBZ |
| Benorylate (paracetamol-ester or aspirin) | Benoral | Winthrop | = ASA, liquid suspension formulation chiefly for paediatric/geriatric use |
| Benzydamine hydrochloride | Benalgin: Benzyrin Dorinamin: Epiroten: Imotryl: Indolin: Ririlim Salyzoron: Ramas: Tantum | Angelini: Palazzo: Fawns McAllan | = ASA, principally topical formulation |
| BPPC | | Syntex | |
| Bufexamic acid | Droxarol: Droxaryl Feximac: Flogocid: Parfenac | Continental Pharma: American Cyanamid | = PBZ |
| Butyl fenamate | Fenazole, Combec | Hokuriku | = PBZ |
| Carprofen | Imadyl: Rimadyl | Roche | = IND |
| Choline salicylate | Actosal: Arret: Arthropan: Atrobione: Mundisal | Various | = ASA |
| Cinmetacin | Cindomet | Chiesi: Lorens: Sanitas: Sam Jin | = IND |
| Clidanac | Indanal: Britai | Bristol Meyers: Takeda | |
| CS-600 | | Sankyo | |
| Diclofenac | Voltaren: Voltarol | Ciba-Geigy | = IND |
| Difenpyramide | Difenax | Zambeletti | |
| Diflunisal | Dolisal: Dolobid Unisal | Merck | = PBZ, non-acetylated salicylates |
| Disalcid (diplosal) | Salsalate | Riker | = ASA, Non-acetylated salicylate |
| Droxicam | | Lab. Dr Esteve | |
| Epirizole | Mebron: Eperizole | Dauchi Seiyaku | |
| Eterylate | Daital | Alter | = ASA |
| Etodolac | Lodine: Romadar | American Home Products: Maggioni: Med Import | = PBZ |
| Etofenamate | | Bayer | = PBZ, topical formulation |
| Fenamole | Bufenid: Cinopal | | |
| Fenbufen | Lederfen: Nabanol Stimsen | American Cyanamid | = PBZ |
| Fenclorac | | Roter | |

Table 1 continued

| Generic (INN) name | Trade mark names | Manufacturer(s) | Rating of therapeutic potency and special notes on use/properties |
|---|---|---|---|
| Fendosal | Alnovin | Hoechst: Roussel Uclaf | = ASA |
| Fenoprofen | Nalfon | Lilly | = PBZ, IBU |
| Fenflumizole | | CDC Life Sciences | |
| Fentiazic | Atilan: Donorest Flogene: Norvedam Regilon | American Home Products: LPB: Niphon Chemiphar: Gist Brocades | |
| Feprazone | Danfenona: Methrazone: Zepelan: Zepelin | Boehringer-Ingelheim: Teijin | = PBZ |
| Flufenamic acid | Archless: Arlef: Fullsafe: Paraflu Parlef: Restogen: Surika: Tecramine | Parke Davis Warner Lambert | = PBZ |
| Flunixin | Banamine | Schering-Plough | |
| Flunoxaprofen | | Ravizza | = PBZ |
| Flurbiprofen | Ansaid: Cebutid Froben | Boots: Smith-Kline: Upjohn | = IND |
| Fluproquazone | Tormosyl | Sandoz | = PBZ |
| Fosfosal | | Uriach | = ASA |
| Flurobufen | | American Home Products | |
| Furofenac | | Alfa Farmaceutici | |
| Glutametacin | Indicin; Indoglucin: Teorema: Teoremec | SIR | = IND |
| Ibuprofen | Brufen | Boots: Upjohn American Home Products | |
| Ibuprofen guaicol-ester | | Lab Angelini | |
| Ibuproxam | Ibudros | Ferrer: Manetti & Roberts | |
| Indomethacin | Amuno: Artrinovo: Artrivia: Conforted: Indomethine: Inacid: Indocid: Indocin: Indomed: Infrocin: Inteban SP: Mezolin Osmosin: Oraflex | Merck | |
| Ionazolac calcium | | Byk Gulden | |
| Isofezolac | | Pharmuka | |
| Isonixin | Nixyn | Hermes | |
| Ketoprofen | Alrheumat: Alrheumen: Orudis Prafenid | Rhone Poulenc/ May & Baker American Home Products | = IND |

Table 1 continued

| Generic (INN) name | Trade mark names | Manufacturer(s) | Rating of therapeutic potency and special notes on use/properties |
|---|---|---|---|
| Ketorolac | | Syntex | |
| Lofemizole | | Farmitas | |
| Loxoprofen sodium | Loxonin | Sankyo | |
| Magnesium salicylate | | Trilisate | = ASA |
| Meclofenamate sodium | Arquel: Meclofen | Warner Lambert/ Parke Davis | = IND |
| Mefenamic acid | Cosland: Lyzalgo: Parkemed: Poustan: Poustel: Poustel: Poustyl: Poutal: Tauston: Vialidon | Warner Lambert/ Parke Davis | = PBZ |
| Methyl salicylate | Various | Various | = ASA |
| Miroprofen | | Yoshimoto | |
| Nabumetone | | Beecham: Ferrosan | = PBZ |
| Naproxen sodium | Anaprox: Flanax: Flanex: Naproxen: Naprozyn-S: Synflex | Syntex | = PBZ |
| Nictindole | | Sanofi | |
| Niflumic acid | Actol: Forenol: Landruma: Nifluril | UPSA | = PBZ |
| Oxametacin | Flogar: Restid | ABC: UBC | = IND |
| Oxaprozin | Duraprox | American Home Products: Talsho | = PBZ |
| Oxepinac | | Daiichi | |
| Parsalmide | Parsal | Sanofi | |
| Perisoxal citrate | Isoxal | Shionogi | |
| Pirazolac | | Schering | |
| Pirprofen | Rengasil | Ciba-Geigy | = IND |
| Pirproxen | Numide | Hosbon | |
| Piroxicam | Feldene | Pfizer; Toyama: Chiesi | ≥ IND |
| Pranoprofen | Niflan | Yoshimoti | |
| Proglumetacin maleate | Afloxan: Protaxil: Proxil | Rorer: Rotta Products | = IND |
| Proquazone | Biarison: Biarson | Sandoz | = PBZ |
| Sfericase | Ponase | Miji Seika | |
| Sodium salicylate | Various | Various | |
| Sulindac | Arthrocine: Clinoril Imberal: Sulindac Udolac | Merck: Banyu | = IND |
| Sulphinpyrazone | Anturan | Ciba-Geigy | = PBZ |

Table 1 continued

| Generic (INN) name | Trade mark names | Manufacturer(s) | Rating of therapeutic potency and special notes on use/properties |
|---|---|---|---|
| Superoxide dismutase | Orgetein | Diagnostic Data: Astra: Bristol-Myers: Toyo Jozo: Zambeletti | Natural product |
| Talniflumate | Somalgen | Bago: Norpro | |
| Tenoxicam | Tilcotil | Roche | = IND |
| Tiabinac | | | |
| Thiazolinobutazone | Deflogix | Almirall: UCB | |
| Tiaprofenic acid | Artiflam: Surgam | Roussel-Uclaf: Eisai | = IND |
| Timegedine | | Leo Denmark | |
| Tioxaprofen | Thioxaprofene | E Merck | |
| Tolfenamic acid | Clotam | Tobisha: Medica: GEA | = IND |
| Tolmetin sodium | Midocil: Tolectin Tolecgin | McNiel Johnson & Johnson | = IND |
| Zidometacin | | Pierrel: Forest | = IND |

based on Rainsford, 1987 (39).
Clinical assessment of therapeutic potency is intended to be a rough guide of the order of effects relative to that of the classic agents aspirin (ASA), ibuprofen (IBU) phenylbutazone (PBZ) and indomethacin (IND). It should be emphasized that this is only a crude estimate and does not include any specific pharmacological effects that might be exhibited by the individual drugs. This scaling is only meant to help in understanding the degree of therapeutic effect.

At the other end there are some drugs which have come under attack[39,40]. Such attacks have come especially from lobbying health groups in the USA, for their untoward safety features and include (a) piroxicam (Feldene®) ulceration in the GI tract[41–44], (b) the overall safety of NSAIDs in the elderly[45]. which in a large part comes from subnormal pharmacokinetic "handling" of some but not all NSAIDs[46,47], and (c) the enormous range and type of rate but severe and invariably fatal adverse reactions which can occur with some of these drugs, much having a hypersensitivity condition as a basis[40,48–51]. This suprasensitive political environment is charged now in the period of 'post-benoxaprofen (Opren)', a drug which was withdrawn following what was considered an unacceptably high number of deaths[40], so that the public, drug regulatory authorities and community agencies alike are ready to jump upon any reports of adverse effects from any drug[39].

Against this background the task here is to address to the fundamental question: What evidence exists for differences in the mode of action, therapeutic efficacy and the pattern and severity of side-effects among the NSAIDs?

For the other group of drugs used more specifically for the treatment

42

of rheumatoid and related seropositive arthritides, the so-called 'disease modifying anti-arthritic drugs' (DMARDs), there are even greater challenges. These drugs can be considered to be more toxic than the NSAIDs even though they have some effects on the arthritic process[3,4,48-51]. Even in this respect, however, they have faced challenges from the relatively high rates of withdrawal through side effects, lack of efficacy, and especially the questionable record of radiological improvement in joint manifestations of rheumatoid arthritis patients receiving these drugs[52]. No doubt these overall conclusions together with the relatively significant proportion of the population presenting with rheumatoid and related arthritic conditions gives much impetus towards the development of safer and more effective DMARDs. One major group of these agents, the gold thiolates, are considered elsewhere in this volume by Haynes and Whitehouse so they will receive only very brief mention here and then in the context of side effects and comparative actions on the events in chronic inflammatory processes. For providing impetus to future development more effective agents some of the current problems in the use of these agents and aspects of more selective therapy learnt from the use of these agents will be considered here.

## II.  NON-STEROIDAL ANTI-INFLAMMATORY DRUGS

### 1.  Differences in pharmacokinetics

One of the major features of the NSAIDs which is of importance in relation to their differing therapeutic actions is that of their pharmacokinetics[53,54]. Details of the pharmacokinetic properties of some commonly used NSAIDs are shown in Table 2. Among the principal features to note are (a) there is a wide range in the rates of absorption reflected by the time to peak plasma levels ($T_{P_{max}}$) and plasma elimination in half lives ($t_{1/2}$) among these drugs, (b) all the drugs except aspirin have plasma binding in excess of 90%, and a volume of distribution, $Vd$, of approximately 0.1–0.15 l/kg with the exception of etodolac ($Vd = 0.4$ h/kg), reflecting confinement to blood compartments, and (c) most if not all acidic NSAIDs are excreted as glucuronide metabolites with or without microsomal $P_{450}$ hydroxylation reactions. One additional and indeed important feature of the NSAIDs in relation to their therapeutic effects is that they accumulate in inflamed tissues and in those organs in which side-effects predominate[54,55]. In respect of (a) and (c) above there are marked differences between the NSAIDs in their quantitative variation as well as in their relative uptake into the GI mucosa and inflamed tissues, especially in synovial fluids. Thus, while synovial fluid concentrations may be at a somewhat lower level the peak values of which are delayed in time with respect to those for the plasma compartment for many drugs this may not be true for a few of the NSAIDs (e.g. diclofenac)[56-60]. In the latter case the synovial concentrations appear the same or appreciably higher than those for plasma values[56,57]. The reasons for this are unclear. Moreover, it is not clear

43

**Table 2** Pharmacokinetic properties and dosage ranges some anti-inflammatory drugs used in arthritic therapy

| Drug | Pharmacokinetic properties | | | Dosage range (mg/day) | Doses per day |
| | $T_{Pmax}$ (h) | $T_{1/2}$ (h) | $C_{pss}$ (mg/l) | | |
| --- | --- | --- | --- | --- | --- |
| Acetylsalicylic acid, | | | | | |
|   aspirin (as ASA) | 0.1–0.5 | 0.2–0.3[1] | | 2400–6000 | 3–4 |
|   (as SAL) | 0.5–3.0 | 2.7–4.5[1] | | | |
| Acemetacin | 1–3 | 4[1] | | 60–180 | 2–3 |
| Azapropazone | 3–5 | 12–17[1,2] | 40–100 | 900–1800 | 2–4 |
| Bumadizone | | 60 | | 300–500 | 2–4 |
| Carprofen | 0.5–1.0 | 9.9–12[1,2] | | 300 | 2–3 |
| Diclofenac (enteric | | | | | |
|   coated tablet) | 2.5[3] | 1.2–1.8[1,2] | 75–150 | | 2–3 |
| Diflunisal | 2–3 | 5–15[1,2] | 150–300 | 250–500 | 2–4 |
| Etodolac | 1–2 | 6–7.4 | | 200–600 | 3–4 |
| Etofenamate | | 8–12[1,3] | | Topical | |
| Fenbufen (Prodrug) | 1–4 | 9–12[1] | | 600–1000 | 2–3 |
| BPAA metabolite: | 6–12 | 9–12[1]) | | | |
| Fenoprofen | | 3–4 | 20–50 | 1200–3000 | 3–4 |
| Flufenamic acid | | 2–3 | (53 μM) | 400–600 | 3–4 |
| Flurbiprofen | 1.5 | 3–4 | 2–12 | 150–300 | 3–4 |
| Ibuprofen | 1–2 | 2–2.5[1] | 25–30 | 600–2400 | 3–4 |
| Indomethacin | 0.5–2.0 | 1–16[1,2,3] | 3.0–3.0 | 50–200 | 3–4 |
| Ketoprofen | 1–2 | = 1.5[1] | 0.5–6.0 | 100–250 | 2–4 |
| | | = 12 | | | (except SR form) = 2 |
| Lonazolac | 2 | 6 | | 600 | 2–3 |
| Meclofenamic acid | 3.0 | 3.3 | (10 μM) | 200–300 | |
| Mefenamic acid | | 2.0 | (41 μM) | 1000 | 3–4 |
| Nabumetone | | | | | |
| Naproxen | 2–4 | 12–15[1,2] | 25–75 | 250–1000 | 2 |
| Niflumic acid | | 3–4 | | 750 | 3–4 |
| Oxaprozin | 3.8 | 40–80 | 17–20 | 1200 | 2 |
| Oxyphenbutazone): | | | | | |
| Phenylbutazone): | 2–5 | 75[1,3] | 50–150 | 100–800 | 1–3 |
| Piroxicam | 2–8[3] | 53[1,2,3] | 3–8 | 10–40 | 1–2 |
| Pirprofen | 1–2 | 5–7[1] | 50 | 800–1200 | 2–3 |
| Salicylate | 0.5–3.0 | 2–3 (low dose) 15–20 (high dose) | 150–300 | 2400–6000 | 3–4 |
| Sulindac, | | | | | |
|   as prodrug | 1 | 7[1,2,4] | 2–6 | 200–400 | 2–4 |
|   as sulphide | 2 | 16–18[1] | | | |
| Tenoxicam | | 70–90 | | 20 | |
| Tiaprofenic acid | 0.5–1.3 | 2[1,2] | | 600–900 | |
| Tolmetin | 0.5–1.0 | 4.5–7[1] | 20–80 | 600–1800 | 3–4 |

44

if this is true for any other NSAIDs because they have not been fully studied over the entire time course. Also, the concentrations of the free drugs in synovial fluid and plasma are lower in rheumatoid and the infectious arthropathies where the most severely affected joints may contain low synovial fluid concentrations[58–60]. The lower synovial fluid concentrations probably occur as a consequence of decreased protein binding of NSAIDs in this compartment from the lower albumen concentrations[58–60].

Further variations occur with the propionic acid derivatives ('profens') which are, with the exception of naproxen, equal mixtures of an active prostaglandin (PG) synthesis inhibitory S( + ) enantiomer and an inactive PG synthesis R(–) isomer; naproxen comprising the active S( + ) isomer alone[61,62]. For the other propionates metabolic conversion of the inactive R(–) isomer occurs to the S( + ) form using the fatty acid coenzyme A thioester enzyme system[61,62]. R(–) and S( + ) enantiomers can have markedly different volumes of distribution[64,65] and protein binding affinities[66]. The rate of conversion may vary considerably among the different propionates as well as with age, sex[63] and renal function[64–67]. Thus, the ester glucuronide of ibuprofen is formed at rates which favour the S( + ) isomer[68]. The clearance of the R(–) ibuprofen is selectively impaired in induced fatty liver degeneration in rats[69]. Hence, abnormal liver function may markedly affect the uptake by the liver and metabolism of the stereo-isomers of ibuprofen as well as possibly other propionates. Renal dysfunction can markedly increase the proportion of unbound S(–)aryl propionate in rabbits[67] and this could have profound consequences for the toxicity of propionates in such conditions.

Recently, it has been shown that the R(–) enantiomer of ibuprofen is, in contrast with the S( + ) isomer, selectively incorporated into the trigly-

---

**Notes on Table 2**

All drugs except aspirin have plasma binding in excess of 90%, and with the exception of etodolac ($Vd = 0.4$ h/kg, Lynch and Brogden, 1986) a volume of distribution, $Vd$, of approximately 0.1–0.15 l/kg (Lin, Cocchetto and Duggan, 1987). Most, if not all, acidic NSAIDs excreted as glucuronide metabolites (Brune and Lanz, 1985)

*Abbreviations:*   $T_{P_{max}}$ = Time for maximal plasma levels
$t_{1/2}$ = Plasma elimination half-life
$Cp_{ss}$ = Steady state plasma levels
SR = Slow (or sustained)-release form
ASA = Acetyl salicylic acid
SAL = Salicylic acid
BPAA = Biphenylacetic acid

*Notes:*
1. Terminal ($t_{1/2}$) half life. Salicylate metabolites are eliminated in a dose-dependent and capacity-limited fashion.
2. Enterohepatic recirculation evident or probable and this will influence elimination.
3. Highly variable.
4. Sulindac and sulindac sulphone excreted but not sulindac sulphide.

Modified from Rainsford, 1988 (Ballière's Clin. Rheumatol., **2**, 485–511).

**Table 3   Drug interactions involving anti-inflammatory drugs**

| Drug combinations | Consequences |
|---|---|
| Aspirin with | |
| alcohol[a] | Increased GI bleeding/ulceration |
| anticoagulants[a] | haemorrhage |
| corticosteroids[a] | GI haemorrhage |
| diclofenac ) | Decreased serum concentration and GI |
| flurbiprofen ) | absorption of diclofenac or flurbiprofen |
| fenoprofen ) | Decreased serum indomethacin or fenoprofen |
| indomethacin ) | from increased elimination |
| insulin | Hypoglycaemia from reduced insulin requirement |
| methotrexate | Serum methotrexate reduced - altered kinetics |
| phenylbutazone ) | Increased serum urate in gout |
| sulfinpyrazone ) | |
| piroxicam | Increased GI bleeding/ulceration |
| sodium valproate | Increased serum valproate |
| Spironolactone | Reversal of natiuresis |
| Azapropazone with | |
| warfarin | Increased hemorrhage from displacement or warfarin from plasma protein-binding sites |
| Diflunisal with | |
| antacids | Variability bioavailability depending on type of antacid |
| warfarin[a] | Decreased plasma warfarin |
| Diclofenac with | |
| lithium salts | Increased plasma (Li) produced increased Li toxicity |
| Fluribiprofen with | |
| flurosemide | Reduced diuretic effect of furosemide |
| nicoumalone (acenocoumarol) | Haemorrhage |
| Ibuprofen with | |
| digoxin | Raised plasma digoxin |
| Indomethacin with | |
| bumetamide[a] ) | Reduced antihypertensive effects |
| captopril ) | Increased free plasma corticosteroid plus |
| corticosteroids ) | reduced elimination |
| flurosemide | Decreased natiuretic effect |
| lithium salts | Increased plasma (Li) with enhanced toxicity |
| oxprenolol | Reduced antihypertensive effects |
| phenylpropanolamine | Enhanced hypertensive effects |
| triamterene | Renal failure |
| warfarin[a] (also with sulindac) | Increased anticoagulant effect |
| Ketoprofen with | |
| probenecid | Decreased plasma-binding and elimination of ketoprofen |

[a]May also be common to other NSAIDs with potent cycloxygenase inhibitory effects
Based on Rainsford, 1987 (40)

cerides *in vivo* following repeated i.p. injection of this form of the drugs to rats[70]. The formation of hybrid triglycerides in adipose tissue was also shown from the normal R/S mixture of the drug under the same conditions and the levels of drug in the adipose tissue was coincident with the previously reported results from orally-administered radiolabelled R/S drug[70]. These observations may have profound consequences for the efficacy of racemic propionic acids and maybe even their toxicity, though with the latter situation there are few obvious possible mechanisms which are evident. Efficacy of R/S propionic acids may be lower than expected simply by conversion of R to S forms by the diversion of R(–) forms into adipose depots. The higher volumes of distribution of the R(–) forms of some[65,67] but not all[64] propionic acids may be a reflection of the greater propensity of the former to undergo triglyceride formation especially in adipose tissue, and thus have reduced efficacy in individuals with appreciable fatty deposits. It may, therefore, be important to consider fat to lean body weights in determining why propionic acid racemates vary in intersubject efficacy.

A few of the NSAIDs are prodrugs (e.g. acemetacin, fenbufen, flupro-quazone, nabumetone, salsalate, sulindac) and like the diastereoisomeric mixtures of propionates their metabolic conversion to active PG synthesis inhibitory drugs as well as the relative rates of uptake into inflamed sites of the active components will affect the therapeutic effects of these drugs.

Some recent studies with nabumetone have shown that elimination rates and other pharmacokinetic parameters were not significantly different for this drug with no evidence of accumulation in elderly compared with younger subjects, despite its inherently complex metabolism[71]. Other prodrugs appear to fulfil their promise of somewhat lower incidence of gastric ulcer side effects but do not eliminate all GI and other side effects[72].

Much variability exists in the rates of absorption and plasma elimination of different NSAIDs[73,74]. This can vary considerably with age and so can be a cause of some concern enabling prediction of therapeutic efficacy and side effects[73,74]. In addition, the combination of age, sex and disease state can influence in different ways the pharmacokinetics of NSAIDs. Variations with different NSAIDs in some of these parameters are reported elsewhere[78]). In many cases the situation is such that complex interactions can occur between all three of these parameters.

Long half life drugs have been selected out for particular concern in few of the incidence of associated side-effects noted with these drugs (e.g. benoxaprofen, isoxicam, piroxicam and tiflimazole)[3,4,6,13,41-7]. The choice of an NSAID with a shorter $t_{1/2}$ in preference to one with a longer $t_{1/2}$ has been proposed for those arthritic patients in which impaired renal elimination of these drugs may occur. This would seem an unattractive suggestion although computer simulation of a three compartment model system comprising gut, plasma and tissue compartments suggests that a shorter $t_{1/2}$ does not predict less drug accumulation[75]. These computer models do not allow for differences the pronounced variations in the drug uptake into specific compartments such as the GI tract (including enterohepatic recirculation which occurs with some, but not all, drugs), liver and kidney where side effects occur as well as in the inflamed tissues in which therapeutic actions occur[58,76-79]. It would seem, therefore, that the simple lumping of these latter compartments under in a generalized tissue compartment in such models is totally unjustified since it does not provide any discrimination of what will happen to drug concentrations in the above mentioned compartments which are of specific importance for the therapeutic and side effects of the NSAIDs.

Differences are evident in pharmacokinetics especially in relation to age and sex within a chemical classes of NSAIDs which influence the therapeutic responses and the safety of these drugs. Also liver and renal disease almost universally result in marked deterioration in the metabolism and elimination of NSAIDs so that in those arthritic states where renal and/or liver dysfunction may be evident (such as rheumatoid arthritis, systemic lupus erythematosus) much care should be taken in compiling dosage regimes and in regular monitoring.

## 2. Differences in pharmacological actions

According to the dogma of the early 1970s[2], the NSAIDs have classically been considered as acting by inhibiting the production of inflammatory prostaglandins (PGs). While the pioneering studies of Vane[2] and many others did show an important role for the inhibition of PGs in the actions of the NSAIDs, there is now convincing evidence[5,6,7,29,30,37] that there are other actions which also contribute to the spectrum of total anti-inflammatory actions. A list of these added actions is shown in Table 4. It will be seen that there are some notable variations in pharmacological actions between different drugs. The challenging question posed at the beginning of this chapter is these differences in action having any influence in the overall anti-inflammatory activities between drugs. In respect of cartilage protection it is likely that variations in the biochemical effects between NSAIDs do have some consequences [see later section 3(4)]. Probably the other effects accounting for an appreciable difference in the overall expression of anti-inflammatory actions between NSAIDs are the differences in effects on (a) oxyradical production/scavenging, (b) polymorph and/or leucocyte migration, (c) control of lysosomal enzyme release, (d) cyclic nucleotide production, (e) calcium movements in and out of cells, and (f) intermediary metabolism[6] (Table 4). The best way of viewing the overall contribution of these latter events compared with PG inhibition in NSAID actions is that there are some weak inhibitors of PG synthesis which exhibit comparable potency to some more potent cyclo-oxygenase inhibitors but through effects on e.g. cell migration (e.g. benoxaprofen), or lysosomal enzyme release and oxyradical inhibition (e.g. azapropazone) appear to manifest anti-inflammatory activity comparable to those NSAIDs with predominantly cyclo-oxygenase activity, i.e. compare the former group of azapropazone, benoxaprofen, fenclofenac,

**Table 4  Comparisons of the actions of some individual NSAIDs**

| Drug | Special chemical/ pharmacological properties | Eicosanoid inhibition | Leucocyte accumul- ation/enzyme release | Proteo- glycan synthesis | Inhibition of generation or action of oxyradicals |
|---|---|---|---|---|---|
| Acetylsali- cyclic acid (ASA = aspirin) | Acetylator of biomolecules incl. cyclo- oxygenase | $\downarrow$ CO ASA > SAL $\downarrow$ 12-LO (in platelets) | $\downarrow$ Enzyme release prob- ably due to salicylate | $\downarrow$ (SAL) | Salicylate scavenges $O_2^-$ to form gentisate ASA weak or inactive depend- ing on system |
| Acemetacin | Indomethacin pro-drug pharma- cological properties as for Indo. | = Ind | ? | | |
| Azapropa- one | Benzotriazine keto-enolate potent lysosomal stabilizer | $\downarrow$ CO (mod.) ?$\downarrow$ 5-LO (weak) | ?$\downarrow$ | $\uparrow$ or no effect | Inhibition of radical production |
| Carprofen | R/S enantiomers complement action | $\downarrow$ AA release $\downarrow$ CO ( = Ind) | | | |
| Diclofenac | Accumulates in synovial fluid > plasma | $\downarrow$ AA release $\downarrow$ CO ( = Ind) Persistant redn. in synovial $PGE_2$ + 5HETE in man | $\downarrow$ | $\uparrow$ | Inhibition at concs higher than for CO inhibition |
| Diflunisal | Non-acetylated bifluorophenyl salicylate mod. long-acting | $\downarrow$ AA release $\downarrow$ CO ( = PB2) ?$\downarrow$ 5-LO (weak) | $\downarrow$ | | |
| Disalcid (Diplosal) | Salicylate dimer pharmacol. as for salicylate | | | | |
| Etodolac | Racemate of a pyranoindole acetate joint damage in adj. arth. | R-enantiomer $\downarrow$ CO ( = Ind) | | | |
| Etofen- amate | Ester of flufenamic acid Topical A-I | as per FFA | | | |
| Fenbufen | Prodrug of biphenyl acetic acid (BPAA) | $\downarrow$ CO (by BPAA only) | | | |
| Fenoprofen | | $\downarrow$ CO ( = PBZ) | | | |
| Flunoxa- profen | Potential propert- ties of benoxa- profen without long plasma $t_{1/2}$ | $\downarrow$ CO ( = PBZ) $\downarrow$ 5-LO | | | |
| Flurbiprofen | | $\downarrow$ CO ( = Ind) No 5-LO activity | $\downarrow$ | | No effect |

49

| Drug | Special chemical/ pharmacological properties | Eicosanoid inhibition | Leucocyte accumul- ation/enzyme release | Proteo- glycan synthesis | Inhibition of generation or action of oxyradicals |
|---|---|---|---|---|---|
| Ibuprofen | R/S enantiomers | ↓ CO ( =PBZ) | | | ?Weak or inactive inhibitor of radical production depending on system |
| Indomethacin | | ↓ AA release ↓ 5 & 12-LO (weak) ↓ CO (potent) | ↓ | ↓ | Weak effect due to blocking of peptide binding to PMNS also with 5-OH metabolite |
| Ketoprofen | R/S enantiomers | ↓ CO ( =Ind) ↓ 5-LO (weak) Persistent ↓ in synovial $PGE_2$ | | | |
| Meclofenamic acid | | ↓ CO ( =Ind) | | ↓ | Oxyradical scavenger |
| Nabumetone | Non-acidic Prodrug AI = fenbufen, naproxen | ↓ CO (v. weak) | ↓ | | |
| Naproxen | S ( +) enantiomer only | ↓ CO ( =PBZ) ↓ 5-LO products (weak) | ↓ | | |
| Oxametacin | Ester of indomethacin, ? same pharmacol. props. | | | | ↓ More potent than Ind |
| Oxaprozin | AI = Ind as R/S enant- iomers | ↓ CO (weak) = ASA | | | |
| Phenylbut- azone | Keto-enolate | ↓ CO ( =IBU) scavenges $Ox^-$ in $PGG_2 \rightarrow PGH_2$ conversion | | ↓ | Inhibitor of radical production |
| Piroxicam | AI > Ind IgMRF T help.supph IL of prodn. | ↓ CO ( >Ind) reversible No 5-LO effects | | ↑ | Inhibits in part by blocking peptide binding |
| Progluta- metacin maleate | Prodrug of indomethacin | | | | |
| Proquazone | Non-acidic pro- drug metabolized to acid | ↓ CO (by active metabolite) | | | |
| Sulindac | Prodrug indene related to indomethacin | ↓ CO by sulphide but renal PGs unaffected | | ↑ | Potent inhi- bition by sulphide but not sulphoxide or sulphone metabolites/forms |

50

| Drug | Special chemical/ pharmacological properties | Eicosanoid inhibition | Leucocyte accumul- ation/enzyme release | Proteo- glycan synthesis | Inhibition of generation or action of oxyradicals |
|---|---|---|---|---|---|
| Sulphasala- zine (salicyl aza-sulpha- pyridine = SASP) | 5-amino Sal/and sulpha- 5-ASA pyridine (SP) may both be active metabolites ESP serum SH CRP | ↓ CO ? ↓ 5- LO by SASP & 5-ASA | ↓ | | SASP inhibits in part by blocking peptide binding SP & 5ASA inactive |
| Tenoxicam | AI = Ind | ↓ CO ( = Ind) | | | |
| Tiaprofenic acid | R/S enantiomer AI = Ind | ↓ CO ( = Ind) | | ↑ | |
| Tolmetin sodium | | ↓ CO ( = Ind) | | | |
| Zidometacin | Indomethacin analogue | as for Ind | | | |

FOOTNOTES

AA = arachidonic acid: CO = cyclo-oxygenase; LO = lipoxygenase (5- and 12- respectively); PGE2 = prostaglan- din E2; 5-HETE = 5-hydroxyeicosatetraenoic acid; ASA = acetylasalicylic acid; Ind = Indomethacin; PBZ = phe- nylbutazone; ↓ = decrease; ↑ = increase

oxaprozin with ibuprofen and naproxen as classic PG cyclo-oxygenase inhibi-tors[6,30]. Since side effects in the GI tract, kidneys and the skin probably re-late in a large part to cyclo-oxygenase inhibition it can be agreed that drugs with actions other than on this system could manifest safer, and a broader spectrum of activity than those which are pure cyclo-oxygenase inhibitors. Clearly as indicated in the previous section the variations in the disposition of the NSAIDs will, combined with these differences in their actions, con-tribute to the overall anti-inflammatory actions of these drugs.

## 3. Important issues – adverse effects

The most frequent side-effects observed with the NSAIDs in controlled clini-cal trials and in reports to drug regulatory authorities of ADRs[3,4,6,40,48–51,80] are shown in Table 5.

The side-effects in the GI tract, kidney and liver appear to exhibit an apparent dose-relatedness. For the majority of other side effects, however, it is not possible to ascribe such a relationship. It appears therefore that cer-tain other factors (e.g. disease state, environmental stressors) may exacerbate the drug effects. The range of possible drug disease or even drug-drug reac-tions is immense. It is, therefore, important that such precipitating factors should be identified so that procedures can be devised to minimize the side effects from these NSAIDs. Also with appropriate animal models incor-porating disease stress conditions it may be possible to use these to screen out the untoward side effects of NSAIDs in their stage of develop-ment[9,11,13,15,81].

51

Table 5  Side-effects of some anti-inflammatory/analgesic drugs

| Drug | GI ulceration and haemorrhage | Other GI | Skin | CNS | Haemato-logical | Liver | Kidney | Other (specified) |
|---|---|---|---|---|---|---|---|---|
| Acetylsalicylic acid | +++ | ++++ | + | + | + | + (SLE) | + (SLE) | + (Respiratory) |
| Azapropazone | + | ± | + | ++ | 0 | 0 | 0 | |
| Benorylate | + | ++ | | ++ | 0 | 0 | 0 | |
| Carprofen | + | ++ | | | | | | |
| Diclofenac | ++ | ++ | + | + | ± | ± | 0 | |
| Diflunisal | ++ | ++++ | + | + | ? | 0 | 0 | |
| Etodolac | ? | + | ++ | | | | | |
| Fenbufen | + | + | + | ++ | + | | + | |
| Fenoprofen | +++ | +++ | + | +++ | 0 | 0 | 0 | |
| Flufenamic acid | +++ | +++ | 0 | +++ | 0 | 0 | 0 | |
| Flurbiprofen | +++ | +++ | 0 | + | + | 0 | 0 | + (Pruritis) |
| Ibuprofen | + | +++ | + | ++ | | 0 | + | + (Respiratory) |
| Indomethacin | +++ | +++ | + | ++ | + | 0 | 0 | |
| Ketoprofen | ++ | +++ | + | 0 | 0 | 0 | 0 | |
| Meclofenamic acid | ++ | +++ | +++ | | | | | |
| Mefenamic acid | + | +++ | ++ | 0 | 0 | | | |
| Naproxen | + | +++ | ++ | ++ | 0 | 0 | 0 | |
| Oxametacin | +++ | +++ | ++ | +++ | | | | |
| Oxaprozin | +++ | | ++ | ++ | ++ | | ? | + (Cardiovascular) |
| Paracetamol | ± | + | | | ++ | | | |
| Phenylbutazone and Oxyphenbutazone | +++ | +++ | 0 | +++ | +++ | + | + | + (Cardiovascular) |
| Piroxicam | +++ | +++ | ++ | +++ | 0 | 0 | 0 | |
| Pirprofen | ++ | +++ | ++ | | 0 | + | | |
| Sulindac | ++ | ++ | ++ | + | + | ± | + | |
| Tolmetin | ++ | + | + | | | | | + (Urticaria, water retention) |

The incidence of the individual side-effects is graded on a scale according to approximate percentage namely, 0.1–5.0% = +, 5.0–10.0% = ++, 10–15% = +++, >20% = ++++. A zero rating denotes that the best clinical evidence indicates that no appreciable numbers of cases have been recorded which give a reliable statistical percentage. ? denotes that the drug may cause the side-effect. ± denotes barely detectable. The absence of any rating means that no adequate data exist to enable a rating to be assessed. It should be emphasised that these are at best only approximate ratings based on clinical trial data from groups of various sizes and studies of varying length of time and methodologies. Based on Rainsford, 1985.

## (1) Gastrointestinal side effects

Ulceration and bleeding, predominantly in the upper region of the GI tract constitute the most serious of all the adverse reactions encountered clinically with the NSAIDs[3,4,8,13,40,45,80]. Estimates of the incidence of GI ulceration associated with use of NSAIDs in arthritis therapy vary somewhat according to the basis upon which the assessments are determined. Of the estimates that have been published recently on a population basis from data derived from governmental regulatory authorities, on admissions of arthritic patients to hospitals for treatment of peptic, gastric or duodenal ulcer[82–88], endoscopic studies in arthritic patients[89,90], or epidemiological survey data on the incidence of upper GI lesions taking NSAIDs[91–100]. A whole range of variables must be considered in determining the percentage incidence and risk of ulcer formation, haemorrhage and perforation. There are some general points which emerge from all these studies, namely:

1.  Upper GI ulceration and haemorrhage are frequent events in arthritic patients taking NSAIDs. In patients referred to hospital for investigation the incidence of NSAID ingestion associated with peptic ulcer disease ranges in some cases between 16–82%[80,82,85,86,90,91]. In cohort studies at community levels this figure is disguised and appears much lower[100] because of the dilution in denominator values for the population numbers.

2.  The incidence of upper GI ulceration and haemorrhage is particularly high amongst patients over 65 years of age, especially women[45,82,86,92,101].

3.  The risks of death from perforated bleeding are relatively low for NSAIDs including aspirin (relative risk odds ratio range in the order of 0.5–2.1 for both categories in one study[99]) but with corticosteroids the risks of mortality are appreciably greater (odds ratio 4.2 ranging from 0.9–25.6).

4.  Upper GI ulcer disease is very common amongst non-aspirin drugs, though with some drugs may be less so than with aspirin[91].

5.  Patients with rheumatoid arthritis might be equally susceptible to the ulcerogenic effects as those with osteoarthritis[91], although the evidence for this is controversial.

*(a) Factors determining GI damage* – Previously it has been considered that NSAIDs only induced injury to the upper GI tract[7,8,13,40,82–91]. Thus peptic and gastric ulcer have been considered the principal pathology in this region[82–91]. The dominance of high drug concentration in the upper GI tract[55,76–79] mucosa obviously relates to the appreciable risk in this region. Such pharmacokinetic factors have been explored extensively[55,76–79]. It is noteworthy that nonacidic NSAIDs which have low gastric irritancy coin-

cidentally do not accumulate in certain cells in the mucosa in direct contrast to acidic drugs (e.g. salicylates, indomethacin) which are classically ulcerogenic[79]. These and other pharmacokinetic features emphasise the importance of this parameter in the upper GI irritancy/ulcerogenicity of NSAIDs[79].

However, it has also now become recognized from animal studies that those NSAIDs which exhibited pronounced enterohepatic recirculation with consequent repeated exposure of the intestinal tract to drug conjugates or from formulation design slowly release the NSAID in the intestinal may cause injury in the lower bowel of rats[102,103]. Evidence is now accumulating that NSAIDs may induce permeability changes and inflammation in the lower intestinal tract in humans[104,105]. At least one NSAID, indomethacin, which has a proven record of causing intestinal perforation in rats has been shown to undergo appreciable biliary elimination in human subjects with T-tubes inserted after cholecystectomy operations[106]. That biliary excretion of the conjugated and free drug is increased in patients with liver disease concomitant with increased plasma levels of the drug[106] is indicative of a mechanism by which liver disease may be responsible for enhanced intestinal injury from this and other NSAIDs in man. The lower intestinal tract could be a particularly treacherous region in which to deliver a drug from slow-release preparations. Such a situation was highlighted by the disaster which occurred with the slow release indomethacin formulation, Osmosin[13].

It is now evident that the mechanism of mucosal injury in the stomach may be quite different to those in the lower intestinal tract[102]. Variations occur in the kinetics of drug absorption from the different regions of the gut and subsequent distribution with individual classes of NSAIDs[102,103]. This is dependent upon their physicochemical properties which are responsible, in part, for their differing ulcerogenic actions in specific regions of the GI tract[107]. There are markedly different physiologic and anatomic properties of these regions which are responsible for variations in the susceptibility of the mucosa towards the ulcerogenic effects of the NSAIDs[102,107]. Hence, acid and pepsin in the stomach obviously contribute to gastric mucosal injury in this region whereas these agents cannot be implicated in damage to the lower intestinal tract because they are just present in this region[102]. However, bile salts and the preponderance of bacteria in the lower intestinal tract appear to contribute considerably to injury in this region whereas both these factors may have less or rather more variable role in the stomach (e.g. as from bile reflux, overgrowth of *Campylobacter* or other bacterial species with achlorhydria)[102]. Hence a variety of physiologic as well as environmental factors contribute to the development of the ulcerogenic potential of a particular NSAID (Table 6)[102]. The physicochemical properties and biochemical actions of these drugs vary considerably not only within particular classes of NSAIDs (e.g. oxicam, fenamates, phenylacetic and phenylpropionic acids) even though they may all have inhibitory effects on the production of the so-called cytoprotective prostaglandins (PGs) $E_2$ and $I_2$, a feature which has been proposed as being most determinative in the ulcerogenic actions of NSAIDs[102,108].

**Table 6a Summary of physiopathologic and biochemical factors implicated in the pathogenesis of GI mucosal injury by NSAIDs**

| Factor | Probable consequences |
|---|---|
| Acidity of drug (organic acid) | Membrane disruption: loss of integrity |
| Inhibition of $PGI_2$ & $PGE_2$ synthesis | Altered blood flow → anoxia |
| | Platelet-vessel adhesion promoted |
| | Microvascular injury |
| | Reduced 'cyto'-protection by: |
| | Decreased mucus production |
| | Decreased $HCO_3^-$ secretion |
| Release of lysosomal hydrolases | Promotes local cellular autolysis |
| Cholinergic activation | Acid/pepsin secretion enhanced (stomach) |
| Histamine release from mast cells | Promotes acid secretion, vasodilation (stomach) |
| Enhanced oxyradical production | Localized tissue destruction |
| Reduced sulphydryls | Loss of reductive protection by mucosal biomolecules against oxyradical damage & perturbed eicosanoid metabolism |
| Enhanced motility (amplitude) | Altered GI transit |
| Inhibition of ATP production | Reduced capacity to resist cell injury from mucus and other synthetic reactions |
| Altered cAMP levels (? from phosphodiesterase inhibition) | Perturbed cell regulation especially of acid secretion (stomach) |
| Inhibition of mucus biosynthesis (at enzyme level) | Reduced mucus surface protection |

It should be emphasized that many of the probable consequences of the abovementioned drug actions are rather speculative at the present state of knowledge.

**Table 6b Summary of pharmacokinetic factors affecting mucosal damaging potential of NSAIDs in specific regions of GI tract**

A. Absorption - dependent upon:
    (a) Dissolution (from tablet, capsule) or release (from sustained release preparations)
    (b) Intrinsic rates of absorption of pure drug related to aquo-/lipo-solubility
    (c) Specific cell accumulation e.g. ASA in parietal cells

B. Metabolism
    (a) Mucosal metabolism of specific drugs e.g. aspirin by esterases to less irritant salicylate, competition with acetylation by salicylate
    (b) Liver or other metabolism:
    Pro-drugs: sulindac → sulindac sulphide interconversion; fenbufen → biphenylacetic acid.
    Glucuronide conjugation: determines 'free' drug concentrations.

C. Distribution
    (a) Extent of enterohepatic recirculation. Where more pronounced this favours propensity for intestinal damage.

D. Elimination
    (a) Plasma or elimination half-life, long half life to drugs result in longer exposure of GI mucosa. Where renal eliminations impaired (as in elderly) these drugs accumulate in systemic circulation.

(b) *Mechanisms of GI ulceration of NSAIDs* – Table 6a gives a summary of the principle biochemical, cellular and physiological actions of NSAIDs which are considered at present to be important in the pathogenesis of mucosal injury in the GI tract.

(i) Inhibition of prostaglandin production. One of the major biochemical effects of the NSAIDs, the inhibition of prostaglandin ($E_2/I_2$) synthesis has been related by some to gastric ulcerogenicity of NSAIDs[108]. However, such relationships do not hold explicitly for all NSAIDs[108]. Thus, even aspirin, a classical cyclo-oxygenase inhibitor given parenterally or orally has been shown to inhibit the production of $PGI_2$ *in vivo* without inducing gastric lesions in rats[109,111]. Furthermore, other NSAIDs when orally administered doses sufficient to achieve inhibition of prostaglandin (PG) synthesis (as assessed from *in vitro* potencies, and from drug absorption data) does not always cause reduction of prostaglandin $E_2$ ($PGE_2$) coincident with the time-course of development of gastric mucosal damage in rats[108,111–114]. Some drugs (e.g. oxaprozin, chloroquine) when orally dosed to rats reduce the content of $PGE_2$ without causing significant signs of gastric mucosal injury (as determined by scanning electron microscopy)[102,114].

Inhibition of PG production may however have specific consequences for the vascular component of mucosal injury[111–113,115]. Evidence in support of this have been summarized recently[116,117].

Enhancement of gastro-irritancy of the NSAIDs has been observed in stressed animal models[8–11,15,81,102,118,119]. It is suggested that the initial inhibition of PG production by the NSAID might be envisaged as a 'priming' effect affecting vascular integrity[15,102,107]. Additional exposure to stressful conditions may, depending on their type and consequent effects, enhance the gastro-irritant actions of the NSAIDs by also affecting blood flow, energy (ATP) metabolism, acid/pepsin secretion, mucus synthesis or mucosal resistance factors[102]. The exact quantitative contribution of each of these biochemical events may vary with the different stressful condition. Whatever the contributions these stress responses may be considered to have 'secondary' effects[102]. Coupling of the initial 'priming' (i.e. inhibition of PG synthesis) with the 'secondary' stress effects and gastric mucosal injury is elicited[102]. This hypothesis though not yet proved may be a useful way of envisaging gastro-ulcerogenesis from NSAIDs[102].

It is of interest that the antimalarial, chloroquine, which is frequently used as a second line anti-arthritic agent reduces the production of gastric mucosal PGs when given orally to rats (presumably as a result of its capacity to inhibit phospholipase $A_2$), but is without any ulcerogenic effects at all[102]. Thus the concept of a relationship between PG synthesis inhibition and GI ulcerogenic effects is again without strict evidence to support it.

(ii) Mucus secretion and synthesis – Comparisons have been made between the gastro-ulcerogenic actions of NSAIDs and their ability to inhibit the biosynthesis *in vivo* of gastric mucus glycoproteins[102–122]. While positive associations have been observed between inhibition of mucus synthesis and the development of gastric damage by NSAIDs[120–122] it could be argued that as mucus secretion is regulated by E-type-PGs[122] these associations derive from a more fundamental control of mucus biosynthesis by PGs. Simply reducing PGs might also decrease the synthetic capacity to produce gastric mucus[123]. While such a possibility exists it is also known from *in vitro* studies that NSAIDs directly inhibit the enzymes involved in the biosynthesis of mucus and related glycoproteins[120,121]. Thus there could be effects of NSAIDs on mucus synthesis unrelated to their actions as inhibitors of PG production[120,121].

Of interest in relation to the specific role of mucus in protecting the mucosa against injury by aspirin and other NSAIDs are the observations that agents which stimulate mucus production (e.g. zolimidine, KL-II, geranyl lactone, sulfalcone) also exert marked protective effects against gastric mucosal damage elicited by the NSAIDs[124–127].

Recent interest has centred on the role of surface phospholipids in the mucus or mucosal barrier in protecting the latter from injury induced by drugs such as aspirin[128,129]. Reduction in surface hydrophobicity due to the phospholipids has been demonstrated with aspirin and the effects are reversed by 16,16-dimethyl $PGE_2$ [128,130]. Exactly how this PGE analogue restores the surface hydrophobicity of the mucosa is not known but it could result from non-specific surface irritant effects well known to be elicited by direct contact of PGs with the gastric mucosa[131,132]. Obviously the connection between reduction in surface hydrophobicity and inhibition of PG production is not proven and may be quite tenuous.

(iii) Consequences of inhibiting prostaglandin synthesis – The evidence cited in the last two sections suggest that the current concept that the main consequence of inhibiting PG $E_2/I_2$ synthesis and production is to reduce the levels of these endogenous 'cytoprotective' agents may be a flawed hypothesis since it implies a negative reaction i.e. a deficiency. An alternative explanation for the effects of inhibiting the PG cyclo-oxygenase enzyme is that there could be diversion of arachidonate through lipoxygenase pathway leading to enhanced production of potent vascular active peptido-leukotrienes as well as an oxyradical species derived from peroxidative attack of HPETEs which have been claimed to have potential cellular injuring effects[133]. This concept can be tested by examining the effects of 5-lipoxygenase (5-LO) inhibitors and peptido-leukotriene (LT) antagonists for their potential to modify the gastro-ulcerogenic effects of NSAIDs[133]. If the hypothesis is valid then these 5-LO inhibitors and LT antagonists would be expected to protect the gastric mucosa against injury by NSAIDs[133]. This hypothesis was examined in a model of NSAID-induced gastro-ulcerogenesis in mice treated with the cholinomimetic, bethanechol, to stimulate acid and pepsin secretion, so enhancing the irritancy of NSAIDs[133]. The results showed that the GI irritant effects of indomethacin when given orally or parenterally, could be prevented by co-administration of a range of 5-LO inhibitors and LT antagonists[133,134]. Further support fro the concept that excess production of 5-

LO products relative to that of the PGs could be a factor in gastric ulcerogenesis is the fact that dual cyclo-oxygenase/lipoxygenase inhibitors (e.g. BW-755c and benoxaprofen) or those drugs exhibiting balanced reduction in products of both pathways (e.g. chloroquine) are notably less ulcerogenic than drugs with equivalent cyclo-oxygenase activity alone[9,11,15,102,111–113,135]. Thus it appears that enhanced production of 5-LO products could be an explanation of some of the consequences of PG cyclo-oxygenase inhibition. It is obviously necessary now to explore these consequences in further detail.

(iv) Recent developments – approaches for reducing GI ulceration – The above discussion on the mechanism of GI ulceration of the NSAIDs has been a prelude to the consideration of procedures for reducing the occurrence of these severe side-effects

(a)  *Improved GI tolerance through molecular design:*

Despite the introduction of newer and in some cases more potent NSAIDs in recent years it is surprising that with a few notable exceptions there have been relatively few attempts with the very potent agents to incorporate in their molecular design some features to reduce GI ulcerogenicity. Extensive studies in laboratory animals have, however, enabled identification of a few of the NSAIDs with somewhat lower gastric irritancy in relation to their anti-inflammatory potency in different animal models[9–11,15,102,111–114,136]. Among these are azapropazone, etodolac, fenbufen (a pro-drug), meclofenamic acid, nabumetone, oxaprozin as well as *benoxaprofen and *fenclofenac which have also proven of low GI irritancy in clinical trials in man[6,8,9–12,14,15,102,111–113].

The selection of these low gastrotoxic drugs has been made possible from studies in special animal models[9–11,15,102,111–113]. These include those in which the animals are exposed to: (a) concurrent arthritic disease, (b) physical stress (which has an appreciable psychologic component), (c) nicotine (replicating the effects of cigarette smoking, and (d) orally administered ethanol (alcohol)[81].

It may therefore be possible in the future to develop less gastrotoxic NSAIDs based on structure-activity analyses to determine the chemical moieties involved in the expression of ulcerogenic effects (e.g. see ref. 137) assayed using the above-mentioned animal model systems. Further investigation of the factors accounting for GI injury by NSAIDs and the mechanisms involved in the cellular pathology of GI injury (Table 6a) will also help in developing less gastric toxic agents.

---

*Now withdrawn because of non-GI side effects

(b)    *Concomitant therapy with anti-ulcer agents:*

A second approach has been to employ agents to protect the mucosa against the ulcerogenic effects of the NSAIDs. Already some successes have been achieved in the application of 'standard' anti-ulcer agents (e.g. histamine $H_2$-, muscarinic $M_1$- and gastrin antagonists, mucoprotectants etc.) for the prevention or treatment of NSAID-induced upper GI mucosal injury[132,138–143]. It must, however, be said that the situation regarding the efficacy, side-effects and safety, as well as cost/benefit ratios of some of these agents is far from ideal[132,138–144].

There are several aspects to be considered in the application of conventional anti-ulcer agents:

(1)    The possibility that different dosage regimes may be required for the *prevention* of GI mucosal injury in those individuals whom are presumably more susceptible to the ulcerogenic effects of these agents (e.g. the elderly frail arthritic patient/compared with those required for treatment of a peptic or gastric ulcer which has presumably *developed* from ingested NSAID(s).

(2)    That cure rates never reach 100% for anti-ulcer agents used in the treatment of established ulcers and, moreover, there are few overall differences between the agents with respect to their cure rates[138,139,141,142].

(3)    While most of the anti-ulcer agents may prevent NSAID induced lesions in both animal model systems and human subjects[132] there have been relatively few studies performed to work out the clinical efficacy cost/benefit ratios and safety in the subjects for whom preventative therapy is contemplated, i.e. the GI-susceptible arthritic patient. There is no doubt that many of the anti-ulcer agents, especially the $H_2$-receptor antagonists are being co-prescribed with NSAIDs in the belief that the anti-ulcer agents work in as preventatives but the efficacy and cost of these has not been established.

(4)    The situation with the prostaglandin analogues, which have recently received special clinical attention, is somewhat controversial. While these agents exhibit impressive 'cytoprotection' (possibly better named G-I protective) effects in preventing ulcers, models induced in animals by NSAIDs and other agents[140,145,149] the fact is that to achieve effective treatment of upper GI ulcers in man or even to prevent their occurrence (given that relatively little data is available in the latter case) doses of the PGs have been appreciably high and approach the level of anti-secretory activity to be effective[139]. Then as will all anti-ulcer agents their effects are not 100%. Moreover, much controversy exists on the true nature of 'cyto-

protection' in that prevention of ulcers induced by NSAIDs and other noxious agents in laboratory animals may not be accompanied by prevention of injury to all mucosal cells[132,145,149]. Furthermore, in human subjects the high frequency of diarrhoea and other side effects poses serious limitations on the application of PG analogues especially as NSAID-ulcer preventative agents for long-term use in susceptible subjects.

In conclusion therefore, the fact that total mucosal protection is not achieved with these rather 'non-specific' anti-ulcer agents is itself recognition of the multiple actions of the NSAIDs in mucosal injury which clearly do not, alone, involve factors such as e.g. acid-secretion or depletion in mucosal prostaglandins alone. It is clear that for more effective prevention of ulcers from NSAIDs procedures will have to be developed to more specifically counteract the biochemical and cellular changes induced by these ulcerogenic agents.

(c)    *Approaches for achieving specific biochemical protection:*

Of the attempts now being vigorously pursued to achieve more specific gastroprotection against NSAID induced ulceration include the combination of NSAIDs with (a) lipoxygenase (LO) inhibitors or leukotriene (LT) antagonists[133,150,151], (b) micronutrients (e.g. amino acids, glucose and certain intermediates or precursors of the tricarboxylate cycle[132,152-159], (c) natural[160] or synthetic[161] phospholipids, (d) gamma-linolenic acid[162], (e) calcium channel blockers[163], (f) antioxidants[164] and (g) cyclic-somatostatin analogues[165] to name but a few of the diverse attempts based on biochemical changes induced by NSAIDs. Each of these has relative gastroprotective efficacy but none totally abolishes the mucosal injury due to the NSAIDs. Of the procedures explored by the author only alkyl-esterification of the acidic NSAID achieves anything approaching total abolition of gastric injury induced by the drugs, without adversely affecting their anti-inflammatory activity[166,167]. In practical terms this approach requires a totally new drug development programme whereas addition of the agents in (a) to (g) above requires much less in the way of development. Each of these procedures in (a) to (d) above has the specific advantage of addition of a naturally-occurring compound, they are inexpensive, and to a considerable extent they attempt to specifically counteract the biochemical abnormalities induced by NSAIDs. While evidence is still needed to support these concepts at least they afford a fresh approach to the problem of GI ulceration from NSAIDs.

Although GI ulceration and haemorrhage present with high morbidity and even appreciable mortality, the incidence of such effects is relatively low[8]. However, dyspepsia, diarrhoea, constipation and other symptomatic effects of the NSAIDs are of relatively high incidence and are among the most frequent reasons for withdrawal from the use of NSAIDs[8,120]. These symptomatic effects present a considerable challenge to the experimentalist to devise procedures or even new drugs to obviate their effects. For dyspepsia and the whole range of painful conditions in the upper GI tract there is really no animal model available to employ in testing these procedures or agents[120]. It is possible to speculate on the physiological basis to such painful states[120]. Thus epigastric pain and heartburn may relate to gastric acidity and certainly antacids and to some extent $H_2$-receptor antagonists give relief of these symptoms[120]. Again, however, it is only possible to speculate on causes but there is no real indication in man what mechanisms might be involved[120]. Likewise, while vomiting and nausea are suggestive of those centres such as the vomit reflex in the central nervous system (CNS) they do not give real indications about possible mechanisms[120]. Clearly the physiological reactions involved in these and other GI symptomatic effects of the NSAIDs require investigation in man possibly in the way of employing pharmacologic agents with known effects on GI motility, e.g. dopamine, alpha receptor antagonists and agonists or other agents to explore the pain-producing, nausea and vomiting symptoms[120]. There might be some limitations on methods which can be applied to the study of such symptomologies especially since they are usually present in already sick patients and, with the exception of NSAID induced diarrhoea and constipation, cannot be usefully explored in laboratory animals or human volunteers[120].

Studies from laboratory animals may help in elucidating the mechanisms of diarrhoea (e.g. by use of the arachidonic acid and various olive or croton oil induced diarrhoea models) and constipation which could also be used in the pharmacological testing of the GI effects of NSAIDs to give clues about the mechanisms of these symptomatic effects[120,168].

## 2.  Renal- and hepato-toxicities: the role of defects of drug metabolism and elimination

The importance is now well-recognised of disease-induced and age-dependent alterations in metabolism of NSAIDs, especially those involving liver, intestinal and renal detoxification, as well as in their renal elimination[3,4,48–57]. These factors contribute markedly to NSAID toxicity in the liver and kidney (see Table 5) as well as in other organ systems[3,4]. Among the most classical examples of this is that concerning the cholestatic jaundice with benoxaprofen which occurred in a group of 14 elderly arthritic patients in Britain during 1982[169,170]. An otherwise relatively safe drug became relatively toxic at what may have been high ingested doses. While the full patient details have yet to be published (because of inevitable restrictions from legal proceedings) the pattern which has emerged is that the benoxaprofen, a drug with long plasma elimination half life, exhibited accumulation in the elderly patients because of sub-normal renal elimination in these individuals[170,171]. The liver drug-metabolizing enzymes became overloaded by the accumulated drug and the jaundice thus ensued[170,171]. In one of the few detailed reports available of a peculiar cluster of five deaths in one area in Northern Ireland, three of the patients were noted to have taken paracetamol at unspecified doses[169]. Combinations of this drug, which is known to have high intrinsic irreversible hepatotoxicity, with that of benoxaprofen may have precipitated the toxic reactions to the latter drug. This leaves open the question of whether or not the other patients who died from cholestatic jaundice were not also receiving paracetamol or other such potentially hepatotoxic drugs. The increased propensity to GI ulceration and haemorrhage was also noted in the elderly with this otherwise low gastrotoxic drug[172,173], may have been a result of depressed renal elimination of the drug in the elderly leading to higher than normal blood levels causing liver dysfunction, which may promote GI mucosal disturbances and/or direct mucosal injury from circulating drug.

Some other examples of NSAID-disease or age interactions are of particular importance clinically[3-5,174]. Thus hepatitis reflected by elevated liver transaminases, occurs somewhat infrequently in arthritic patients taking NSAIDs[3-5,174]. This problem is notably frequent on children with rheumatic fever or juvenile rheumatoid arthritis taking aspirin[175,176] as well as in adults with arthritis[177,178].

Hepatotoxicity induced by NSAIDs has been extensively investigated in laboratory animals as well as in cell culture systems. Some NSAIDs (e.g. benoxaprofen and indomethacin) have been found to affect the clearance of bromosulphophthalein (BSP)[179]. Liver concentrations of ATP are influenced by the clearance liver of salicylate and other xenobiotics[5,180]. It could be that uncoupling reactions of the NSAIDs (e.g. salicylates, phenylbutazone and indomethacin) on mitochondrial ATP production could deplete levels of this high energy intermediate required for hepato-biliary transport of bile and other conjugates[5,180,181]. It is also known that mitochondrial functions are abnormal in the livers of adjuvant arthritic rats, so the effect of this disease could enhance the uncoupling actions of the NSAIDs on mitochondria[181]. Liver toxicity from NSAIDs could also result from other metabolic perturbations from the arthritic disease process, e.g. sub-normal microsomal drug metabolism, albumin or other plasma protein, oxyradical production[181-183], which can also be influenced by environmental and genetic variables[182]. Drug interactions can also influence the development of hepatotoxicity, those of most concern are the interactions between paracetamol and aspirin[184,185] (or vice versa). That NSAIDs have intrinsic cytotoxic properties to hepatocytes has been demonstrated in primary cultures of rat cells[186]. In such systems indomethacin and benoxaprofen show pronounced leakage of lactase dehydrogenase at very high concentrations (500-1000 μmol/l) concomitant with reduced variability which ibuprofen and aspirin showed appreciably low toxicity[186]. While the concentrations required for effect are very high the cytotoxic effects of the two former drugs are in agreement with their known action in impair and clearance of BSP in rats, a functional index of *in vivo* viability[179]. Such *in vitro* culture systems may prove useful in rapidly screening the intrinsic toxicity of NSAIDs, especially the effects of drug combinations, disease status (e.g. in cells derived from arthritic rats or humans) and exposure to other agents. Such rapid screening procedures may be useful in establishing at an early stage of drug development the intrinsic hepatotoxicity of new drugs and combinations with other therapeutic agents.

Of interest in relation to the pharmacological effects of NSAIDs influencing their hepatotoxic actions has indirectly come from observations of the protective effects of 16,16-dimethyl-$PGF_{2\alpha}$ in reversing the depressed cytochrome $P_{450}$ enzyme system induced by indomethacin[187]. It is possible that depressed circulating levels of endogenous PGs produced by NSAIDs could contribute to the depressed drug metabolism of NSAIDs. This protective effect of the PG analogue might be explored as a means of restoring subnormal drug metabolizing enzyme capacity to normal.

Impaired renal function with nephrotic syndrome is associated with the NSAIDs. This is evident in those individuals with certain arthritic conditions (e.g. systemic lupus erythematosus, rheumatoid arthritis) and then only in those patients with particularly severe disease[3,4,18,19,188,189]. It appears depletion of the production of vasodilatory PGs may allow for the enhanced activity of renin-angiotensin system and noradrenaline to elicit vasoconstrictor effects without appropriate or normal counter-regulation by the PGs[18,19,188]. Enhanced effect of angiotensin II activity and of noradrenaline are produced in stress conditions[18,19,188]. Some patients with particularly severe arthritic disease which are under chronic stress may have enhanced renin-angiotensin activity[18,19,188]. It is important however, to determine the extent of responses to the stress conditions and relate them to the effects of NSAIDs on renal malfunction following the intake of these drugs. Claims of renal sparing effects of sulindac[16,17] are probably critically related to dose of the drug and the presence of pre-existant renal disease[18,19].

In summary, therefore,

(1)     NSAIDs may exhibit pronounced hepato-renal toxicity if given to elderly and other individuals with subnormal renal eliminating capacity for these drugs. Those drugs with long plasma elimination half lives may be especially hazardous in such individuals if the dosage is not properly optimized[46,47].

(2)     Monitoring of renal function is clearly a means of reducing the likelihood of untoward effects from the NSAIDs in the elderly not only from the point of view of hepatorenal toxicity but also that affecting other organ systems. The development of accurate nomograms to adjust dosage for age and surface area in the elderly may also be one way of minimizing the risk of NSAID associated side effects.

(3)     There may be no truly 'renal-sparing' NSAID currently available although weak sparing effects may be evident with sulindac.

(4)     Combinations of cyclosporin, gold thiolates and D-penicillamine with NSAIDs are bound to lead to enhanced toxicity since these groups of drugs are all potentially hepatotoxic if only by different mechanisms[3,4,6,39,46]. If such combinations cannot be avoided then clearly rigorous monitoring of renal and hepatic function is mandatory in subjects receiving such combinations. Applying the choice of NSAID to minimizing the likelihood of such combinations producing effects would probably rely on the use of a weak PG synthesis inhibitor (e.g. azapropazone, fenbufen, sulindac) since the inhibition of PG synthesis might be expected to exacerbate the effects of the DMARDs.

(5)     The development of drugs with less hepato-renal toxicity might come from screening using the above-mentioned tissue culture systems. At least this is a quick and economical means of selecting out potentially toxic drugs. Also the use of animal models of disease activity in man might be justified (e.g. adjuvant-arthritic rat) especially where studies are combined with therapeutic investigations.

A footnote to these thoughts comes from a recent report that the FDA has, after 5 years, finally approved the use of diclofenac (Voltaren®) in the USA but only on condition that an approved labelling should include warnings that this drug is associated with significant elevations of liver enzymes and that periodic monitoring is recommended[190]. Why this should be a specific issue for this drug alone is hard to establish from the report[190] but such warnings might well be applied to all other NSAIDs since it is well-known that all will produce elevated liver transaminases is a proportion of arthritic subjects.


## 3.    Skin and related hypersensitivity reactions

*(a) Extend and pathology of dermatological reactions* Dermatologic side effects, especially rashes, are statistically among the most frequent and are also the most diverse of the adverse reactions encountered with the NSAIDs[3,4,6,48–51](Table 7).

Of these events, rashes occur with greatest frequency and are often reason for withdrawal from therapy[3,4,5,48,51,191]. Rashes form part of the spectrum of inflammatory skin disorders associated with the NSAIDs which are collectively termed *Dermatitis medicamentosa* or so-called 'Drug Eruptions'[192].

The manifestations of drug eruptions can be categorized as follows[192,193]:

-   Erythematous rash
-   Urticaria

64

- Morbilliform or macupapular eruptions
- Mucocutaneous reactions grading in severity to bullous-type, e.g. Stevens–Johnson syndrome
- Toxic epidermal necrolysis
- Photosensitivity reactions
- Fixed drug eruptions
- Lichen plannus and lichenoid eruptions
- Purpura

While the occurrence of rashes *per se* from NSAIDs may have relatively mild outcomes, i.e. being more inconvenient and unpleasant to live with, it is important to recognise that these manifestations may have, in but a few individuals with undefined susceptibility, potentially severe consequences, e.g. toxic epidermal necrolysis, and Steven's-Johnson syndrome, which are frequently fatal (Table 7). The grading of pathology between rashes and other more severe skin reactions is variable and may even include a variety of reactions in one individuals[193].

NSAIDs appear to vary in their propensity to produce rashes but alclofenac*, aspirin, azapropazone, benoxaprofen*, fenclofenac*, fenbufen, feprazone*, gold salts, isoxicam, D-penicillamine, piroxicam and tiaprofenic acid feature particularly as being most frequently associated with these reactions (Table 7)[3,4,48–51]. In the case of alclofenac, fenclofenac and feprazone the occurrence of these and related adverse effects was sufficiently high as to necessitate withdrawal or suspension of these drugs from the market, while with benoxaprofen there were other added factors as well.

The effect of isoxicam is apparently related to the presence of a manufacturing impurity (Compound 533) encountered in certain batches of the drug in France though this may not entirely explain all the instances of Lyell's syndrome produced by the drug which necessitated its withdrawal[195].

*(b) Hypotheses for the mechanisms of NSAID-associated skin rashes* – Most mild rashes from NSAIDs are essentially reversible inasmuch as the condition abates upon cessation of therapy. Thus, aside from the inconvenience to the patient, the problem is manageable. Simple erythematous rashes and associated urticarial conditions are probably Type I immediate-type hypersensitivity reactions, of Gell and Coombs type involving the B-cell production of IgE which upon binding to mast cells and subsequent sensitization yields histamine and leukotrienes[193]. Thus antihistamines find predominant place in treatment of these states though in general this therapy is often limited or ineffective. Drug-induced rashes may also have a non-allergic basis as a result of accumulation in high concentrations of drugs in the skin; as seen by autoradiography in rats NSAIDs have been shown to have a specific propensity to accumulate in this tissue[193].

---

*Now withdrawn

Table 7  Dermatological side effects associated with NSAIDs

| Type | Frequency | Nature |
|---|---|---|
| Skin rashes | High, especially with penicillamine (pemphigis type - sometimes fatal) also with fenbufen, fenclofenac, feprazone, azapropazone, gold salts | Mild, but in cases of benoxaprofen, fenclofenac and feprazone, a major reason for withdrawal of these drugs; often with photo-toxic component |
| Erythema multiforme with variants, i.e. Stevens–Johnson syndrome, Lyell's syndrome (toxic epidermal necrolysis) | Rare, but noted especially with phenyl-butazone, oxyphenbutazone, benoxaprofen, piroxicam, clobuzarit (Clozic), rarely with zomepirac, sulindac, meclofenamate | Severe, often with fatal outcome; Stevens-Johnson syndrome associated with clobuzarit (Clozic) and isoxicam was major reason for withdrawal |
| Photosensitivity reactions | High, especially with phenylpropionic acids, indomethacin, piroxicam | Normally related to sun exposure and spectral properties of drugs |
| Miscellaneous | | |
| aspirin-induced urticaria | Relatively frequent | Variable |
| benign morbilliform eruptions | Noted with phenylalkanoic acids; phenylbutazone, oxyphenbutazone | Variable |
| vasculitis | Noted especially with alclofenac | |
| anaphylactoid conditions | Noted especially with zomepirac, ibuprofen | Can be fatal; reasons for withdrawal of zomepirac |
| Lupus-like syndrome | Specifically seen with penicillamine | Severe |

Source: based on ref 40

Types III and IV delayed-type hypersensitivity reactions manifest respectively in formation of immune complexes which induce complement-activated tissue damage (vasculitis, agranulocytosis and anaphylactoid reactions), or of production of sensitized T-cells which elaborate lymphokines[193]. These states commonly underly the development of most other drug-associated skin reactions aside from simple rashes and urticarial conditions[193].

The underlying chemical features and biochemical actions responsible for the initiation of the range immunologic reactions responsible for NSAID-induced rashes and related reactions can essentially be considered as being due to:

1.  The development of a photo-degradation product(s). The best studied examples are the phototoxic products derived from benoxaprofen[194,196], and piroxicam[197]. In both these cases a photo-degradation product has been identified and cellular reactions identified (Table 8).

**Table 8  Reactive products obtained from ultraviolet exposure or metabolism of NSAIDs with proven skin toxicity, and associated cellular responses**

| Drug | Cellular responses identity/ structure of toxic product(s) | Cellular responses studied |
|------|------------------------------------------------------------|----------------------------|
| Benoxa-profen[10,22] | **Photoproducts:** (1) 2,-(4-dichlorophenyl-5-ethyl benzoxazole (DPEB) (2) Superoxide, singlet oxygen and hydroxyethyl radicals from UV + $O_2$. Possibility of hydroxy-ethyl peroxyl radical as inter-mediate during UV activation of benoxaprofen | (1) UV-A treatment induces intense itching and burning later with urticaria in sensitized individuals (2) Cell lysis of human erythrocytes exposed to benoxaprofen, $O_2^{\cdot-}$ and $O_2$ and UV ("photohaemolysis"). Reaction induced also by the photoproduct, DPEB (3) Release of histamine from rat peritoneal mast cells treated with benoxaprofen, $O_2$ and UV (but this was also evident with the drug alone) |
| Piroxicam[12] | **Metabolite "C"; UV-A-induced phototoxicity** | (1) Direct phototoxic effect not demonstrable; only metabolite C induces phototoxicity (2) Photoallergy to C demonstrated in guinea pigs and C3H mice exposed to UV-A (3) Photohaemolysis assay (as for benoxaprofen) (4) Reduction to tritiated thymidine in lymphoblastoid cells by metab-olite but not by piroxicam (5) Phototoxicity of human mono-nuclear cells exposed to metab-olite C + UV-A |

2.  The eliciting of non-self antigen production by the reaction of photo-product(s) with self proteins which could then set up the immunologic reactions[198]. Thus for example, photodegradation of azapropazone and its 8-hydroxymetabolite has been demonstrated[198] and it has been suggested that a non-self antigen derived from the reaction of the photoproduct (as yet undefined) with self proteins.

3.  Direct *chemical modification* has been proposed. Thus the hypersensitivity reactions attributed to aspirin, some of which involve skin reactions have been attributed to formation of (a) aspirinyl or salicyl antibodies, or (b) acetylation of biomolecules by aspirin[5]. Likewise the skin rashes produced by tablets and to a lesser extent, capsules of alclofenac[199] can be attributed to manufacturing impurities which could be bioreactive (i.e. covalently interact with biomolecules to form non-self antigens). Alternatively the epoxide metabolite is produced by alclofenac[200]. However, to the authors' knowledge no skin reactions of this alkyl-epoxide metabolite have been demonstrated although it is hepatotoxic[200].

4.  The diversion of arachidonic acid through the lipoxygenase (LO) pathway following cyclo-oxygenase inhibition by the NSAID; the excess LO products being presumed to affect Langerhans cell reactions in the skin by known mechanisms of action of products e.g. leukotriene $B_4$ induced leukocyte accumulation[201–203]. It has been shown that the release of histamine by peritoneal cells induced by exposure to UV-A radiation and treated with NSAIDs, is accompanied by elevation of leukotriene $B_4$ ($LTB_4$)[204]. Interestingly, the release of $LTB_4$ was not induced by the treatment of the cells with NSAIDs alone suggesting that the UV exposure was required to elicit release of arachidonic acid, which then induced inflammatory reactions[202,203].

5.  Disease-related sensitivity to the skin reactions elicited by NSAIDs could be due to their secondary effects on the control of interleukin-1 production resulting from their effects on cyclo-oxygenase activity. While this hypothesis has not been tested it has been shown that:
    (a)  Enhanced IgG production occurs by treatment of mononuclear cells from patients with systemic lupus erythematosus with interleukin-1 (IL-1)[205].
    (b)  The subnormal production of IL-1 in mononuclear cells from patients with scleroderma is markedly increased by indomethacin[206]. This and other studies[22] indicates that cyclo-oxygenase inhibitors enhance mononuclear IL-1 production.
    (c)  The keratinocytes and reticular-histocytic, presumably Langerhans cells produce IL-1 in abundant quantities[208,209].
    (d)  UV radiation, notably that by UV-B induces expression of membrane-associated IL-1 by rat macrophages[210].

68

(e)     Langerhans cells can elicit cytotoxic T-cell responses against normal epidermal cells[211].

It is, therefore, postulated that skin reactions induced by toxic metabolites or photoproducts of NSAIDs could, with exposure to UV radiation, elicit immunological reactions in the skin by enhanced production of IL-1 which leads to production of IgG, increased IL-2 production to cause T-cell proliferation with consequent cytotoxic reactions by the latter on keratinocytes. The frequent, though variable association of HL-A bearing mononuclear-lymphocytes with skin manifestations of D-penicillamine and gold salts, for example, may be a reflection of the predisposition of the patients bearing these haplotypes towards developing skin reactions; phenomena which again show the importance of the monocyte/macrophage/Langerhans cell interactions with T-lymphocytes that could be dependent on the production and actions of IL-1 at the level of skin cells. Other inflammatory mediators (e.g. PAF[212], C5a[213]) could also be of considerable importance in aiding the generally promoting these responses in skin, and these, with other mediators (e.g. eicosanoids) would be a consequence of leukocyte infiltration.

Disease related propensity could also be due to sensitivity of lymphocytes to UV as exemplified by studies in patients with systemic lupus erythematosus[214]. The basis of this sensitivity resides in the inherent production of superoxide anions by lymphocytes of these patients. The consequence of this could be that this leads to superoxide-induced production of a presumptively skin toxic drug metabolite.

Clearly, studies on the mechanisms of NSAID-induced skin rashes and other hypersensitivity states could serve as a basis for defining assays to screen out these effects in newly developed drugs. Further studies are needed to also define the mode of action of these agents in producing these side effects in different disease states and so enable rational procedures to be devised to prevent these as well as the more serious dermatological reactions in man from the current NSAIDs.

## (4)  Destruction or protection of cartilage and bone with NSAIDs?

A number of studies[28] have implicated indomethacin in exacerbating cartilage and bone destruction in osteoarthritis (OA), since the initial observations by Cox in 1967[215]. Recently, suggestions have been made an international symposia, notably those sponsored by certain drug companies, that cartilage destruction might be related to the *in vitro* and *in vivo* inhibition by some NSAIDs of proteoglycan biosynthesis[20,34,33–36]. Claims have been extended to imply that some NSAIDs may not exhibit this biochemical effect and so may be regarded as cartilage protective. While these aspects are of interest especially in elucidating the suggestion that there may be some NSAIDs more suitable for pain relief in OA because they lack effects on proteoglycan synthesis it should be noted that nearly all the studies on the biochemical effects of the NSAIDs have been performed on normal i.e. non-diseased tissues and the pattern of drug effects may not be the same as that in tissues from arthritic animals or patients.

Moreover, inhibition of proteoglycan synthesis might be conceived as being potentially harmful in osteoarthritis, this may however be of benefit in rheumatoid arthritis where there is proliferation of proteoglycan containing connective tissues. Thus, if differences do exist in the effects of different NSAIDs on connective tissue metabolism, including proteoglycan synthesis, this may have an important bearing on the appropriate choice of NSAIDs for the therapy of specific arthritic conditions.

## (5) Improving the safety of NSAIDs

With all the concerns now evident about the occurrence and severity of adverse effects from NSAIDs, it is of considerable importance to define the conditions and mechanisms involved in their development. Thus it should be possible to devise procedures to prevent the occurrence of these untoward effects by modifying therapeutic regimes, employing preventative or prophylactic agents, or designing drugs devoid of these effects.

What are the lessons which can be learnt from observations on the mechanism of NSAID side-effects? Some principle features include:

(a)     The fundamental importance of relating the pattern of drug biodisposition and pharmacokinetics to toxic effects in laboratory animal systems as well as in man,

(b)     The need to evaluate drug-disease interactions both in relation to pharmacokinetics and toxic reactions in laboratory animal models (e.g. adjuvant arthritic rat, MRL-mouse) so as to more accurately predict the likely toxicity in arthritic patients of newly developed as well as even some established NSAIDs,

(c)     The importance of investigating the role of impairment of the renal elimination of NSAIDs by elderly arthritic patients and,

(d)     The role of concomitant intake of other NSAIDs or analgesics which might be expected to compete with renal elimination and drug detoxification mechanisms.

*(a) Enhancing the predictability of preclinical studies* – Of the side-effects of the NSAIDs only those involving GI ulceration, hepatic, renal and haematological disorders can be predicted with any element of certainty from short or long term toxicological studies in laboratory species. The general approach in toxicological screening for evaluation of a drug for regulatory purposes is crude and essentially 'legalistic' in approach. The usual procedure in long-term toxicity trials is to establish from dosing drugs at a series of levels in cer-

70

tain species (one of which should be a non-rodent) with certain 'end points' i.e. doses at which a clear toxic effect is recorded. This process is exhaustive since it is considered that some of the rarer reactions may only be evident after a relatively long period of exposure to a particular drug.

However, a detailed analysis of data submitted by drug companies from the UK, FGR and Switzerland on short and long term toxicity of 40 pharmaceutical agents showed that *no new salient toxicological features were observed after 1-3 months in 31/62 case studies* and in a further 17 case studies then only after 6 months of drug exposure[216]. Thus short term toxicity studies in their present crude form have just as good a chance of predicting eventual long-term effects so why prolong the time of study?

Furthermore, the reliability of estimates of these studies being dose-response related and so serve as a guide to predict their occurrence in man is poor. This is due to the simple 'end point' read out from such studies, i.e. that an effect with occur at roughly such a dose after a given period of time, being highly variable.

The overall poor predictability of toxicity studies in animals can be attributed to a number of important factors, including:

(a)   The studies being performed in *normal* animals and not those having a form of the disease which can be considered representative of that in man.

(b)   Few if any reports incorporate common drug-drug interactions (not even with the most ubiquitous of all drugs, ethanol).

(c)   The toxicological profile of a drug not being always related to its pharmacokinetics and drug metabolism in the animal species especially those with an inducable inflammatory disease with those in man, often the studies are not strictly comparable (i.e. in respect of time or dosage).

(d)   More often no attempt is made to fully explore a known side effect for its mechanistic basis in a species of appropriate choice.

Some approaches should therefore be employed to improve the toxicological testing of NSAIDs and so achieve a more *Rational Toxicology*, for example:

(a)   Perform short-term studies in appropriate arthritic animal models to fully explore the dose-related toxic effects and explore the mechanisms of any drug-disease interaction(s) which may be apparent.

(b)   Relate dose-effects in animal toxicity at an early stage to drug metabolism and pharmacokinetics of the drug in appropriate species. Some predictive drug metabolism and pharmacokinetic studies should be performed with related compounds or predicted from theoretical analysis by computer model simulation to represent the situ-

71

ation in man to establish the organs in which the drug concentrations are highest and where active metabolites are formed. Since drug effects are most manifest in those organs where the drug or its active metabolites are present in highest concentration, it should be possible to identify the drug concentration in these organs and more rigorously relate this to drug toxic effects.

(c)     To more fully explore the more common drug interactions (e.g. with ethanol, β-blockers, calcium antagonists, nicotine and diuretics) in the animal models outlined above.

Overall, a more thorough mechanistic approach is required to understand and more accurately predict the toxicity of newly developed drugs for arthritis. A major effort is required to unhinge the current ties to a legalistic framework of drug safety requirements imposed largely by large, slow, clumsy and financially crippling bureaucracies which by virtue of the domination of some countries in the market place have a disproportionate control of the drug safety evaluation in the world today.

## III.   Slow-acting or disease-modifying anti-arthritis drugs for rheumatoid and related arthropathies

These comprise a heterogenous collection of agents for which the term 'slow acting' has aptly described the onset of their actions, but whether they can be considered to be truly 'disease-modifying' is very debatable. Nonetheless they constitute about the best available drugs likely to control the rheumatoid disease process. The major issues concerning the therapy with DMARDs are:

(1)     What are the real long-term benefits of these drugs?

(2)     How can their benefits be reckoned against the wide range of what are really quite severe and long lasting side effects?

(3)     What aspects of their mode(s) of action An be considered relevant to true disease-modifying activity, and thus what leads can be determined as a basis for future drug developments?

This section attempts to address to these specific issues. A comprehensive coverage of the literature is not envisaged, for this the reader can refer to several recent reviews or papers on their therapeutic[6,30,53,217-21] (see also Haynes and Whitehouse, this volume) and side effects[3,4,40,48-51].

## 1.   Benefits/risks

The 'sharp-edge' or 'bottom line' of the issues concerning long-term benefits of DMARDs has been criticised by an eminent rheumatologist, Professor Harry Paulus[222], who summarized the situation by pointing out the 'fall out' rate for therapy with these agents for 1–5 years is extraordinarily high (see also Tables 10 and11). This he attributes to being a lack of therapeutic response and an unacceptably high incidence of adverse effects in an appreciable number of patients.

Moreover, the dilemmas in assessing what are meaningful biochemical measures of disease-modifying activity which can be used as leads for future drug therapy have been well-expressed by the conclusions drawn in a recent review by Pullar and Capell[52]:

> "The message to be gained from recent studies is that currently used second-line treatment can slow radiological progression but in most cases does not. Why is this the case? If control of acute phase proteins is the major goal the continuing search for more effective second-line drugs or more effective ways of using those currently available should bear fruit."

and

> "The final uncertainty relates to parameters (i.e. the acute phase reactants, e.g. C-reactive protein ( + CRP) that are not readily measured yet may influence outcome."

Some attempts to move closely define the responses to 'second-line' therapies from gold salts have come from recent attempts to sub-group analyses of responders and non-responders[52]. Overall, the outcome from these studies can be summarised:

(1)     If comparisons are made in a group of individuals with high initial values of ESR and CRP (i.e. presumptive high disease activity), then those in which ESR and CRP are markedly reduced (i.e. to values of ESR < 30 mm/h and CRP < 20 mg/l) will show evidence of no radiological deterioration[223]. That is to say that in the group most likely to be considered as 'responders' biochemically-speaking, will show no evidence of improvement but will not obviously deteriorate either. In other words, the most that can be expected is slowing down of the process of deterioration.

(2)     For other groups showing no major response to ESR and CRP the outcome is marginal at best[52,223].

(3)     The only drugs showing convincing reversal of radiologically observed progression are by cyclophosphamide and azathioprine[224]. With these there are real problems of toxicity, in the case of cyclophosphamide which can be regarded as so severe as to be unacceptable.

(4)     The impression is that if selection for entry to second line DMARD therapy is made more rigorously on the basis of high CRP and ESR values then the outcome is, for treatment with gold salts and D-peni-

cillamine, likely to be at best the most favourable and then only a delaying process. For other categories it may not be justified to employ this class of thiolates, because the benefits/risk ratio may prove unfavourable.

## 2. Mode of action of thiolates relevant therapeutically

The impression from the above analysis of the actions of thiolates relevant to their potential to control the radiological progression of joint manifestations in rheumatoid arthritis is the link of therapeutic actions of these drugs to their ability to modify the acture phase reactants.

To understand how this may occur it is necessary to review the controls of the production of acute phase proteins (APPs) and indicate or perhaps speculate how these may be modified by DMARDs and what relevance this may have, for the ultimate therapeutic outcome the control of joint damage. While considerable information is available on the molecular biology of the production of APPs in inflammation[225] especially that involving interleukins (ILs) 1 and 6, practically nothing is known about the molecular aspects of modifying APP production except that some thiolates may modify the production or action of IL-1.

The second level of action of the thiolates is at the level of the lymphocyte populations and especially the modification of macrophage/monocyte production of cytokines that influence lymphocyte proliferation[219,220] (see also gold thiomalates by Haynes and Whitehouse, this volume).

Table 9   Summary of side-effects from SARDS/DMARDS

| |
|---|
| *Gold salts; D-penicillamine: usually major reason for withdrawal* |
| Renal: proteinuria |
| Skin: rashes |
| GI: diarrhoea (Au especially AF), upsets |
| Haematological:      agranulocytosis |
|                                  thrombocytopenia |
|                                  leucopenia |
| Neuromuscular system: myasthenia (Pn) |
| Oral: taste, lichen planus (Pn) |

Abbreviations: Au = gold salts, AF = auranofin, Pn = D-penicillamine
Based on refs 3-6, 30, 48-51

The third level which thiols such as D-penicillamine could act is in the control of connective tissue metabolism have been studied extensively[217]. Recent interest has surrounded the modification of IL-1 production and responses and the link with inflammatory cell accumulation[227]. At this level D-penicillamine has pronounced effects in reducing cartilage degradation in the Willoughby-Sedgwick air pouch model of cartilage resorption[227].

Table 10    Frequency of adverse effects observed in D-penicillamine treatment

| Adverse effect | High dose > 750 mg/d (Frequency in %) | | Low dose < 750 mg/d (Frequency in %) | |
|---|---|---|---|---|
| | Overall | Withdrawal | Overall | Withdrawal |
| Mucocutaneous toxicity | | | | |
| Skin rashes | 16 | 9 | 15 | 9 |
| Mouth ulcers | 11 | | 6 | 4 |
| Taste impairment | 26 | 1 | 12 | |
| Gastrointestinal toxicity | 20 | 11 | 13 | 5 |
| Renal toxicity | | | | |
| Proteinuria | 16 | 11 | 10 | 10 |
| Haematuria | | | | |
| Haematological | | | | |
| Thrombocytopenia | 12 | 3 | 9 | 5 |
| Neutropenia | 3 | 2 | 3 | 2 |
| Eosinophilia | | 0.5 | — | |
| Autoimmune syndromes | | | | |
| Systemic lupus | | | | |
| erythematosus | < 1 | Apparently not dose dependent | | |
| Myasthenia gravis | < 1 | | | |
| Goodpasture | < 1 | | | |
| Alveolitis | | | < 1 | |
| Hepatic dysfunction | | | < 1 | |

based on Howard-Lock, Lock, Mewa & Kean, 1986

The problem of thiol reactivity has attracted much interest over the years[217]. Thus serum sulphydryl (SH) reactivity is improved by D-penicillamine but other NSAIDs and presumptive DMARDS, such as salazopyrine, also influence SH activity. Linkage of serum SH reactivity with the production of albumin as well as $\alpha$ and $\beta$-globulins/components and copper and zinc ion status of the acute phase response has been shown in the adjuvant arthritis model, thus providing a link between acute phase response and thiol reactivity. The molecular controls underlying this association are not known but metallothionein synthesis which is important in metal-thiol interactions, undergoes modulation by gold thiomalate and auranofin by an acquired resistance[232–234].

At the level of lymphocyte proliferation and T-cell mediated cytotoxicity, sulphydryl group reactivity is a critical regulant. It is therefore not difficult to envisage the potential for thiolate DMARDs to modify these lymphocyte responses, which are obviously central to modifying the rheumatoid disease process.

The major difficulty with thiolates is in determining how much of the thiol drug reaches the sites of action on or in cells in the form which is presumed to be pharmacologically active. The extensive thiol interchange which occurs including the modification of albumin leaves open the question of how much drug reaches cells in the 'free', i.e. thiol form or whether or not this is the active form? Thus, some evidence exists for drug disulphides having actions[226].

Some novel thiol compounds have been developed for therapy of rheumatoid arthritis (reviewed in ref. 237). S-Adenosyl methionine (SAM) is a naturally-occurring thiol recently developed as a drug treatment for osteoarthritis[2238], a situation which is interesting in that there is a thiol drug being applied for an arthropathy hitherto thought unresponsive to thiol compounds. In addition to inhibiting synthesis of PGE and $TXA_2$ like materials[239], SAM seems to act by stimulating proteoglycan synthesis by isolated chondrocytes[240]. This drug may therefore present a novel development by controlling local PG related inflammatory responses which at the same time stimulate 'remodelling' at the level of cartilage metabolism. Clearly, further studies are needed to determine the clinical significance of these and other biochemical effects.

Recently thiolates including D-penicillamine have been shown to inhibit myelopoiesis *in vitro*[241] and this opens up another level of attack by these drugs of potential significance in the control of immune reactions in chronic inflammation.

## IV. CYTOKINES AS THERAPEUTIC TARGETS

Collectively the interleukins (ILs) by the extensive control of lymphocyte growth and proliferation, haematopoiesis, connective tissue and bone metabolism, fever and the acute phase responses to inflammatory insult represent an enormous potential for therapeutic modulation[207,225]. Their production variously by leucocytes, endothelial cells, fibroblasts (among many cells) coupled with the high degree of specificity of their production by inflammatory stimuli and potency of their responses makes them unique. Their predominance as mediators being produced by inflammatory cells and those cells which are involved in inflammation essentially embraces many of the components of chronic reactions. They are linked extensively with lymphocyte growth and proliferation and control the proliferation of cells of the monocyte lineage. Thus, as monocyte-lymphocyte cell cooperativity is an expression of chronicity of inflammation and the ILs are so much involved in the expression or controls between these cells then they obviously play a central role in chronic inflammation.

This rather superficial overview, meant more to give a conceptual framework for discussion in this section, disguises many of the complexities underlying the control of the expression of the six or possibly even more ILs which are produced by a range of different cellular stimuli and their targeted actions. The emphasis in this section will be to illustrate how current anti-arthritic drugs can control the production and actions of the ILs, principally IL-1, IL-2 and IL-6 (*syn.* B-cell stimulatory growth factor (BSF)/hepatic 2 stimulating factor (HSF)), and of tumour necrosis factor alpha

(TNF)[207,225,259]. The discussion is confined to these cytokines because more pharmacological studies on cytokines have been done on these mediators. Some aspects of the role of eicosanoids, principally the prostaglandins (PGs), on the production and actions of IL-1 will also be discussed as a means of illustrating the limited control by PG synthesis inhibitory NSAIDs in comparison with the potential for pharmacological control of other cytokines. These and other points will then serve as a basis for suggestions for future therapeutic developments.

## 1. Effects of NSAIDs and glucocorticoids on production of IL-1

Glucocorticoids almost universally inhibit the production of IL-1 $\alpha$ and $\beta$ *in vitro* by monocytes/macrophages, fibroblasts, synoviocytes, explants of synovial tissues in organ culture (Table 11 - see ref. 207). These drugs also appear to inhibit IL-1 production in *in vivo* models[243]. They are, therefore, essentially, a universal standard for experimental investigation even though little is known how they regulate IL-1 production, nor indeed if this has therapeutic significance for the mode of anti-inflammatory actions of these drugs.

By comparison, the actions of NSAIDs are much more complex (Table 11)[37]. There are considerable complications in interpretations of studies reported arising from different assay methodologies, variations in the purity and source of IL-1 preparations and the paucity of information on the rates of drug uptake into the cells or tissue systems under investigation[207]. Given these limitations the summary in Table 11 shows that NSAIDs regardless of whether they are simply cyclo-oxygenase (CO), or lipoxygenase (LO) or mixed CO-LO inhibitors show disparate effects on monocyte/macrophages *in vitro* compared with the effects on synovial IL-1 production. However, IL-1 induced resorption is blocked by chloroquine and related anti-malarials as well as by auranofin[32,242–247].

Likewise the products of eicosanoid metabolism have different effects showing that there may be important regulatory differences of eicosanoids metabolism on macrophage/monocytes (especially also as these influence cytokine actions on T- and B-cells - see Fig. 1) compared with that of synovial cells[243].

The actions of IL-1 in cartilage resorption also appear quite different to those on lymphocytes (Fig. 1). Thus, NSAIDs have virtually no effects on proteoglycan resorption by IL-1 and neither do the products of eicosanoid metabolism (PGs, LTs etc.)[244–247]. However, the latter products do modulate lymphocyte responses to IL-1 directly (Fig. 1) as well as through regulating IL-1 release from monocyte/macrophages. The lack of effects of NSAIDs and of eicosanoids on IL-1 induced cartilage protoglycan resorption[244,245] is intriguing in view of the activation by IL-1 of phospholipase $A_2$ in chondrocytes and production of PGs and other eicosanoids[248,249]. The major site for control of IL-1 induced resorption is that of transcription[242,245] and this may represent the site for chloroquine and auranofin[32,242,245].

**Table 11  Modulation of the release of interleukin-1 (like) activity[31,32,37,38,207,242-247]**

| Drug | System | |
|---|---|---|
| | Monocytes/macrophages | Synovial tissue |
| Corticosteroids | ↓ | ↓ |
| NSAIDs: Potent CO inhibitors, e.g. | | |
|       indomethacin, piroxicam | ↑ | ↓ |
|     Modest CO inhibitors, e.g. | | |
|       ibuprofen, aspirin | 0 | ?0,↓ |
| Dual CO/LO inhibitors:  ) | | |
|     BW 755c  ) | | |
|     ETYA  ) | ↓ | ↑ |
|     Benoxaprofen ) | | |
| D-penicillamine | | |
| Gold salts | | |
| Gold thiomalate | | 0 |
| Auranofin | | ↓ |
| Prostaglandins: | | |
|     PGE$_2$, PGI$_2$ | ↓ | |
|     PGF$_{2\alpha}$ | ↑ | |
| Ouabain (Na$^+$/K$^+$ ATPase inhibitor) | ↓ | |
| Actinomycin D | ↓ | ↓ |
| Echinomycin | | ↓ |
| Various inhibitor proteins | ?↓ | ↓ |
|   (ca. 20–40 kD) from cartilage, | | |
|   bone marrow, leukocytes) | | |

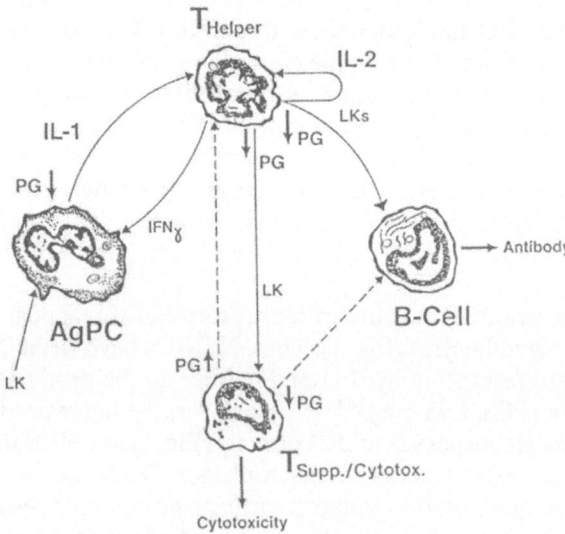

**Figure 1**  Modulation of T- and B-cell functions by prostaglandin E (PG), lymphokines (LK), interleukins (IL) 1 and 2, and γ–interferon (γ–INF). Leukotriene B$_4$ also modulates these lymphocyte functions.

At the level of IL-2 activity and especially the effects on receptors for this cytokine much interest has been shown on the effects of cytoclosporin A which has potent effects on these processes[250]. Auranofin has also been shown to effect proliferative responses of T-cells to IL-2. An interesting synergy has been recently noted between the *Streptomyces* derived drug, FK-506 and cyclosporin A on T-cell proliferation[250], which in view of the toxicity of cyclosporin A, (but nonetheless valuable therapeutic actions of this drug[253,254]) may be potentially useful combinations in the future.

An alternative approach to modulating IL-1 and IL-2 production has been afforded by the immunostimulator, OKY 432, which stimulates production of both these cytokines[255]. In rheumatoid arthritis immuno-stimulants such as levamisole have proven useful (although the latter drug has considerable side-effects which mitigate against its use). It is possible to consider steps of the rheumatic disease process which may benefit from immunostimulants. Thus, drugs such as OKY 432 and Wy18,251[256] may prove useful in rheumatoid arthritis by acting at the level of IL-1 and IL-2 production.

While it is possible to ascribe many immunoregulatory actions of the abovementioned drugs to their actions on IL-1 and IL-2 it should be noted that these drugs have other actions equally important on lymphocyte functions, e.g. cyclosporin A control of the expression of HLA-DR[257–258].

Finally, the actions of IL-6 have been shown to be regulated by glucocorticoids. While several drugs are known to be under investigation for effects as IL-6 induced APP production[259] the hepatocyte stimulating factor HSF effect[260], full reports of these are still to come.

## V. CONCLUSIONS

The studies reviewed in the latter section show how future progress may come from an intense investigation of the control of production and actions of cytokines known to be of significance in rheumatoid and related arthropathies. Perhaps too it may be possible to understand some of the actions of glucocorticoids in respect of their immunosuppressive effects. This may give leads for the development of drugs with steroid like actions without the inherent toxicities of their drugs.

## References

1. Buchanan, WW and Kean, WF (1987). Current non-steroidal anti-inflammatory drug therapy in rheumatoid arthritis, with emphasis on use in the elderly. In Lewis, AJ and Furst, DE (eds) *Nonsteroidal Anti-inflammatory Drugs. Mechanisms and Clinical Use*, pp. 9-29. (Marcel Dekker: New York and Basel)
2. Vane, JR (1971). Inhibition of prostaglandin biosynthesis as a mechanism of action of aspirin-like drugs. *Nature New Biol*, **231**, 232-5
3. Rainsford, KD and Velo, GP (eds)(1984). *Side Effects of Anti-inflammatory/Analgesic Drugs*. (Raven Press: New York)
4. Rainsford, KD and Velo, GP (eds)(1987). *Side Effects of Anti-inflammatory Drugs, Vols. I and II*. (MTP Press: Lancaster)

5.    Rainsford, KD (1984). *Aspirin and the Salicylates*. (Butterworth: London)
6.    Rainsford, KD (1985). *Anti-inflammatory and Anti-rheumatic Drugs, 3 Vols*. (CRC Press: Boca Raton, FI)
7.    Pemberton, RE and Strand, LJ (1979). A review of upper gastro-intestinal effects of newer non-steroidal anti-inflammatory drugs. *Dig Dis Sci*, **24**, 53-62
8.    Rainsford, KD (1982). An analysis of the gastro-intestinal side-effects of non-steroid anti-inflammatory drugs, with particular reference to comparative studies in man and laboratory species. *Rheumatol Internat*, **2**, 1-11
9.    Rainsford, KD (1981). Comparison of the gastric ulcerogenic activity of new non-steroid anti-inflammatory drugs in stressed rats. *Br J Pharmacol*, **73**, 79c-80c
10.   Rainsford, KD (1982). A comparison of the gastric ulcerogenic activity of benoxaprofen with other non-steroid anti-inflammatory drugs in rats and pigs. *Europ J Rheumatol Inflamm*, **5**, 148-64
11.   Dearden, JC and Nicholson, RM (1984). Correlation between gastric irritancy and anti-inflammatory activity of non-steroidal anti-inflammatory drugs. *J Pharm Pharmacol*, **36**, 713-5
12.   Greenberg, BP and Bernstein, J (1985). Fenbufen. In Rainsford, KD (ed) *Anti-Inflammatory and Anti-rheumatic Drugs, Vol. II*, pp. 87-103. (CRC Press: Boca Raton, FL)
13.   Rainsford, KD (1985). Anti-inflammatory drugs and the gastro-intestinal mucosa. *Gastroenterol Clin Biol*, **9**, 98-101
14.   Mangan, FR (1987). Nabumetone. In Lewis, AJ and Furst, DE *Nonsteroidal Anti-inflammatory Drugs*, pp439-72. (Marcel Dekker: New York and Basel)
15.   Rainsford, KD (1987). Gastric ulcerogenicity of non-steroidal anti-inflammatory drugs in mice with mucosa sensitized by cholinomimetic treatment. *J Pharm Pharmacol*, **39**, 669-72
16.   Bunning, RD and Barth, WF (1982). Sulindac: A potentially renal-sparing nonsteroidal anti-inflammatory drug. *J Am Med Assoc*, **248**, 2864-7
17.   Ciabattoni, G, Cinotti, GA and Pierucci, A (1984). Effects of sulindac and ibuprofen in patients with chronic glomerular disease. Evidence for the dependence of renal function on prostacyclin. *N Engl J Med*, **310**, 279-83
18.   Arroyo, V, Gines, P, Rimola, A and Gaya, J (1986). Renal function abnormalities, prostaglandins and effects of nonsteroidal anti-inflammatory drugs in cirrhosis with ascites. *Am J Med*, **81** (Suppl. 2B), 104-22
19.   Clive, DM and Stoff, JS (1984). Renal syndromes associated with nonsteroidal anti-inflammatory drugs. *N Engl J Med*, 563-72
20.   Ishioka, T (1987). Is tiaprofenic acid different from other NSAIDs with regard to renal function in the elderly? In Huskinsson, EC and Shiokawa, Y (eds) *Focus on Tiaprofenic Acid. Proceedings of the International Symposium on Rheumatology, Tokyo 1987*, pp. 159-68. (Excerpta Medica: Amsterdam)
21.   Palmoski, MJ and Brandt, KD (1980). Effects of some nonsteroidal anti-inflammatory drugs on proteoglycan metabolism and organization in canine articular cartilage. *Arth Rheum*, **23**, 1010-20
22.   Palmoski, MJ and Brandt, KD (1983). Benoxaprofen stimulates proteoglycan synthesis in normal canine knee cartilage *in vitro*. *Arth Rheum*, **26**, 771-4
23.   Brandt, KD and Palmoski, MJ (1984). Effects of salicylates and other non-steroidal anti-inflammatory drugs on articular cartilage. *Am J Med*, **77**, 65-9
24.   Herman, JH and Hess, EV (1984). Nonsteroidal anti-inflammatory drugs and moclulation of cartilagenous changes in osteoarthritis and rheumatoid arthritis. Clinical implications. *Am J Med*, **77**, 16-25
25.   Cooke, TDV (1985). Mechanisms of cartilage degradation: relation to choice of therapeutic agent. *Sem Arth Rheum*, **15**, 16-23
26.   Palmoski, MJ and Brandt, KD (1985). Proteoglycan depletion, rather than fibrilation, determines the effects of salicylate and indomethacin on osteoarthritis cartil-

age. *Arth Rheum*, **28**, 548-53

27. Kirkpatrick, KJ, Mohr, W, Wildfeyer, A and Hafercamp, O (1983). Influence of non-steroidal anti-inflammatory agents on lapine articular chondrocyte growth *in vitro. Z Rheumatol*, **42**, 58-65

28. Newman, NM, Ling, RSM (1985). Acetubular bone destruction related to non-steroidal anti-inflammatory drugs. *Lancet*, **2**, 11-4

29. Annenfield, M, Raiss, R and Cleres, C (1984). Einfluss steroidaler und nichtsteroidaler Antiphlogistika auf die Ultrastruktur von Chondrozyten der Ratte. *Arzneim Forsch*, **34**, 1763-5

30. Lewis, AJ and Furst, DE (eds)(1987). *Nonsteroidal Anti-inflammatory Drugs. Mechanisms and Clinical Use*. (Marcel Dekker: New York and Basel)

31. Rainsford, KD (1985). Preliminary investigations on the pharmacological control of catabolin-induced cartilage destruction *in vitro. Agents and Actions*, **16**, 55-7

32. Rainsford, KD (1986). Effects of anti-malarial drugs on interleukin 1-induced cartilage proteoglycan degradation *in vitro. J Pharm Pharmacol*, **38**, 829-33

33. Kagiwara, T, Mitsui, K, Fuju, K and Murota, K (1987). Effects of NSAIDs and synovial fluid on proteoglycan metabolism. In Huskisson, EC and Shiokawa, Y (eds) *Focus on Tiaprofenic Acid. Proceedings of the International Symposium on Rheumatology, Tokyo, Japan*, pp. 14-23. (Excerpta Medica: Amsterdam)

34. Carney, SL (1987). A study of the effects of NSAIDs on proteoglycan metabolism in cartilage explant cultures. In Huskisson, EC and Shiokawa, Y (eds) *Focus on Tiaprofenic Acid. Proceedings of the International Symposium on Rheumatology, Tokyo, Japan*, pp. 24-34. (Excerpta Medica: Amsterdam)

35. Iwata, H (1987). Effect of anti-arthritic drugs for articular cartilage and synovial fluid. In Huskisson, EC and Shiokawa, Y (eds) *Focus on Tiaprofenic Acid. Proceedings of the International Symposium on Rheumatology, Tokyo, Japan*, pp. 35-46. (Excerpta Medica: Amsterdam)

36. Shinmei, M, Kikuchi, T, Masuda, K and Shimomura, Y (1987). Effects of interleukin 1 and anti-inflammatory drugs on the degradation of human articular cartilage. In Huskisson, EC and Shiokawa, Y (eds) *Focus on Tiaprofenic Acid. Proceedings of the International Symposium on Rheumatology, Tokyo, Japan*, pp. 33, 47-59. (Excerpta Medica: Amsterdam)

37. Rainsford, KD (1987). Effects of anti-inflammatory drugs on the release from porcine synovial tissue *in vitro* of interleukin-1 like cartilage degrading activity. *Agents and Actions*, **21**, 328-40

38. Rainsford, KD (1988). Inhibition by cartilage and bone marrow fractions of cartilage resorption induced by interleukin 1 and tumour necrosis factor. *Agents and Actions*, **23**, 67–68

39. Rainsford, KD (1987). Introduction and historical aspects of the side effects of anti-inflammatory analgesic drugs. In Rainsford, KD and Velo, GP (eds) *Side Effects of Anti-inflammatory Drugs, Part 1*, pp. 3-26. (MTP Press: Lancaster)

40. Rainsford, KD (1987). Toxicity of currently used anti-inflammatory and anti-rheumatic drugs. In Lewis, AJ and Furst, DE (eds) *Non-steroidal Anti-inflammatory Drugs. Mechanisms and Clinical Use*, pp. 215-44. (Marcel Dekker: New York)

41. Anonymous (1986). Pfizer on NSAI ADRs. *Scrip*, **1079**, 22

42. Anonymous (1986). FDAs NSAI GI warning. *Scrip*, **1163**, 11

43. Anonymous (1986). Feldene hearing evidence. *Scrip*, **1084**, 18-20

44. Wolfe, SM (1986). Safety of Piroxicam. *Lancet*, **2**, 808-9

45. Anonymous (1987). CSM on ADRs in the Elderly. *Scrip*, **1084**, 25

46. Orme, M (1985). Pharmacokinetics of non-steroidal anti-inflammatory drugs in the elderly. In Brooks, P and Day R (eds) *Non-steroidal Anti-inflammatory Drugs. Basis for Variability in Response. Agents and Actions*, (Suppl. 17), pp. 135-40. (Birkhauser: Basel)

47. Lamy, PP (1987). Non-steroidal anti-inflammatories in the elderly. In Rainsford, KD

and Velo, GP *Side Effects of Anti-inflammatory Drugs*, pp. 151-172. (MTP Press: Lancaster)

48. O'Brien, WM and Bagby, GF (1985). Rare adverse reactions to nonsteroidal anti-inflammatory drugs. Pt. I. *J Rheumatol*, **12**, 13-20

49. O'Brien, WM and Bagby, GF (1985). Rare adverse reactions to non-steroidal anti-inflammatory drugs. Pt. II. *J Rheumatol*, **12**, 347-53

50. O'Brien, WM and Bagby, GG (1985). Rare adverse reactions to non-steroidal anti-inflammatory drugs. Pt. III. *J Rheumatol*, **12**, 562-7

51. O'Brien, WM and Bagby, GG (1985). Rare adverse reactions to non-steroidal anti-inflammatory drugs. Pt. IV. *J Rheumatol*, **12**, 785-90

52. Pullar, T and Cappell, HA (1986). Can treatment really influence the radiological progression of rheumatoid arthritis? *Br J Rheumatol*, **25**, 2-4

53. Day, RO (1985). Variability in response to NSAID. In Brooks, P and Day, R (eds), *Non-Steroidal Anti-inflammatory Drugs. Basis for Variability in Response*, pp. 15-9. (Birkhauser: Basel)

54. Famaey, J-P (1987). Synovial anti-inflammatory and anti-rheumatic drug levels: importance in therapeutic efficacy. In Lewis, AJ and Furst, DE (eds), *Nonsteroidal Anti-inflammatory Drugs, Mechanisms and Clinical Use, Chapter 13*, pp. 201-14. (Marcel Dekker: New York and Basel)

55. Rainsford, KD, Schweitzer, A and Brune, K (1981). Autoradiographic and biochemical observations on the distribution of non-steroidal anti-inflammatory drugs. *Arch Int Pharmacodyn*, **250**, 180-94

56. Fowler, PD, Shadforth, MF, Crook, PR and John, VA (1983). Plasma and synovial fluid concentrations of diclofenac sodium and its major hydroxylated metabolites during long-term treatment of rheumatoid arthritis. *Europ J Clin Pharmacol*, **25**, 389-94

57. Liauw, L, Moscaritola, JD and Burcher, J (1987). Diclofenac. In Lewis, AJ and Furst, DE (eds), *Nonsteroidal Anti-inflammatory Drugs, Mechanisms and Clinical Use, Chapter 19*, pp. 329-47. (Marcel Dekker: New York and Basel)

58. Wanwimolruk, S, Brooks, PM and Birkett, DJ (1983). Protein building of non-steroidal anti-inflammatory drugs in plasma and synovial fluid of arthritic patients. *Br J Clin Pharmacol*, **15**, 91-4

59. Wallis, WJ and Simpkin, PA (1983). Anti-rheumatic drug concentrations in human synovial fluid and synovial tissue. Observations on extravascular pharmacokinetics. *Clin Pharmacokinet*, **8**, 496-522

60. Lin, JH, Cocchetto, DM and Duggan, DE (1987). Protein building as a primary determinant of the clinical pharmacokinetic properties of non-steroidal anti-inflammatory drugs. *Clin Pharmacokinet*, **12**, 402-32

61. Hutt, AJ and Caldwell, AJ (1983). The metabolic conversion of 2-aryl propionic acids - a novel route with pharmacological consequences. *J Pharm Pharmacol*, **35**, 693-704

62. Hutt, AJ and Caldwell, AJ (1984). The importance of stereochemistry in the clinical pharmacokinetics of the 2-aryl propionic acid non-steroidal anti-inflammatory drugs. *Clin Pharmacokinet*, **9**, 371-3

63. Jamali, F (1988). Research methodology in NSAID monitoring: plasma concentrations of chiral drugs. *J Rheumatol*, **15** (suppl. 17) 71–78

64. Hayball, PJ and Meffin, PJ (1987). Enantioselective disposition of 2-aryl propionic acid nonsteroidal anti-inflammatory drugs. III. Fenoprofen distribution. *J Pharmacol Exp Therap*, **240**, 631-6

65. Abas, A and Meffin, PJ (1987). Enantioselective disposition of 2-aryl propionic acid nonsteroidal anti-inflammatory drugs. IV. Ketoprofen distribution. *J Pharmacol Exp Therap*, **240**, 637-41

66. Jones, ME, Sallustio, BC, Purdie, YJ and Meffin, PJ (1986). Enantioselective disposition of 2-aryl propionic acid nonsteroidal anti-inflammatory drugs. II. 2-phenylpropionic acid protein binding. *J Pharmacol Exp Therap*, **238**, 288-94

67. Meffin, PJ, Sallustio, BC, Purdie, YJ and Jones, ME. Enantioselective disposition of 2-aryl propionic acid nonsteroidal anti-inflammatory drugs. I. 2-phenyl propionic acid disposition. *J Pharmacol Exp Therap*, **238**, 280-7

68. Lee, EJD, Williams, K, Day, R, Graham, G and Champion, D (1985). Stereoselective disposition of ibuprofen enantiomers in man. *Br J Clin Pharmacol*, **19**, 669-74

69. Cox, JW, Cox, SR, Van biessen, G and Ruivart, MJ (1985). Ibuprofen stereoisomer hepatic clearance and distribution in normal and fatty *in situ* perfused rat liver. *J Pharmacol Exp Therap*, **232**, 636-43

70. Williams, K, Day, R, Knihinicki, R and Duffield, A (1986). The stereoselective uptake of ibuprofen enantiomers into adipose tissue. *Biochem Pharmacol*, **35**, 3403-5

71. McMahan, FG, Vargas, R, Ryan, JR and Fitts, DA (1987). Nabumetone kinetics in the young and elderly. *Am J Med*, **83**, (Suppl. 4B), 92-5

72. Thomson, CM (1987). Recent developments in the formulation of anti-inflammatory drugs. In Williamson, WRN (ed), *Anti-inflammatory Compounds*, pp. 303-22. (Marcel-Dekker: New York and Basel)

73. Day, RO (1985). Variability in response to NSAID. In Brooks, P and Day, R (eds), *Non-Steroidal Anti-inflammatory Drugs. Basis for Variability in Response*, pp. 15-9. (Birkhauser: Basel)

74. Cox, NL and Doherty, SM (1987). Non-steroidal anti-inflammatories: outpatient audit of patient preferences and side-effects in different diseases. In Rainsford, KD and Velo, GP (eds), *Side Effects of Anti-inflammatory Drugs*, pp137-53. (MTP Press: Lancaster)

75. Sebaldt, R-J (1986). A shorter plasma half life does not predict less drug accumulation. *J Rheumatol*, **13**, 1185-6

76. Brune, K (1974). How aspirin might work: a pharmacokinetic approach. *Agents and Actions*, **4**, 230-2

77. Brune, K, Rainsford, KD and Schweitzer, A (1980). Biodistribution of mild analgesics. *Br J Clin Pharmacol*, **10**, 279S-84S

78. Brune, K and Lanz, R (1985). In Bonta, IL, Bray, MA and Parnham, MJ (eds), *Handbook of Inflammation, Vol.5: The Pharmacology of Inflammation*, pp. 413-49. (Elsevier: Amsterdam)

79. McCormack, K and Brune, K (1987). Classical absorption theory and the development of gastric mucosal damage associated with non-steroidal anti-inflammatory drugs. *Archiv Toxicol*, **60**, 261-9

80. Rainsford, KD (1984b). Side-effects of anti-inflammatory/analgesic drugs: epidemiology and gastrointestinal tract. *Trends Pharmacol Sci*, **5**, 156-9

81. Rainsford, KD (1988). Animal models for the assay of gastrointestinal toxicity of anti-inflammatory drugs. In Greenwald, RA and Diamond, HS (eds), *CRC Handbook of Animal Models for Arthritis Research*, in press. (CRC Press: Boca Raton, FI)

82. Collier, D St J and Pain, JA (1985). Anti-inflammatory drugs and upper gastrointestinal ulcer perforation. *Clin Rheumatol*, **4**, 389-91

83. Duggan, JM, Dobson, AJ, Johnson, H and Fahey, P (1986). Peptic ulcer and non-steroidal anti-inflammatory agents. *Gut*, **27**, 929-33

84. Collins, AJ and DuToit, JA (1987). Upper gastrointestinal findings and faecal occult blood in patients with rheumatic diseases taking nonsteroidal anti-inflammatory drugs. *Brit J Rheumatol*, **26**, 527-32

85. Armstrong, CP and Blower, AL (1987). Non-steroidal anti-inflammatory drugs and life threatening complications of peptic ulceration. *Gut*, **28**, 527-32

86. Collier, D St J and Pain, JA (1987). Anti-inflammatory drugs and upper gastrointestinal perforation. In Rainsford, KD and Velo, GP (eds), *Side Effects of Anti-inflammatory Drugs*, pp. 285-93. (Lancaster: MTP Press)

87. Beard, K (1987). Nonsteroidal anti-inflammatory drugs and hospitalization for gastroesophageal bleeding in the elderly. *Arch Intern Med*, **147**, 1621-3

88. Sladen, G (1986). Peptic ulcer, nonsteroid anti-inflammatory drugs and the rheu-

matic diseases. *Brit J Rheumatol*, **25**, 330-2

89.    Caruso, I and Bianchi Porro, G (1980). Gastroscopic evaluation of anti-inflamma-
       tory agents. *Brit Med J*, **180**, 75-7

90.    Collins, AJ, Davies, JF and Dixon, A St J (1986). Contrasting presentations and find-
       ings between patients with rheumatic complaints, taking non-steroidal anti-inflam-
       matory drugs and a general population referred for endoscopy. *Br J Rheumatol*, **25**,
       50-3

91.    Malone, DE, McCormick, PA, Daly, L, Jones, B, Long, A, Breshirihan, B, Malony,
       J and O'Donogue, DP (1986). Peptic ulcer in rheumatoid arthritis - intrinsic or re-
       lated to drug therapy? *Br J Rheumatol*, **25**, 342-44

92.    CSM Update (1986). Non-steroidal anti-inflammatory drugs and serious gastroin-
       testinal adverse reactions, Parts 1 and 2. *Br Med J*, **292**, 614 and 1190-1

93.    Weber, JCP (1986). Epidemiology in the United Kingdom of adverse drug reactions
       from non-steroidal anti-inflammatory drugs. In Rainsford, KD and Velo, GP (eds),
       *Side Effects of Anti-inflammatory drugs, Part 1*, pp. 27-34. (MTP Press; Lancaster)

94.    Inman, WHW and Rawson, NSB (1987). Prescription-event monitoring of five non-
       steroidal anti-inflammatory drugs. In Rainsford, KD and Velo, GP (eds), *Side Ef-
       fects of Anti-inflammatory drugs, Part 1*, pp. 111-123. (MTP Press; Lancaster)

95.    Jick, H (1987). Incidence of serious side effects from non-steroidal anti-inflamma-
       tory drugs (NSAIDs) in the USA. In Rainsford, KD and Velo, GP (eds), *Side Effects
       of Anti-inflammatory drugs, Part 1*, pp. 47-52. (MTP Press; Lancaster)

96.    Wiholm, BE, Myrhed, M and Eckman, E (1987). Trends and patterns in adverse drug
       reactions to non-steroidal anti-inflammatory drugs reported in Sweden. In Rains-
       ford, KD and Velo, GP (eds), *Side Effects of Anti-inflammatory drugs, Part 1*, pp. 55-
       70. (MTP Press; Lancaster)

97.    Langman, MJS (1987). Anti-inflammatory drugs and gastrointestinal disease. Rea-
       sons for the failure of adverse reaction reporting and surveillance systems to detect
       a significant association. In Rainsford, KD and Velo, GP (eds), *Side Effects of Anti-
       inflammatory drugs, Part 1*, pp. 303-306. (MTP Press; Lancaster)

98.    Haglund, U, Frost, L and Wiholm, BE (1987). An evaluation of the frequency of anti-
       inflammatory drug intake among patients with acute gastrointestinal bleeding. In
       Rainsford, KD and Velo, GP (eds), *Side Effects of Anti-inflammatory drugs, Part 1*,
       pp. 309-314. (MTP Press; Lancaster)

99.    Henry, DA, Johnston, A, Dobson, A and Duggan, J (1987). Fatal peptic ulcer com-
       plications and the use of non-steroidal anti-inflammatory drugs, aspirin and corticos-
       teroids. *Br Med J*, **295**, 1227-9

100.   Carson, JL, Strom, BL, Soper, KA, West, SL and Morse, ML (1987). The association
       of non-steroidal anti-inflammatory drugs with upper gastrointestinal bleeding. *Arch
       Intern Med*, **147**, 85-8

101    Walt, R, Katshinsky, B, Logan, R, Ashley, J and Langman, M (1986). Rising fre-
       quency of ulcer perforation in elderly people in the United Kingdom. *Lancet*, **1**, 489-
       92

102.   Rainsford, KD (1987). Mechanisms of gastric contrasted with intestinal damage by
       non-steroidal anti-inflammatory drugs. In Rainsford, KD and Velo, GP (eds), *Side
       Effects of Anti-inflammatory Analgesic Drugs, Part 2*, pp. 3-26. (MTP Press; Lancas-
       ter)

103.   Brune, K, Dietzel, K, Nürnberg, B and Schneider, Th (1988). New insights into the
       mechanism of gastrointestinal tract ulcertations. In Lewis, A, Ackerman, N and Ot-
       terness, I (eds), *New Perspectives in Anti-inflammatory Therapies. Advances in Inflam-
       mation Research, Vol. 12*, pp. 239-245. (Raven Press: New York)

104.   Bjarnason, I, Zanelli, G, Prouse, P, Williams, P, Gumpel, MJ and Levi, AJ (1986).
       Effect of non-steroidal anti-inflammatory drugs on the human small intestine. *Drugs*,
       **32**, (Suppl. 1), 35-41

105.   Jenkins, RT, Rooney, PJ, Jones, DB, Bienenstock, J and Goodacre, RL (1987). In-

creased intestinal permeability in patients with rheumatoid arthritis: a side-effect of oral non-steroidal anti-inflammatory drug therapy? *Br J Rheumatol*, **26**, 103-7

106.    Terhaag, B and Hermann, U (1986). Biliary elimination of indomethacin in man. *Eur J Clin Pharmacol*, **29**, 691-5

107.    Rainsford, KD (1987). Drug induced mucosal damage. In Rees, WDW (ed), *Peptic Ulcer Disease. Proc. 7th BSG. SK and F International Workshop 1986*, pp. 7-12. (Smith Kleine & French Labs: Welwyn Garden City)

108.    Rainsford, KD (1988). Interplay between anti-inflammatory drugs and eicosanoids in gastrointestinal damage. In Hillier, K (ed), *Eicosanoids and the Gastrointestinal Tract*, pp111-28. (MTP Press: Lancaster)

109.    Ligumsky, M, Golanska, EM, Hansen, DG and Kaufmann, GL (1985). Aspirin can inhibit mucosal cyclo-oxygenase without causing lesions in the rat. *Gastroenterology*, **84**, 756-61

110.    Whittle, BJR (1981). Temporal relationship between cyclooxygenase inhibition, as measured by prostacyclin biosynthesis, and the gastrointestinal damage induced by indomethacin in the rat. *Gastroenterology*, **80**, 94-8

111.    Rainsford, KD and Willis, C (1982). Relationship of gastric mucosal damage induced in pigs by anti-inflammatory drugs. *Dig Dis Sci*, **27**, 624-35

112.    Rainsford, KD, Fox, SA and Osborne, DJ (1984). Comparative effects of some non-steroidal anti-inflammatory drugs on the ultrastructural integrity and prostaglandin levels in the rat gastric mucosa: relationship to drug uptake. *Scand J Gastroenterol*, **19**, (Suppl. 101), 55-68

113.    Rainsford, KD, Fox, SA and Osborne, DJ (1985). Relationship between drug absorption, inhibition of cyclo-oxygenase and lipoxygenase pathways and the development of gastric mucosal damage by non-steroidal anti-inflammatory drugs in rats and pigs. In Bailey, MJ (ed), *Advances in Prostaglandins, Leukotrienes and Lipoxins*, pp. 639-653. (Plenum Press: New York)

114.    Rainsford, KD. Comparative irritancy of oxaprozin on the gastrointestinal tract of rats and mice: relationship to drug uptake and effects *in vivo* on eicosanoid metabolism. *Aliment Pharmacol Therap*, **2**, 439-450

115.    Rainsford, KD (1983). Microvascular injury during gastric mucosal damage by anti-inflammatory drugs in pigs and rats. *Agents and Actions*, **13**, 457-60

116.    Szabo, S, Spill, WF and Rainsford, KD (1988). Non-steroidal anti-inflammatory drug-induced gastropathy: mechanisms and management. *Medical Toxicology*, in press

117.    Pihan, G and Szabo, S (1988). Effect of eicosanoids on gastrointestinal blood flow and microcirculation. In Hiller, K (ed), *Eicosanoids and the Gastrointestinal Tract*, pp. 163-94. (MTP Press: Lancaster)

118.    Shriver, DA, Dove, PA, White, CB, Sandor, A and Rosenthale, ME (1977). A profile of the gastrointestinal toxicity of aspirin, indomethacin, oxaprozin, phenylbutazone and fentiazic in arthritic and normal Lewis rats. *Toxicol App Pharmacol*, **42**, 75-83

119.    Rainsford, KD (1978). The role of aspirin in gastric ulceration. Some factors involved in the development of gastric mucosal damage induced by aspirin in rats exposed to various stress conditions. *Am J Dig Dis*, **23**, 521-30

120.    Rainsford, KD (1978). The effects of aspirin and other non-steroid anti-inflammatory/analgesic drugs on the gastrointestinal mucos glycoprotein biosynthesis *in vivo*: relationship to ulcerogenic actions. *Biochem Pharmacol*, **27**, 877-85

121.    Rainsford, KD (1982). Effects of anti-inflammatory drugs on mucus production: relationship to ulcerogenesis. In Pfeiffer, CJ (ed), *CRC Handbook "Drugs and Peptic Ulcer Disease"*, Vol. 2, pp. 227-236. (CRC Press Inc)

122.    Berrisford, RG, Wells, M and Dixon, MF (1985). Gastric epithelial mucus - a densetometric histochemical study of aspirin-induced damage in the rat. *Br J Exp Path*, **66**, 27-33

123.    Allen, A, Garner, A, Hunter, AC and Keogh, JP (1988). The gastrointestinal mucus

barrier and the place of eicosanoids. In Hillier, K (ed), *Eicosanoids and the Gastrointestinal Tract*, pp. 195-213. (MTP Press: Lancaster)

124. Ezer, E and Szporny, L (1970). Prevention of experimental gastric ulcer in rats by a substance which increases biosynthesis of acid mucopolysaccharides. *J Pharm Pharmacol*, **22**, 143-44

125. Corinaldesi, R, Casadio, R, Sovera, A, Girotti, A, Practico, A, Paparo, GF and Barbara, L (1980). Zolimidine: protection against aspirin damage in man. *Drugs Exptl Clin Res*, **2**, 55-60

126. Murakami, M, Oketani, K, Fujisaki, H, Wakabayashi, T and Ohgo, T (1982). Effects of the anti-ulcer drug geranyl-geranylacetone on aspirin-induced gastric ulcers in rats. *Jap J Pharmacol*, **32**, 299-306

127. Muramatsu, M, Arai, I, Isobe, Y, Hirose, H, Usaki, C and Aihara, H (1986). Effect of sofalcone on acute gastric mucosal lesions induced by aspirin and ethanol in reference to the biosynthesis of gastric mucosal glycoprotein. *Res Commun Chem Path Pharmacol*, **54**, 321-37

128. Hills, BA, Butler, BD and Lichtenberger, LM (1983). Gastric mucosal barrier: hydrophobic lining to the lumen of the stomach. *Am J Physiol*, **244**, G561-G568

129. Lichtenberger, LM, Grazian, LA, Dial, EJ, Butler, BD and Hills, BA (1983). Role of surface-active phospholipids in gastric cytoprotection. *Science*, **219**, 1227-9

130. Lichtenberger, LM, Richards, JE and Hills, BA (1985). Effect of 16,16-dimethyl prostaglandin $E_2$ on the surface hydrophobicity of aspirin-treated canine gastric mucosa. *Gastroenteroly*, **88**, 308-14

131. Rainsford, KD (1979). Prostaglandins and the development of gastric mucosal damage by anti-inflammatory drugs. In Rainsford, KD and Ford-Hutchinson, AW (eds), *Prostaglandins and Inflammation*, pp. 193-210. (Birkhauser: Basel)

132. Rainsford, KD (1989). The biochemical protective mechanisms against anti-inflammatory drug-induced GI mucosal damage. *Acta Physiologica Hungarica*, in press

133. Rainsford, KD (1987). Effect of 5-lipoxygenase inhibitors and leukotriene antagonists pathway on the development of gastric mucosal lesions induced by anti-inflammatory drugs in cholinomimetic treated mice. *Agents and Actions*, **21**, 316-9

134. Young, JM and Tomdonis, AJ (1987). Diphenylsulfide inhibits indomethacin-induced ulcerogenesis in rats. *Agents and Actions*, **21**, 314-5

135. Whittle, BJR, Higgs, GA, Eakins, KE, Moncado, S and Vane, JR (1980). Selective inhibition of prostaglandin production in inflammatory acidates and gastric mucosa. *Nature*, **284**, 271-3

136. Rainsford, KD (1978). Comparative studies of gastric ulcerogenesis by non-steroid anti-inflammatory drugs: effects of fenclofenac. *Proc Roy Soc Med*, **70** (Suppl. 6), 4-10

137. Rainsford, KD (1978). Structure-activity relationship of non-steroid anti-inflammatory drugs. I. Gastric ulcerogenic activity. *Agents and Actions*, **8**, 587-605

138. Hawkey, CJ and Rampton, DS (1985). Prostaglandins and the gastro-intestinal mucosa: are they important in its function, disease or treatment? *Gastroenterology*, **89**, 1162-88

139. Hawkey, CJ and Walt, RP (1986). Prostaglandins for peptic ulcer: a promise unfulfilled. *Lancet*, **II**, 1084-6

140. Londong, W (1986). Anti-ulcer drugs in anti-secretory doses for 'cytoprotection' in arthritic patients? *Klin Wochenschr*, **64** (Suppl. VII), 32-4

141. McLean, AJ, Harcourt, DM, McCarthy, PG, Dudley, GJ and McNeil, JJ (1987). Relative effectiveness and costs of anti-ulcer medications as a basis for rational prescribing. *Med J Aust*, **146**, 431-8

142. Malchow-Moller, A (1987). Treatment of peptic ulcer induced by non-steroidal anti-inflammatory drugs. *Scand J Gastroenterol*, **22** (Suppl. 127), 87-91

143. Konturek, SJ (1988). Clinical uses of prostaglandins in peptic ulcer disease. In Hillier, K (ed), *Eicosanoids and the Gastrointestinal Tract*, pp. 46-74. (MTP Press: Lan-

caster)

144. Boyd, EJS and Wormsley, KG (1987). Gastrointestinal side-effects of prostaglandins. In Rainsford, KD and Velo, GP (eds), *Side Effects of Anti-inflammatory Drugs, Vol.2*, pp. 143-149. (MTP Press: Lancaster)

145. Robert, A, Lancaster, C, Davis, JP, Field, SO and Nezamis, JC (1984). Distinction between anti-ulcer effect and cytoprotection. *Scand J Gastroenterol*, **19** (Suppl. 101), 69-72

146. Miller, TA (1983). Protective effects of prostaglandins against gastric mucosal damage: current knowledge and proposed mechanisms. *Am J Physiol*, **245**, G601-G623

147. Robert, A (1984). Mechanisms of cytoprotection. In Paton, W, Mitchell, J and Turner, P (eds), *Proceedings of the 9th International Congress of Pharmacology, IUPHAR, London, Vol. 3*, pp. 355-359. (Macmillan: London)

148. Wilson, DE (1986). Therapeutic aspects of prostaglandins in the treatment of peptic ulcer disease. *Dig Dis Scie*, **31** (Suppl.), 42S-46S

149. Szabo, S and Szelenyi, I (1987). 'Cytoprotection' in gastrointestinal pharmacology. *Trends Pharmacol Sci*, **8**, 149-55

150. Young, RN, Zamboni, R and Leger, S (1987). Preparation and formulation of 2-substituted quinolines as antagonists of leukotrienes and inhibitors of leukotriene biosynthesis. Europ Patent Appl EP219,307, 22 Apr 1987. US Patent Appl 788,180, 16 Oct 1985. *Chem Abstr*, **107**, 39645S

151. Young, RN and Zamboni, R (1987). Preparation and formulation of 2-(phenoxymethyl)-quinolines as anti-allergic, anti-asthmatic, anti-inflammatory and cytoprotective agents. US Patent 4,661,499, 28 Apr 1987. *Chem Abstr*, **107**

152. Okabe, S, Takeuchi, K, Nakamura, K and Takagi, K (1974). Inhibitory effects of L-Glutamine on the aspirin-induced lesions in the rat. *J Pharm Pharmacol*, **26**, 605-11

153. Okabe, S, Takeuchi, K, Nakamura, K and Takagi, K (1976). Effects of various aminoacids on gastric lesions induced by acetylsalicylic acid (ASA) and gastric secretion in pylorus-ligalidrates. *Arzneim-Forsch*, **26**, 534-7

154. Rainsford, KD and Whitehouse, MW (1980). Biochemical gastro-protection from acute ulceration induced by aspirin and related drugs. *Biochem Pharmacol*, **29**, 1281-9

155. Rainsford, KD and Whitehouse, MW (1980). Are all aspirins alike? A comparison of gastric ulcerogenicity and bioefficacy in rats. *Pharmacol Res Commun*, **12**, 85-95

156. Mersereau, WA and Hinchey, EJ (1982). Prevention of phenylbutazone ulcer in the rat by glucose: role of a glycoprivic receptor system. *Am J Physiol*, **242**, G429-G432

157. Whitehouse, MW, Rainsford-Koechli, V and Rainsford, KD (1984). Aspirin gastrotoxicity: protection by various strategies. In Rainsford, KD and Velo, GP (eds), *Side Effects of Anti-Inflammatory/Analgesic Drugs*, pp. 77-87. (Raven Press: New York)

158. Rainsford, KD (1987). Prevention of indomethacin-induced gastrointestinal ulceration in rats by glucose-citrate formulations: role of ATP in mucosal defences. *Br J Rheumatol*, **26** (Abstr. Suppl. 2), Abstr. 144, 81

159. Walker, FS, Pritchard, MH, Jones, JM, Owen, GM and Rainsford, KD (1987). Inhibition of indomethacin-induced gastrointestinal bleeding, both immediate and persistent, in man by citrate-glucose formulations. *Br J Rheumatol*, **26** (Abstr. Suppl. 2), Abstr 20, 12

160. Swarm, RA, Ashley, SW, Soybel, DI, Ordway, FS and Cheung, LY (1987). Protective effect of exogenous phospholipid on aspirin-induced gastric mucosal injury. *Am J Surg*, **153**, 48-52

161. Leyck, S, Huther, AM and Parnham, MJ (1987). Polyene phosphatidylcholine: an inhibitor of NSAID gastric toxicity which increases impaired mucosal $PGE_2$ synthesis. In Rainsford, KD and Velo, GP (eds), *Side Effects of Anti-Inflammatory Drugs, Pt. II*, pp. 163-164. (MTP Press: Lancaster)

162. Huang, YS, Drummond, R and Harrobin, DF (1987). Protective effect of gamma linolenic acid on aspirin-induced gastric haemorrhage in rats. *Digestion*, **36**, 36-41

163. Ghanayem, BI, Mathews, HB and Maronpot, RR (1987). Calcium channel blockers protect against ethanol- and indomethacin-induced gastric lesions in rats. *Gastroenterology*, **92**, 106-11

164. Von Kolfschoten, AA, Hagelin, F and van Noordwijk, J (1984). Butyl hydroxy toluene antagonizes the gastric toxicity but not the pharmacological activity of acetylsalicylic acid in rats. *Naunyn Schmiedeberg's Arch Pharmacol*, **325**, 283-5

165. Goldenberg, MI and Keller, DL (1984). Anti-inflammatory/analgesic combination of cyclo-(N-methyl-ala-tyr-D-trp-lys-val-phe) and a selected non-steroidal anti-inflammatory drug (NSAID). *US Patent No. 4,474,766*, 2 Oct 1984

166. Rainsford, KD and Whitehouse, MW (1980). Anti-inflammatory/anti-pyretic salicylic acid esters with low gastric ulcerogenic activity. *Agents and Actions*, **10**, 451-6

167. Whitehouse, MW and Rainsford, KD (1980). Esterification of acidic anti-inflammatory drugs suppresses their gastrotoxicity without adversely affecting their anti-inflammatory activity in rats. *J Pharm Pharmacol*, **32**, 795-6

168. Donowitz, M, Wicks, J, Cusolito, S and Sharp, GWG (1984). Pharmacotherapy of diarrheal diseases: an approach based on physiologic principles. In *Mechanisms of Intestinal Electrolyte Transport and Regulations by Calcium*, pp. 329-359. (Alan R Liss)

169. Taggard, H McA and Alderdice, JM (1982). Fatal cholestatic jaundice in elderly patients taking benoxaprofen. *Br Med J*, **284**, 1372

170. Del Favero, A (1983). Anti-inflammatory analgesics and drugs used in rheumatoid arthritis and gout. In Dukes, MNG and Elis, J (eds), *Side Effects of Drugs Annual 7, Chapter 10*, pp. 104-125. (Excerpta Medical: Amsterdam)

171. Prescott, LF and Leslie, PJ (1982). Side effects of benoxaprofen. *Br Med J*, **284**, 1783

172. Stewart, IC (1982). Gastrointestinal haemorrhage and benoxaprofen. *Br Med J*, **284**, 163-4

173. Halsey, JP and Cardoe, N (1982). Benoxaprofen: side-effect profile in 300 patients. *Br Med J*, **284**, 1365-8

174. Babany, G and Pessayre, D (1984). Heptatites dues aux nouveaux anti-inflammatoires non-steroidiens. *Gastroenterol Clin Biol*, **8**, 523-429

175. Hamdan, JA, Manasra, K and Ahmed, M (1985). Salicylate-induced hepatitis in rheumatic fever. *Am J Dis Child*, **139**, 453-5

176. Bernstein, BH, Singsen, BH, King, KK and Hanson, V (1977). Aspirin-induced hepatotoxicity and its effect on juvenile rheumatoid arthritis. *Am J Dis Child*, **131**, 659-63

177. Scaman, WE, Ishak, KG and Plotz, PH (1974). Aspirin-induced hepatotoxicity in patients with systemic lupus erythematosus. *Ann Intern Med*, **80**, 1-8

178. Saltzman, DA, Gall, EP and Robinson, SF (1976). Aspirin-induced hepatic dysfunction in a patient with adult rheumatoid arthritis. *Am J Dig Dis*, **21**, 815-20

179. Rossi, F, Filipelli, W, Guarino, V, Russo, S, Magliulo, R and Marmo, E (1985). Organ tolerance of non-steroidal anti-inflammatory drugs: effect on liver cells. *Drugs Exptl Clin Res*, **11**, 511-6

180. Bullock, GR, Delaney, VB, Sawyer, BC and Slater, TF (1970). Biochemical and structural changes in rat liver resulting from the parenteral administration of a large dose of sodium salicylate. *Biochem Pharmacol*, **19**, 245-53

181. Whitehouse, MW (1977). Some biochemical complexities of inflammatory disease affecting drug action. In Bouta, IL (ed), *Recent Developments in the Pharmacology of Inflammatory Mediators, Agents and Actions, Suppl. 2*, pp. 135-147. (Birkhauser: Basel)

182. Parke, AL and Parke, DV (1987). Genetic and environmental aspects of drug metabolism relevant to side-effects in arthritic disease. In Rainsford, KD and Velo, GP (eds), *Side-Effects of Anti-Inflammatory Drugs, Pt. I*, pp. 241-255. (MTP Press: Lancaster)

183. Whitehouse, MW (1987). Drug disease interactions: utility of the conditional con-

cept for experimental pharmacology and toxicology in the context of inflammation. In Rainsford, KD and Velo, GP (eds), *Side-Effects of Anti-Inflammatory Drugs, Pt. I*, pp. 259-271. (MTP Press: Lancaster)

184. Zimmerman, HJ (1981). Effects of aspirin and acetaminophen on the liver. *Arch Intern Med*, **141**, 333-42

185. Douidar, SM, Boor, PJ and Ahmed, AE (1985). Potentiation of the hepatotoxic effect of acetaminophen by prior administration of salicylate. *J Pharmacol Expt Therap*, **233**, 242-8

186. Sorensen, EMB and Acosta, D (1985). Relative toxicities of several non-steroidal anti-inflammatory compounds in primary cultures of rat hepatocytes. *J Toxicol Environ Health*, **16**, 425-40

187. Burke, MD, Falzon, M and Milton, AS (1983). Decreased hepatic microsomal cytochrome $P_{450}$ due to indomethacin: protective roles of 16,16-dimethyl prostaglandin $F_{2\alpha}$ and inducing agents. *Biochem Pharmacol*, **32**, 389-97

188. Dunn, MJ (1984). Non-steroidal anti-inflammatory drugs and renal function. *Ann Rev Med*, **35**, 411-28

189. Unsworth, J, Sturman, S, Lunec, J and Blake, DR (1987). Renal impairment associated with non-steroidal anti-inflammatory drugs. *Ann Rheum Dis*, **46**, 233-6

190. Anon (1988). Voltaren "approvable" in the US: FDA caution on NSAI labelling. *Scrip*, **1311**, 25 May, 22

191. Cox, NL and Doherty, SM (1987). Non-steroidal anti-inflammatories: outpatient audit of patient preferences and side effects on different diseases. In Rainsford, KD and Velo, GP (eds), *Side-Effects of Anti-Inflammatory Drugs, Pt. I*, pp. 137-148. (MTP Press: Lancaster)

192. *The Merck Manual of Diagnosis and Therapy, 15th Edn* (1987), pp. 2287-8 and 2024-5. (Merck, Sharp & Dohme Res Labs: Rahway, NJ)

193. Bork, K (1988). Cutaneous side effects of drugs. (WB Saunders: Philadelphia)

194. Reszka, K and Chignell, CG (1983). Spectroscopic studies of cutaneous photosensitizing agents - IV. The photolysis of benoxaprofen, an anti-inflammatory drug with phototoxic properties. *Photochem Photobiol*, **38**, 281-91

195. Anon (1987). Isoxicam - a scientific 'whodunnit'. *Rheumatol Pract*, Sept 1987, 21

196. Sik, RH, Pasehall, CS and Chignell, CF (1983). The phototoxic effect of benoxaprofen and its analogs on human erythrocytes and rat peritoneal mast cells. *Photochem Photobiol*, **38**, 411-5

197. Kochevar, IE, Morison, WC, Lamm, JL, McAuliffe, DJ, Western, A and Hood, AG (1986). Possible mechanisms of piroxicam-induced photosensitivity. *Archiv Dermatol*, **122**, 1283-7

198. Jones, RA, Navaratnam, S, Parsons, RJ and Philips, GO (1987). Photosensitivity due to anti-inflammatory analgesic drugs: a laser flash photolysis study of azapropazone. In Rainsford, KD and Velo, GP (eds), *Side-Effects of Anti-Inflammatory Drugs, Pt. II*, pp. 345-354. (MTP Press: Lancaster)

199. Hort, JF (1975). Adverse reactions to alclofenac. *Curr Med Res Opin*, **3**, 333-7

200. Ford-Hutchinson, AW (1980). Personal communication

201. Aked, D, Foster, SJ, Howarth, A, McCormick, ME and Potts, HC (1986). The inflammatory responses of rabbit skin to tropical arachidonic acid and its pharmacological modulation. *Br J Pharmacol*, **89**, 431-8

202. Chang, J, Carlson, RP, O'Niell-Davis, L, Lamb, B, Sharma, RN and Lewis, AJ (1986). Correlation between mouse skin inflammation induced by arachidonic acid and eicosanoid synthesis. *Inflammation*, **10**, 205-14

203. Aked, DM and Foster, SJ (1987). Leukotriene and prostaglandin $E_2$ mediate the inflammatory responses of rabbit skin to intradermal arachidonic acid. *Br J Pharmacol*, **92**, 545-52

204. Ring, J, Przybilla, B and Ruzicka, T (1987). Nonsteroidal anti-inflammatory drugs induce UV-dependent histamine and leukotriene release from peripheral human

leukocytes. *Int Arch Allergy Appl Immunol*, **82**, 344-6

205.   Jaudl, RC, George, JL, Dinarello, CA and Schur, PH (1987). The effect of interleukin 1 on IgG synthesis in systemic lupus erythematosus. *Clin Immunol Immunopathol*, **45**, 384-94

206.   Sandborg, CI, Berman, MA, Andrews, BS and Friou, GJ (1985). Interleukin-1 production by mononuclear cells from patients with scleroderma. *Clin Exp Immunol*, **60**, 294-302

207.   Hunneyball, I (1988). Pharmacological regulation of interleukin 1. In Glauert, AM (ed), *Control of Connective Tissue Degradation*, in press. (Elsevier: Amsterdam)

208.   Gahring, LC, Buckley, A and Daynes, RA (1985). Presence of epidermal-derived thymocyte activating factor/interleukin 1 in normal human stratum corneum. *J Clin Invest*, **76**, 1585-91

209.   Hsu, S-M and Zhao, X (1987). Localization of interleukin-1 in normal or reactive lymphoid tissues and skin: abundance of IL-1 in interdigitating reticulum cells. *Lymphokine Res*, **6**, 13-8

210.   Lange-Wantzin, G, Rotheim, R, Kahn, J and Faanes, RB (1987). Effect of UV irradiation on expression of membrane IL-1 by rat macrophages. *J Immunol*, **38**, 383-3807

211.   Faure, M, Dezutter-Dambuyant, C, Schmitt, D, Gaucherand, M and Thivolet, J (1985). Langerhans cell induced cytotoxic T-cell responses against normal epidermal cell targets: *in vitro* studies. *Br J Dermatol*, **113** (Suppl. 28), 114-7

212.   Morley, J, Sanjar, S, Page, CP and Bretz, U (1985). The role of circulating cells in skin reactions. *Br J Dermatol*, **113** (Suppl. 28), 86-90

213.   Yancey, KB, Hammer, CH, Harvath, L, Kenfer, L, Frank, MM and Lawley, TS (1985). Studies on human C5a as a mediator of inflammation in normal skin. *J Clin Invest*, **75**, 486-95

214.   Emerit, I and Michelson, AM (1981). Mechanisms of photosensitivity in systemic lupus erythematosus patients. *Proc Natl Acad Sci*, **78**, 2537-40

215.   Cox, H (1967). Long term indomethacin therapy of coxarthrosis. *Ann Rheum Dis*, **26**, 346-57

216.   Walker, SR, Schuetz, E, Schuppan, D and Gelzer, J (1984). A comparative retrospective analysis of data from short- and long-term toxicity studies on 40 pharmaceutical compounds. *Arch Toxicol, Suppl 7*, 485-87

217.   Lyle, H (1986). Penicillamine. In Rainsford, KD (ed), *Anti-inflammatory and Antirheumatic Drugs, Vol. III*, pp. 3-30. (CRC Press: Boca Raton, Fl)

218.   Walters, MT, Smith, JL, Moore, K, Evans, PR and Midcawley. An investigation of the action of disease modifying antirheumatic drugs on the rheumatoid synovial membrane: reduction in T lymphocyte subpopulations and HLA-DR and DQ antigen expression after gold or penicillamine therapy. *Ann Rheum Dis*, **46**, 7-16

219.   Arrigoni-Martelli, E, Binderup, L and Bramm, E (1977). Role of macrophages in D-penicillamine-induced stimulation of DNA synthesis in lymph node cells. In Willoughby, DA, Giroud, JP and Velo, GP (eds), *Future Trends in Inflammation*, pp. 295-301. (MTP Press: Lancaster)

220.   Binderup, L, Bramm, E and Arrigoni-Martelli, E (1978). D-Penicillamine and macrophages modulation of lymphocyte transformation by concanavalin A. *Scand J Immunol*, **7**, 259-64

221.   Lyle, H (1987). Side effects of penicillamine. In Rainsford, KD and Velo, GP (eds), *Side Effects of Anti-inflammatory Drugs, Pt. 2* pp. 171–181. (MTP Press: Lancaster)

222.   Paulus, HE (1985). Slowly acting anti-rheumatic drugs (SARDS) rarely improve the outcome of rheumatoid arthritis patients. XVIth International Congress of Rheumatology, Sydney, Australia, 19–25 May 1985, Abstract R35.

223.   Davies, PT, Fowler, PD, Clarke, S et al (1986). Rheumatoid arthritis: treatment which controls the C-reactive protein and ESR reduces the radiological progression. *Br J Rheumatol*, **25**, 44-9

224.   Cooperating Clinics Committee of American Rheumatism Association (1970). A

controlled trial of cyclophorphamide in rheumatoid arthritis. *New Engl J Med*, **283**, 883-9

225. Gordon, AJ and Koj, A (eds)(1985). *The Acute Phase Response to Infection and Immunity*. (Elsevier: Amsterdam)

226. Merryman, PF, Nowakowski, J and Jaffe, IA (1978). Alteration of lymphocyte response by sulfydral and disulfide compounds. *Biochem Pharmacol*, **28**, 2297-302

227. Sedgwick, AD, Moore, AR, Sin, YM, Al-Daub, AY, Lansdon, B and Willoughby, DA (1984). The effect of therapeutic agents on cartilage degradation *in vivo. J Pharm Pharmacol*, **36**, 709-10

228. Pickup, ME, Dixon, JS and Bird, HA (1980). On the effects of antirheumatic drugs on protein sulphydryl reactivity in human serum. *J Pharm Pharmacol*, **32**, 301-2

229. Castell, M, Moreno, JJ, Oliva, JC, Queralt, J and Castellote, MC (1987). Serum sulfhydryl group levels in experimental chronic inflammation. *Rev Esp Fisiosy*, **43**, 19-24

230. Olivia, JC, Castell, M, Queralt, J and Castellote, C (1987). Effect of chronic inflammation on copper and zinc metabolism. *Rev Esp Fisiol*, **43**, 25-32

231. Butt, TR, Sternberg, EJ, Mirabelli, CK and Crooke, ST (1986). Regulation of metallothionein gene expression in mammalian cells by gold compounds. *Molec Pharmacol*, **29**, 204-10

232. Glennas, A and Rugstad, HE (1985). Acquired resistance to auranofin in cultured human cells. *Scand J Rheumatol*, **14**, 230-8

233. Glennas, A and Rugstad, HE (1986). Cultured human cells acquire resistance to the antiproliferative effect of sodium aurothiomalate. *Ann Rheum Dis*, **45**, 389-95

234. Glennas, A, Hunziker, PE, Garvey, JS, Kagi, JHR and Rugstad, HE (1986). Metallothionein in cultured human epithelial cells and synovial rheumatoid fibroblasts after *in vitro* treatment with auranofin. *Biochem Pharmacol*, **35**, 2033-40

235. Broome, JD and Jeng, MW (1973). Promotion of replication in lymphoid cells by specific thiols and disulfides *in vitro. J Exp Med*, **138**, 574-92

236. Thorne, KJ, Free, J and Franks, D (1982). Role of sulphydryl groups in T lymphocyte-mediated cytotoxicity. *Clin Exp Immunol*, **50**, 644-50

237. Gilman, SC and Lewis, AJ (1985). Immunology drugs in the treatment of rheumatoid arthritis. In Rainsford, KD (ed), *Anti-inflammatory and Anti-rheumatic Drugs, Vol. III*, pp. 127-154. (CRC Press: Boca Raton, FI)

238. Various authors (1987). Proceedings of a symposium, osteoarthritis: the clinical picture, pathogenesis, and management with studies on a new therapeutic agent. S-adenosyl-methionine. *Am J Med*, **83**, Suppl, 5A

239. Gualano, M, Stramentimoli, G and Berti, F (1983). Anti-inflammatory activity of S-adenosyl-L-methionine: interference with the eicosanoid system. *Pharmacol Res Commun*, **15**, 683-96

240. Harmand, M-F, Vilamitjana, J, Maloche, E, Duphil, R and Ducasson, D (1987). Effects of S-adenosylmethionine on human articular chrondrocyte differentiation. *Am J Med*, **83**, (Suppl. 5A), 48-54

241. Hamilton, JA and Williams, N (1985). *In vitro* inhibition of myelopoiesis by gold salts and D-penicillamine. *J Rheumatol*, **12**, 892-6

242. Rainsford, KD (1989). Doxorubicin (Adriamycin{R}) is a potent inhibitor of interleukin-1 induced cartilage resorption *in vitro. Agents and Actions*, **21**, 337-40

243. Connolly, KH, Stecher, VJ, Davis, E, Pruden, DJ and La Brie, T. (1988). Alteration of interleukin-1 activity and the acute phase response in adjurant arthritic rats treated with disease - modifying antirheumatic drugs. *Agents and Actions*, **25**, 94–105

244. Rainsford, KD (1988). Effects of anti-inflammatory drugs and pharmacological agents which modify intracellular events in inflammation on interleukin-1 induced cartilage proteoglycan resorption *in vitro*. Submitted for publication

245. Rainsford, KD (1989). Effects of anti-inflammatory drugs on interleukin-1 induced cartilage proteoglycan resorption *in vitro*: inhibition by aurothiophosphines but no influence from perturbed eicosanoid metabolism. *J Pharm Pharmacol*. In press

246. Rainsford, KD (1988). Actions of auinoline antimalarials in control of cartilage resorption by interleukin-1 and *E. coli* lipopolysaccharide. Abstracts 4th Int. Conference of the Inflammation Research Association, White Haven, PA, Oct 23–27 (1988)

247. Rainsford, KD (1985). Preliminary investigations on the pharmacological control of catabolin-induced cartilage destruction *in vitro*. *Agents and Actions*, **16**, 55-7

248. Chang, J, Gilman, SC and Lewis, AJ (1986). Interleukin 1 activates phospholipase $A_2$ in rabbit chondrocytes: a possible signal for IL-1 action. *J Immunol*, **136**, 1283-7

249. Carroll, GJ (1986). A study of the effects of catabolin on cyclic adenosine monophosphate biosynthesis and prostaglandin $E_2$ secretion in pig articular chondrocytes. *Br J Rheumatol*, **25**, 359-65

250. Zeevi, A, Duquesnoy, R, Eiras, G, Rabinowich, H, Todo, S, Makowka, L and Starzi, TE (1987). Immunosuppressive effect of FK-506 on *in vitro* lymphocyte alloactivation: synergism with cyclosporine A. *Transp Proc*, **19**, 40-1

251. Wolf, RE and Hall, VC (1988). Inhibition of *in vitro* proliferative response of cultured T lymphocytes to interleukin-2 by gold sodium thiomalate. *Arth & Rheum*, **31**, 176-81

252. Lee, JC, Rebar, L, Demuth, S and Hanna, N. Suppressed IL-2 production and response in AA rats: role of suppressor cells and the effect of auranofin treatment. *J Rheumatol*, **12**, 885-91

253. Weinblatt, ME, Coblyn, JS, Fraser, PA, Anderson, RJ, Spragg, J, Trentham, D and Austen, KF (1987). Cyclosporin A treatment of refractory rheumatoid arthritis. *Arthritis and Rheumatism*, **30**, 11-17

254. Van Rijthoven, AWAM, Dijkmans, BAC, Goeithe, HS, Hermans, J, Montnor-Beckers, ZLMB, Jacobs, PCJ and Cats, A (1986). Cyclosporin treatment for rheumatoid arthritis: a placebo controlled, double blind, multicentre study. *Ann Rheum Dis*, **45**, 736-31

255. Ichimura, O, Suzuki, S, Saito, M, Sugawara, Y and Ishida, N (1985). Augmentation of interleukin 1 and interleukin 2 production by OK-432. *Immunopharmacol*, **7**, 263-70

256. Gilman, SC, Carlson, RP, Daniels, JF, Datko, L, Berner, PR, Chang, J and Lewis, AJ (1987). Immunological abnormalities in rats with adjuvant-induced arthritis - II. Effect of antiarthritic therapy on immune function in relation to disease development. *Int J Immunopharmacol.* **9**, 9-16

257. Marder, P and Schmidtke, JR (1985). Cyclosporin A inhibits helper/inducer surface antigen expression on activated human lymphocytes. *Int J Immunopharmacol*, **7**, 165-75

258. Palacios, R and Moller, G (1981). Cyclosporin A blocks receptors for HLA-DR antigens on T cells. *Nature*, **290**, 792-4

259. Gauldie, J. (1989) Interleukin 6 in the inflammatroy response. In: Therapeutic Control of Inflammatory Diseases. 4th Int. Conference Inflammation Research Association, White Haven, PA, Oct 23–27, 1988. Plenum Press, *in press*

260. Andus, T, Geiger, T, Hirano, T, Kishimoto, T, Tran-Thi, T, Decker, K and Heinrich, PC (1988). Regulation fo synthesis and secretion of major rat acute-phase proteins by recombinant human interleukin-6 (BSF-2/IL-6) in hepatocyte primary cultures. *Europ J Biochem*, **173**, 287-93

# 4
# Animal models of arthritic disease: influence of novel compared with classical antirheumatic agents

I M Hunneyball[*], M E J Billingham[**] and K D Rainsford[***]
[*]The Boots Company PLC, Nottingham NG2 3AA, UK, [**]Lilly Research Centre, Eli Lilly & Co, Windlesham, Surrey GU20 6PH, UK
[***]Strangeways Research Laboratory, Worts Causeway, Cambridge CB1 4RN, UK

## I. INTRODUCTION

To be of real value, models of arthritis should be close enough to the human diseases to enable rational drug discovery for halting or even reversing these crippling afflictions. Unfortunately this is not yet totally so, and our existing models of arthritis are frequently criticized for both their failure to replicate the human condition, and to reliably demonstrate the disease-modifying qualities of gold and penicillamine, the mainstays of human therapy. Clearly we live in an imperfect world; nevertheless penicillamine has been found active in one model of arthritis, after considerable, patient experimentation[1], and clobuzarit (Clozic® ICI), a molecule with the ability to slow down the erosive progression of rheumatoid arthritis, is active in various models of polyarthritis in the rat[2]. Precedent has therefore been set, and this success, though limited, is sufficient to justify optimism that further refinement of arthritis models will lead to disease-modifying therapy for arthritic disease.

Historically, the criticisms of the current models as outlined have led medicinal chemists and pharmacologists to pursue the inhibition of inflammatory mediators as a means to achieving the goal of disease-modifying therapy. As with the modelling approach, the mediator approach has also been largely unsuccessful, except in the symptomatic treatment of disease, and its critics point to the narrowness of the view that any single mediator will be omnipotent in the mediation of the chronicity of the arthritic process. This is reinforced with the current awareness of the potential role in arthritis for the new wave of polypeptide mediators, cytokines, lymphokines and growth factors, whose pleomorphism and overlapping properties highlight the problems surrounding selection of the key mediator, and where and when to in-

*New Developments in Antirheumatic Therapy.* Rainsford, KD and Velo, GP (eds), Inflammation and Drug Therapy Series, Volume III.

hibit it, as has been so succinctly discussed by Sporn and Roberts recently[3].

The dilemma facing scientists searching for potential disease-modifying therapy still remains. Should they delve ever more deeply into the complexity of the activity and interactions between lymphokines, cytokines, growth factors and acute inflammatory mediators, often by way of *in vitro* systems? Or, conversely, should they rely on the possibility that such complex mediation occurs in some animal model of arthritis in a manner relevant to human disease? There is no simple answer to this. Commenting on the mediator approach, Sporn and Roberts[3] suggest, with particular reference to growth factors, that they should not be viewed as single entities, but will only be understood as part of a cascade involving interactions with other polypeptides, interleukins and interferons, and lipid products in the totality of signals which operate within and between cells during defence and repair processes, and in chronic diseases. Such an understanding is becoming possible through the availability of increasing numbers of recombinant interleukins, lymphokines and growth factors which, at the least, does allow contemplation of relevant *in vitro* systems as paradigms of arthritic destruction, and hence drug discovery. In models of arthritis, not only are growth factors operating, but also interleukins, interferons and other lymphokines which possess the ability to drive the destructive process; by their very nature models offer the virtue of having relevant cells and mediators present in a suitable environment for the demonstration of drug activity. Nowadays a combination of both approaches to drug discovery is probably optimal.

This review will concentrate on the various models of arthritis which are available, the molecules which have emerged from their use and their potential or actual efficacy against human arthritic disease. For this review it must be borne in mind that the drugs discussed, whether under evaluation pre-clinically or in the clinic, will have been discovered between 5 and 15 years ago. Many new techniques have evolved in the meantime which will impact on the discovery process. Simple measurements of foot volume are probably not sensitive enough to detect potentially relevant drug-induced changes, though monitoring of immune function and biochemical parameters such as the acute phase response are increasingly being undertaken. Advances being made in molecular biology, i.e. *in situ* hybridization and the application of monoclonal antibodies, will find their way into drug discovery programmes involving arthritis models, and future generations of drugs will have benefited from these advances.

## II. HISTORICAL PERSPECTIVES

The first and most widely studied model of arthritis was essentially found by accident. Stoerk and his colleagues[4], in 1954, discovered a model of polyarthritis whilst studying the reaction to spleen extracts, emulsified in Freund's complete adjuvant, injected into the rat. Instead of the desired autoimmunity to the spleen extracts, a polyarthritis developed 2–3 weeks later, which Pearson[5] demonstrated in 1955 was due simply to the mycobacterial component of Freund's adjuvant; a seed for drug discovery had been sown. Newbould[6] developed the model as a drug screen in 1963, and it remains a popular model even now, some 25 years later, despite the development of other polyarthritis models based on the theme of Gram-positive cell walls or extracts.

A separate approach was developed around the same time, in 1962, by Dumonde and Glynn[7] who, viewing arthritis as an immune problem, produced a mono-articular model of arthritis by injecting antigen into one joint cavity of previously immunized rabbits. An erosive arthritis developed subsequently in the challenged joint, and this model became amenable to wider screening and drug discovery in 1977 when Brackertz *et al.*[8] described a similar model in mice.

Autoimmunity to some self-component has been widely proposed, over the years, as a means of induction and maintenance of human arthritic process. Trentham and his colleagues[9] gave this hypothesis considerable momentum in 1977 when they reported that polyarthritis could be induced in the rat following immunization with homologous and heterologous type II collagen, the major cartilage phenotype. Subsequently, type II collagen was shown to induce arthritis in mice by Courtenay *et al.*[10], and type XI collagen, another cartilage phenotype, has also been found capable of inducing arthritis[11]. Finally on this theme, a separate cartilage component, the proteoglycan core protein, was found to induce arthritis in mice, interestingly as a paraphenomenon during attempts to produce monoclonal antibodies[12].

Models of arthritis with the potential for drug discovery have thus been in existence for over 30 years, sometimes found by chance but more often through validation of an hypothesis. Induction, pathogenesis and measurement of the various models have been extensively reviewed previously[13] and will not be given here in any detail; readers requiring this information are referred to the earlier literature (see reference 13).

The objective of the use of arthritis models has been the discovery of disease-modifying drugs, the value of which is aptly summarized by Wright and Amos[14] in an earlier discussion of which drugs may alter the course of rheumatoid arthritis: "Probably the best method to detect unequivocal progression of rheumatoid arthritis is radiological assessment...." Of all the laboratory tests available, only the ESR and the measurement of C-reactive protein have been correlated with radiological progression. Measurement of the ESR and acute phase reactants is easy, and this may distinguish those drugs that might be expected to have an effect on the outcome of RA from those that almost certainly do not".

The paucity of such useful molecules emerging from our models undoubtedly reflects both our ignorance of the human disease and an oversimplistic use of the models. There has been too much emphasis on paw swelling and too little on detailed biochemical and immunological analysis of pertinent, drug-induced changes; this is reflected in the discussions of each model.

95

## III. MODELS OF POLYARTHRITIS IN RODENTS

A diverse collection of materials, both antigenic and non-antigenic, lead to the expression of a polyarthritis in the rat which tends to have a broadly similar histopathology, regardless of the initating arthritogen[13]. Thus many species of mycobacteria, certain streptococcal species, *Nocardia asteroides* and *Corynebacterium rubrum* can induce arthritis, and peptidoglycan fractions extracted from these and other species of Gram-positive bacteria are also arthritogenic. The key element for mycobacteria appears to be muramyl dipeptide, which is itself non-antigenic, unlike the peptidoglycans and whole cell walls, and can induce an arthritis essentially identical to that produced by the intact mycobacterium[15]. The non-antigenic, synthetic interferon inducer from Pfizer, CP20961 [N,N-dioctadecyl-N′,N′-bis(2-hydroxyethyl) propanediamine] also induces a polyarthritis "morphologically identical"[16] to classical adjuvant arthritis. Types II and XI collagen evoke a polyarthritis which in one of the author's experience (MEJB) has a similar histological appearance to that of the other models, involving considerable periostitis and new bone formation, and had led to the suggestion that a common pathological process is triggered in the rat by the various arthritogenic materials[2,13]. This possibility, of a common pathology, has important implications concerning the use of rat polyarthritis models for drug discovery, in that the same agents will essentially be found active in each model.

### (1) Adjuvant-induced polyarthritis

An understanding of the pathogenesis of a disease model has considerable importance when viewing the activity, or not, of any drug in that model. For whilst the pathogenesis of the human disease remains a matter for speculation, drug activity can give clues to the human condition through a realization of the mechanisms operating in the disease model. The pathogenesis of adjuvant disease has been unravelled to a considerable degree over the past decade, and the current understanding is given as a prelude to describing the activity of drugs.

The key experiments along the pathway to unravelling the mechanisms were those of Kohashi *et al.*[15] and Chang and his colleagues[16], respectively demonstrating the arthritogenicity of the non-antigenic materials muramyl dipeptide (MDP) and CP20961. Comparison of the effect of MDP in euthymic rats, with their athymic litter mates, demonstrated that the full polyarthritic syndrome involving extensive periostitis only developed in the euthymic rats[17]; this clearly established a role for thymus processed (T) lymphocytes in the pathogenesis of the arthritis. T-lymphocyte involvement was elegantly confirmed by the adoptive transfer of arthritis with T-lymphocytes obtained from rats primed with mycobacteria and the non-antigenic arthritogen CP20961[18]; such lymphocytes were of the CD4 positive helper/inducer subset. The work of Cohen and his colleagues[19] with T-lymphocyte lines derived from rats with adjuvant arthritis again confirmed the necessity of T-lymphocytes for establishment of this model of arthritis. Finally, to complete the picture, monoclonal antibodies to the CD4 positive subset of T-helper lymphocytes have been found to be very effective inhibitors of the development of classical adjuvant arthritis, and the adoptive transfer of the disease with primed T-lymphocytes[20].

The fact that non-antigenic materials can induce polyarthritis in the rat suggests that they activate reactivity against some self-component, or epitope. Van Eden and his colleagues[21] have suggested that this may reside on the link protein, which binds proteoglycan to hyaluronic acid in the cartilage matrix, since a nonapeptide epitope shares considerable homology with a similar sized peptide on a 65 kD protein found in mycobacteria. They also showed[21] that these small peptide epitopes induced proliferation of their arthritogenic T-lymphocyte lines and that the 65 kD mycobacterial protein could induce tolerance to arthritis development.

Whether or not the whole story revolves around this particular epitope remains to be confirmed, but it is clear that rat polyarthritis models are driven by T-lymphocyte reactivity against some self-component/s. It is becoming clearer that the human disease has a considerable T-lymphocyte involvement[22,23], and this, amongst other factors, has been the impetus in a search for immunomodulatory molecules via models of polyarthritis in the rat.

### (a) Therapy of adjuvant arthritis

Much of the earlier work with non-steroidal anti-inflammatory drugs (NSAI), and the known disease-modifying drugs has been reviewed previously[13,24], and need not be included here again. Suffice it to say that NSAI, and steroids by and large, are effective inhibitors of adjuvant arthritis, but, with the exception of certain gold salts, the clinically used disease-modifying drugs are unimpressive in models of rat polyarthritis and may even exacerbate this disease, as reported for levamisole[25] and penicillamine[26].

A new era heralded, however, with the arrival of cyclosporin A, discovered by Borel and his colleagues in 1976[27]. This molecule was found to have a marked suppressive effect on lymphocyte proliferation and lymphokine release without being toxic to the haemopoietic system; autoimmune diseases were clearly a target for this molecule. Borel et al.[27] demonstrated that cyclosporin A could very effectively inhibit the development of classical adjuvant disease, and that it was effective therapeutically against the established disease, a property not shared by earlier cytotoxic and cytostatic immunosuppressive drugs. These results and the variable but strongly positive positive results seen with levamisole in the clinic, against rheumatoid arthritis, ushered in the class of immunomodulatory agents which are currently under investigation. Cyclosporin A has now been demonstrated to have some effect clinically[28,29], though renal toxicity is proving to be a problem with rheumatoid patients.

Chronologically, bredinin, a nucleoside antibiotic isolated from *Eupenicillium brefeldiaum*[30], was amongst the first of these newer immunomodulatory agents to be shown to possess anti-arthritic activity against adjuvant disease, particularly the secondary lesion development. Around the same time, in 1977, Ohsugi and his colleagues[31] reported on the activity of N-(2-carboxyphenyl)-4-chloroanthranilic acid (CCA, Lobenzarit®) in adjuvant disease; this molecule lacked both anti-inflammatory and immunosuppressive properties, and later studies[32] led the authors to suggest that a potential mechanism was through the enhancement of immunosuppression via T-suppressor lymphocytes. Clinical studies have demonstrated a positive effect against rheumatoid arthritis[33], but definite disease-modifying activity, associated with a fall in the erythrocyte sedimentation rate and acute phase proteins has yet to be established.

BM41,332 a 2-cyanaziridine derivative, is another agent considered to enhance suppressor lymphocyte activity. Bicker[34] in 1982 described the activity of this molecule against developing adjuvant arthritis, and suggested that its mode of action probably lay in its ability to increase the percentage of T-suppressor lymphocytes whilst reducing the percentage of T-helper lymphocytes. Somewhat similar claims have been made for TE1-3096, a thiazolopyrimidine[35], which also inhibits adjuvant disease without possessing conventional NSAI activity. These two agents have not, however, been reported to influence established arthritis, unlike cyclosporin, and their effectiveness in the clinic remains to be determined.

Bender and his colleagues[36] have adopted another approach, of combining the anti-inflammatory properties of flumizole with the immunomodulatory properties of levamisole, in an attempt to discover a hybrid pharmacophore. A series of 5,6-diaryl-2,3-dihydroimidazo[2,1-b]thiazoles was synthesized which are effective inhibitors of both developing and established adjuvant arthritis; clinical studies are awaited.

Other immunomodulatory molecules with anti-arthritic activity have emerged during the last few years. Binderup[37] has demonstrated some activity for isoprinosine in adjuvant arthritis, and SA96 (N-(2-mercapto-2-methyl-propanoyl)-1-cysteine has also been claimed to be effective[38]. Detailed studies on the effectiveness of an isoxazole, HWA486, against adjuvant arthritis have been reported by Bartlett and Schleyerbach[39], and further studies discriminated the immunomodulatory properties of this compound from those of cyclophosphamide and cyclosporin A[40]. HWA486 is a very effective inhibitor of developing adjuvant arthritis, and as is common with this whole group of immunomodulatory compounds, restored the depressed cellular immune reactivity, which occurs as arthritis develops, towards normal values. Effectiveness of HWA486 against established disease has yet to be reported, and its effect in the clinic also remains to be determined.

The Wyeth Company has been searching for immunomodulatory

Oxaprozin

SR 41 319

Ebselen

DIAM 4

BW 755C

Lobenzarit

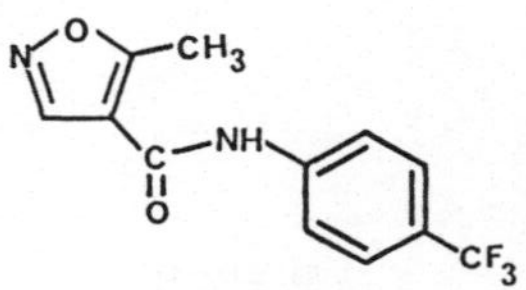

Mizoribine (bredinin)

FUT-175

LS 2616

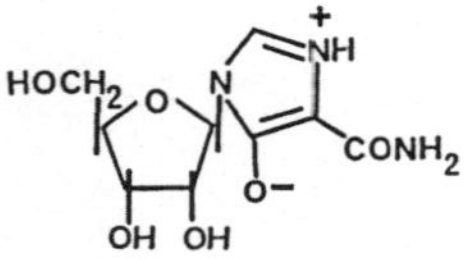

Zimet-3164

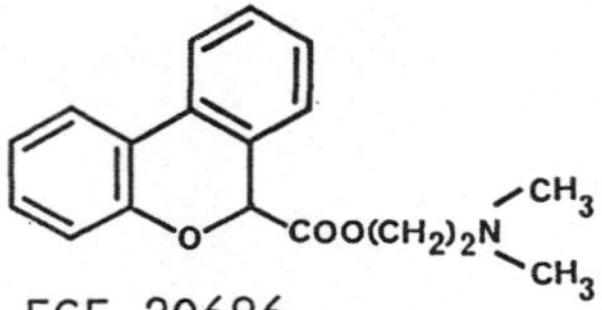

FCE 20696

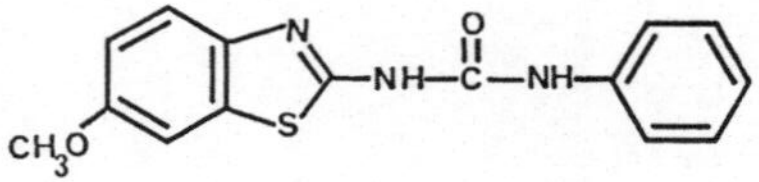

HWA 486 (leflunomide)

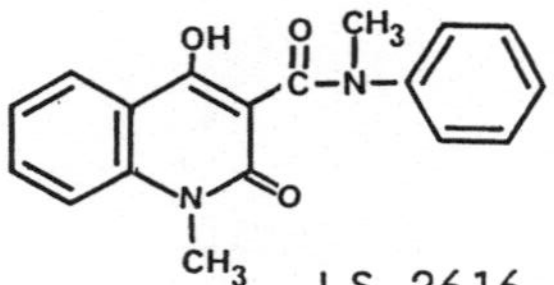

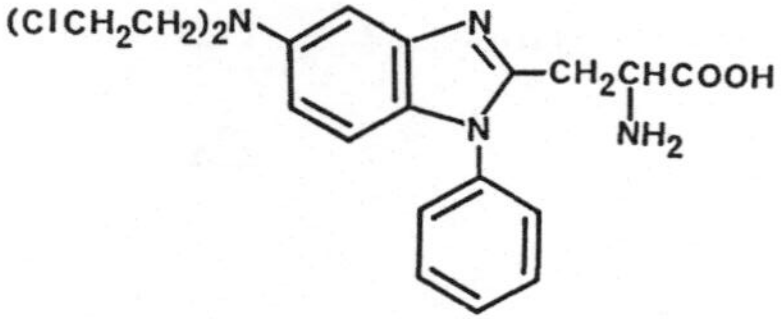

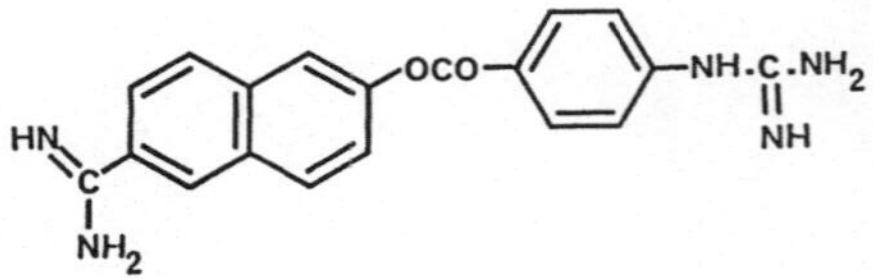

Frentizole

100

compounds for some time[41-43] and now has one molecule in the clinic, Wy-18,251(3-(p-chlorophenyl)thiazolo[3,2-a]benzimidazole-2-acetic acid), also known as tilomisole. This molecule is effective against both developing and established adjuvant arthritis[42], again restoring depressed immune function in the model. Tilomisole also possesses prostaglandin synthetase inhibitory activity but this is not considered to account for all the anti-arthritic activity since drugs such as indomethacin do not restore the depressed immune reactivity of adjuvant disease. A suggested mode of action[42] is that the T-cell stimulatory properties of tilomisole elevate T-suppressor cell function. Preliminary evidence suggests an effect in the clinic against rheumatoid arthritis[43] and further clinical studies are under way to determine the disease-modifying potential of this interesting molecule.

Finally on the theme of immunomodulation, Cohen and his colleagues in Israel[44] have isolated a clone of T-lymphocytes which both induces resistance to arthritis development, and reverses established disease. Larsson *et al.*[45] have shown that pan T monoclonal antibodies delay development of adjuvant disease, and Billingham and his colleagues[20] have found that anti-CD4 monoclonal antibodies can completely prevent the development of adjuvant disease and reduce the established disease.

Clearly, modulation of the immune response has considerable potential to influence the course of rheumatoid arthritis, if this can be achieved safely.

## (b) Other types of agents

Very few compounds have emerged from adjuvant arthritis with the potential for disease modification in man, and which are not immunomodulatory. Some of these have been reviewed previously[13], and included alclofenac, benoxaprofen, clobuzarit and fenclofenac. Only clobuzarit was shown, however, to slow down X-radiographic progression of human rheumatoid arthritis (ref. 2 for review). Whereas molecules such as fenclofenac and benoxaprofen possessed some cyclooxygenase activity which could contribute to the anti-arthritic activity in arthritis model and man, clobuzarit was devoid of cyclooxygenase, anti-inflammatory and immunomodulatory activities. Clobuzarit was able to reduce the effects of cytokine activity, as seen as a fall in acute phase proteins, in several models of rat polyarthritis, in line with therapeutic response, and could achieve the same effect in two distinct chronic connective tissue disease of man, rheumatoid arthritis and atherosclerosis[2]. As with other compounds mentioned above, clobuzarit was withdrawn from the clinic due to the appearance of side effects, so its full therapeutic potential was never established and neither was its mechanism of action determined. However, another molecule, Ro31-3948 (2[[2-(4-chlorophenyl)-4-methyl-5-oxazolyl]-methoxy]-2-methyl propionic acid), with a similar profile of pharmacological activity to clobuzarit is about to enter clinical trial. In addition to inhibiting rat models of polyarthritis, Ro31-3948 inhibits some of the effects of IL1 such as the rise in serum levels of amyloid P and fibroblast activation[46].

Certain proprionitriles have also been found active in adjuvant arthritis, but which lack conventional anti-inflammatory properties; these are benzoyl acetonitrile[47] and Primidone[48], a triethanolamine salt of a pyrrole proprionitrile compound, which in preliminary clinical studies[49] has demonstrated effects similar to established disease-modifying drugs.

Clearly, the adjuvant arthritis models are capable of the discovery of disease-modifying activity against the human disease, but careful attention to rat strain and the monitoring of biochemical parameters and immune function are important for a reasonable chance of success. It should be remembered that classical NSAI have very good disease-modifying activity in these arthritis models, but not in man.

## (2) Streptococcal cell wall arthritis

This was originally described by Cromartie and colleagues[50] in 1977, but has not been extensively used for drug discovery, perhaps because the process of treating these cell walls to render them arthritogenic is less convenient than the use of mycobacteria simply ground up in oil. Interestingly, aqueous suspensions of streptococcal cell walls can induce the arthritis; this is not the case for adjuvant disease where such administration of mycobacteria would only produce tolerance to arthritis induction.

Not all strains of rat develop this model of arthritis, though the Lewis strains are particularly susceptible, and certain aspects of the histopathology, particularly the periostitis and bone remodelling, are reminiscent of adjuvant arthritis. The arthritis does not develop in athymic rats[51], as in the case with adjuvant disease, but further unravelling of the T-lymphocyte sub-sets involved has not been reported. A few reports of drug studies are available, and it has been convincingly demonstrated that cyclosporin A is an effective inhibitor of this model of arthritis[52]. A synthetic retinoid, 4-hydroxyphenyl-retinamide, produces a dose-dependent suppression of both the development of the arthritis and the established form of the disease[53], though it was noted that the drug was less effective in well-advanced disease. Classical disease-modifying agents such as penicillamine and gold thioglucose were found to be inactive[54], though methotrexate was moderately inhibitory.

Overall this model has not had the attention of other rat models such as adjuvant disease or type II collagen arthritis; this may well be an omission on the part of arthritis scientists.

## (3) Type II collagen arthritis in the rat

This model was also described for the first time in 1977 by Trentham and his colleagues[9]. In histopathological terms the model has considerable similarity with adjuvant arthritis, though in some strains of rat the collagen is directly attacked, and cartilage may be completely stripped from the bone. Not all strains show this picture, and with some rat strains the cartilage is essentially untouched, as is invariably the case with the adjuvant diseases. The disease is T-lymphocyte dependent, since it can be passively transferred between in-bred rats[55], but the full syndrome, involving periostitis, cannot be induced by immune serum. This T-lymphocyte dependency is similar to the situation with adjuvant arthritis, but overall experience is that the disease is milder and less reproducible than adjuvant disease. This may account for some of the differences seen with disease-modifying drugs in this model, in comparison with their effects on adjuvant arthritis.

As with adjuvant disease, most reports on NSAI indicate that they are effective inhibitors of both developing and established phases of type II collagen arthritis in the rat[56–58], possess a disease-modifying effect in terms of producing a reduction of acute phase protein levels[57,59]; steroids and classical immunosuppressants are also good inhibitors of this experimental arthritis[56,60]. In these respects type II collagen arthritis resembles adjuvant arthritis in susceptibility to therapy, and likewise a good therapeutic response is usually associated with an effective inhibition of the periostitis and bone re-modelling which accompanies development of arthritis[58].

Where type II collagen arthritis differs from adjuvant disease is in relation to the effect of the human disease-modifying drugs. The earliest studies were those of McCune et al.[61] in 1980, who found that sodium aurothiomalate and levamisole were totally without effect against collagen arthritis. By contrast Sloboda[56] and his colleagues found that the same drugs actually enhanced the arthritis; with penicillamine it was however reported to inhibit the radiographic destruction of bone. Using haptoglobin levels to measure the biochemical response to therapy, Gilbertsen[59] confirmed the effectiveness of NSAI, and again found that the human disease-modifying drugs, gold thioglucose, auranofin and chloroquine, enhanced the disease. Retinoids have also been found to enhance the severity of this polyarthritis[64].

Studies with cyclosporin A have provided some interesting results. Two groups have reported that the drug is an effective inhibitor of the development of collagen arthritis[62,63], with such inhibition being accompanied by a reduction of both cell-mediated and humoral immunity to the collagen. Treatment for just the first 6 days in fact was sufficient to produce a marked inhibition of the arthritis[63], but Kaibara and his colleagues[63] also found that cyclosporin A could exacerbate collagen arthritis when administered to the established disease; this was accompanied by an elevation of delayed-type hypersensitivity and a suppression of humoral immunity to the type II collagen. They suggested that these paradoxical results may be due to differential effects on separate populations of regulatory T-cells.

Certain other treatments, such as oestrogen therapy[65] and a variety of immunological manipulations, have been found to modulate collagen arthritis. Passive transfer of T-cells from rats in the early, inductive phase of the arthritis has been shown to inhibit collagen arthritis development[66], and certain T-cell lines have the same effect[67], akin to the work of Cohen and his colleagues with adjuvant disease[44]. Heterologous anti-idiotypic antibodies to the anti-collagen antibodies[68] have also been reported to suppress development of this polyarthritis, as has prior gastric administration of the type II collagen[69].

Type II collagen arthritis thus shares some features with adjuvant arthritis, in terms of susceptibility to some drugs and immunological manipulation. Its major difference is the greater tendency for disease exacerbation with, particularly, the human disease-modifying drugs. As mentioned earlier, this may be a reflection of the generally milder nature of this polyarthritis in comparison with adjuvant disease.

## (4) Type II collagen arthritis in the mouse

Of all the models of polyarthritis in experimental animals, type II collagen-induced arthritis in the mouse is perhaps the most strain-specific, and only a few strains of mice are susceptible. Arthritis is associated with marked T-lymphocyte and humoral antibody responses to the type II collagen, but there is still debate as to which component is the dominant force for arthritis induction and maintenance. Passive transfer with immune serum generally results in a transient synovitis, but in B10 D2/new line mice[70] passive transfer of purified anti-type II collagen antibodies resulted in a degree of erosive arthritis, involving macrophages and osteoclasts. Both arms of the immune response may well be working in the model, but the overall histopathology is reminiscent of the T-lymphocyte-driven processes active in other models of polyarthritis. Further evidence for a major T-cell influence comes from observations that the polyarthritis does not develop in athymic mice, but can be adoptively transferred with type II collagen reactive T-cell lines[71]. Treatment of recipient mice with radiation levels sufficient to kill mature lymphocytes, as a prelude to adoptive transfer of arthritis with these T-cell lines, resulted in the development of arthritis in the absence of antibody-producing B-lymphocytes[71]. Finally, two groups have demonstrated that monoclonal antibodies directed against the $CD_4$ helper subset of T-lymphocytes prevented the development of arthritis[72,73], and that anti-pan T antibodies could inhibit progression of the established disease[73]. In these latter respects, type II collagen polyarthritis in the mouse has considerable similarity to the rat models of polyarthritis.

Only a few reports of drug effects in the model have appeared to date. The first was by Phadke and her colleagues[74], in 1985, where it was found that a number of NSAI, including benoxaprofen, naproxen and aspirin, and the long-standing antirheumatic drugs gold, chloroquine, levamisole and D-penicillamine, were without effect. Interestingly, penicillamine treatment led to an earlier onset of the arthritis[74]. Only the steroid paramethasone and cyclophosphamide had activity in Phadke's hands[74]. A little later Paska and his group[75] largely confirmed the earlier findings that steroids and cyclophosphamide inhibit the disease, and that penicillamine exacerbated the arthritis. However, gold in the form of auranofin was found to enhance the disease and, in further contrast to Phadke's findings, benoxaprofen and indomethacin, as representatives of the NSAI, were found to inhibit the developing paw inflammation[75]. Another NSAI, etodolac, has been found active against the developing arthritis[76], but had no effect on the established disease. Cyclosporin A has been reported to inhibit the developing arthritis, and the immune response to collagen, but interestingly did not affect the clinical course of the disease when used therapeutically[77]. The incidence and severity of the disease have also been shown to be inhibited by long-term oestrogen therapy[78], and an interesting study by Waites and Whyte[79] has demonstrated the influence of pregnancy on the disease process. Female mice becoming pregnant during the induction phase of arthritis all showed an earlier onset of arthritis, during the post-partum period, in comparison to non-pregnant mice. If they became pregnant with established arthritis, the arthritis went into remission but flared again post-partum. This situation is somewhat similar to the human situation, and may provide further insight into the pregnancy remission phenomenon.

The slow onset of this model of arthritis, overall, and the present situation with drug activity, make the mouse model an interesting variant on the other forms of polyarthritis; time will tell whether this model has real advantages in the search for disease-modifying drugs.

## IV. ANTIGEN-INDUCED ARTHRITIS IN RABBITS

The Dumonde and Glynn model of arthritis in rabbits[7] is arguably the closest model of rheumatoid arthritis to the clinical condition. However, it is not used very widely for pharmacological investigations because of the size of the animals and the consequent cost implications. Nevertheless, the principal disease-modifying antirheumatic agents have been investigated in the model[80] and a few groups of workers have used the model for investigating novel compounds.

The arthritis is induced by sensitizing rabbits to a foreign protein antigen (usually ovalbumin, bovine serum albumin or human fibrin) emulsified with Freund's complete adjuvant and subsequently giving a single challenge injection of the antigen in saline into the knee joint. The arthritis is characterized by an acute inflammatory reaction which lasts for approximately 7–10 days and is followed by a chronic inflammatory phase which persists indefinitely. Erosive changes generally begin to appear 2–3 weeks after the intra-articular injection and increase progressively with time.

Both prophylactic and therapeutic schedules have been investigated with established drugs in this model of arthritis. In the former case, drug treatment commences on the day of intra-articular injection; in the latter case, treatment schedules commencing either 14 days or 35 days after intra-articular injection have been used (i.e. after the acute phase has subsided).

There is general agreement that the classical NSAIDs have no effect on the erosive disease in this model as judged by histopathology[81,82]. The only exception to this is ketoprofen which at the high dose of 60 mg/kg reduced the histopathological changes[81]. Ketoprofen, indomethacin and naproxen have been shown to reduce joint swelling and synovial fluid cell count[81]; indomethacin also reduced joint surface temperature[83].

The anti-inflammatory corticosteroids prednisolone and methylprednisolone effectively inhibit both the symptomatic changes and the underlying erosive disease. A variety of treatment schedules have been used and reductions have been observed in joint swelling, synovial fluid cell count, gross erosive changes, histopathological changes, synovial antibody levels and synovial β-glucuronidase levels[80]. Systemic immune responsiveness was also reduced during treatment. Intra-articularly injected corticosteroids are also effective in this model of arthritis. Triamcinolone hexacetonide (2 mg/injection, injected on three occasions at 14-day intervals) reduced joint swelling, gross erosive changes and histopathological changes[84]. Rimexolone (Org 6216) and prednisolone-t-butylacetate (5 mg/injection) also reduced joint swelling; unfortunately, the histopathological changes were not measured in this study[85]. More recently, two esters of dexamethasone, namely the hexanoate and the t-butyl acetate (2 mg/injection) were shown to reduce both joint swelling and histopathological changes[86].

The rabbit model of arthritis is dependent on cell-mediated immune responses. Consequently, it is not surprising that the arthritis can be suppressed by treatment with the cytotoxic immunosuppressants azathioprine and cyclophosphamide. Both drugs have been shown to suppress the histopathological changes with concomitant suppression of immune responses using a variety of dosing regimens (reviewed in ref 80). Furthermore, the novel selective immunosuppressive agent 2-(4-chloroanilino)quinazoline-4(3H)-thione (US Patent 4,079,057) has been shown to suppress the arthritic symptoms when administered using either prophylactic or therapeutic schedules; unfortunately there is no indication as to whether or not the histopathological changes were suppressed under these conditions.

The major established slow-acting antirheumatic drugs have been investigated in the rabbit arthritis model. Chloroquine had no significant effect at doses similar to those used clinically (5 mg/kg), although higher doses (10–

2-(4-chloroanilino)quinazoline-4(3H)-thione

100 mg/kg for 4 weeks) have been shown to suppress the synovial fluid cell count and histopathological changes but not joint swelling or macroscopic indices of inflammation[80,81]. D-penicillamine has been shown to reduce joint circumference and histopathological parameters in rabbits with established arthritis; however, this has only been demonstrated in New Zealand White (NZW) rabbits with long-term treatment (15–30 mg/kg for 30 weeks). Arthritis induced under the same conditions in Old English rabbits appears to be refractory to the drug (A. Blackham; personal communication). Short-term treatment (4 weeks) of either Old English or NZW rabbits appears to have no effect on the arthritis[81]. The suppression of the arthritis by D-penicillamine in NZW rabbits was accompanied by a reduction in cell-mediated immune responsiveness as well as a restoration of serum IgA levels to normal[80].

Both the currently available gold compounds, sodium aurothiomalate and auranofin, have been investigated in the rabbit model. Long-term intramuscular injection of sodium aurothiomalate (1 mg/kg/week for 20 weeks or 3 mg/kg/week for 10 weeks) has been shown to suppress the histopathological changes without affecting the inflammatory symptoms such as joint swelling[80,87]. In contrast, short-term treatment (2.5 mg/kg twice per week for 4 weeks) was found to suppress symptomatic parameters without affecting the histopathology[81]. Auranofin at the high dose of 25 mg/kg daily for 17 days reduced the histopathological changes and immunological parameters, but this may have been due to gross toxicity of the compound[82]. Reducing the dose to 12.5 mg/kg resulted in lack of efficacy. Thus it seems that when gold compounds are administered in high doses in the short term, or at lower doses over longer periods, they may affect the inflammatory symptoms and/or the histopathology, albeit to only a moderate extent.

Using a sequential, increasing dosing schedule over the range 1–30 mg/kg/day, over a 4-week period, Blackham and Radziwonik[81] failed to demonstrate any effect on either symptomatic or histopathological parameters of arthritis in rabbits as a result of treatment with levamisole. Similarly, treatment with sulphasalazine at a dose of 30 mg/kg/day for 10 weeks failed to have any effect on either symptomatic or histopathological parameters (I. M. Hunneyball, unpublished observations).

The size of the rabbit knee joint enables intra-articular injection with relative ease. Consequently rabbit models of arthritis have been used for the investigation of various novel intra-articular drug delivery systems. Initial studies of this nature employed a model of arthritis induced by intra-articular injection of a poly-D-lysine-hyaluronate complex. Using this model, Dingle et al.[88] showed that the potency of anti-inflammatory steroids could be markedly enhanced by their incorporation into liposomes. Unfortunately, this effect was relatively short-lived and in this respect this formulation did not compare very favourably with commercially available long-acting steroid esters such as triamcinolone hexacetonide[84]. Nvertheless, this work was extended to incorporation of radioisotopes into liposomes by means of a lipophilic chelator 3-cholesteryl-6[N'iminobis-(ethylenenitrilo) tetra-acetic acid] hexyl ether[89]. These liposomes have been used to retain both [51]chromium and [177]lutetium within the synovium; in the latter case the loss of radioactivity from the synovium being less than 1% per day over a 47-day period[90]. The [177]lutetium produced a reduction in joint diameter, joint sur-

$(HO_2CCH_2)_2NCH_2CH_2NCH_2CH_2N(CH_2)_6O$

$CH_2CO_2H$

$CH_2CO_2H$

3-cholesteryl-6[N′iminobis-(ethylenenitrilo) tetra-acetic acid hexyl ether

face temperature and synovitis as judged by histopathology.

Studies with liposomes have also been performed in the Dumonde and Glynn model. Foong and Green[91] showed that entrapment of methotrexate into liposomes improved the retention of the drug within the joint; however, most of the drug appeared in the synovial fluid rather than the synovial membrane, indicating poor uptake of the liposomes by the synovial cells. Further studies of this nature have involved investigation of the effect of linking daunorubicin to protein molecules such as bovine serum albumin in order to improve its retention within the joint[92]. Although daunorubicin itself (50 g injected 1 week after induction or arthritis) was effective in reducing joint swelling (but not joint temperature), daunorubicin linked to bovin serum albumin had a delayed and more prolonged effect on joint swelling[92].

Foong and Green[93] have also investigated the effect of intra-articular yttrium-90 and chlorambucil on the Dumonde and Glynn rabbit model. A single injection of 500 μCi [90]Y given 1 week after induction of the arthritis produced a reduction in joint swelling and surface temperature for up to 5 weeks following the injection; however when the animals were sacrificed 7 weeks after the injection there was no difference between control and treated animals histologically. Established arthritis of 3 weeks duration was less responsive to [90]Y injection. In contrast, Meier-Ruge et al.[94] have previously shown a single injection of 200 μCi [90]Y to be effective in established arthritis of 15 weeks duration, as judged by histopathology. Intra-articular injection of chlorambucil (1 mg) 1 week after induction of arthritis produced a reduction in joint swelling which was sustained up to the time of sacrifice (8 weeks after injection). Furthermore, histopathological changes to the synovium and cartilage were also suppressed at this time point[93].

## V. ANTIGEN-INDUCED ARTHRITIS IN MICE

Antigen-induced arthritis can be produced in mice[95] using comparable procedures to those used in rabbits by Dumonde and Glynn[7]. The principal methodological differences are that in mice a potent cationic antigen, such as methylated BSA, is required and *Bordetella pertussis* is required as a secondary adjuvant. This mouse model parallels its rabbit equivalent in several respects, including hypertrophy and hyperplasia of the synovial lining cells together with infiltration of the synovial subintima by lymphocytes, plasma cells and macrophages forming pannus which produces marked erosive changes in the articular cartilage and subchondral bone[95,96]. Furthermore, both mouse and rabbit models are dependent on T-cell function.

Because of the small size of the mouse knee joint, measurement of symptomatic parameters such as joint swelling is very difficult. As a result, the pharmacological studies in this model have utilized joint histopathology as the sole assessment of drug effects on the disease progress. Although this is labour-intensive and difficult to quantitate, it still represents the most meaningful assessment of disease activity after drug treatment. Both prophylactic (commencing on the day of arthritis induction) and therapeutic (commencing 14 days after arthritis induction) treatment schedules have been investigated in this model. In the former case, treatment is continued for 6 weeks, in the latter case 4 weeks[96–98]. With certain classes of drugs (e.g. NSAIDs, corticosteroids, cytotoxic immunosuppressants) the arthritis in mice responds in a similar manner to that in rabbits. However, differences occur with the slow-acting antirheumatic agents.

Three classical NSAIDs, indomethacin, ibuprofen and flurbiprofen, have been investigated in this mouse model over a wide dose range employing both prophylactic and therapeutic treatment schedules; none of these drugs had any significant effect on either synovitis or erosions, although minor changes in the synovial fluid differential cell count were observed with ibuprofen and indomethacin[96]. Preliminary studies with the dual cyclo-oxygenase/lipoxygenase inhibitor BW 755C (3-amino-1-[m-(trifluoromethyl phenyl]-2-pyrazolone) indicate that this compound also has no significant effect on the disease process (Hunneyball *et al.*, unpublished observations).

The anti-inflammatory corticosteroids prednisolone (1–10 mg/kg) and dexamethasone (0.5–2.5 mg/kg) produced a dose-dependent suppression of the arthritis when administered daily for a period of at least 14 days at any time during the course of the disease. Parallel suppression of synovitis and erosions was observed histopathologically. This suppression did not appear to be due to a generalized suppression of immunological responsiveness since circulating antibody levels and leukocyte counts (both total and differential) were not affected by treatment with these drugs[96].

The cytotoxic agents azathioprine and methotrexate have been investigated under both prophylactic and therapeutic dosing schedules. Azathioprine (20 mg/kg daily) produced significant suppression of arthritis under

109

both schedules, although a greater degree of suppression was achieved with prophylactic treatment. However, at the effective doses, there was evidence of bone marrow aplasia indicating a close relationship between activity and toxicity. Methotrexate (1.5–2.0 mg/kg daily) also showed evidence of suppression of the arthritis under both treatment schedules but this only reached statistical significance with the prophylactic schedule[97,98].

Most of the currently used slow-acting antirheumatic drugs have been investigated in this model of arthritis. Neither D-penicillamine (3–100 mg/kg daily) nor chloroquine (1–30 mg/kg daily) has been shown to have any effect using either prophylactic or therapeutic treatment schedules. Tiopronin (N-(2-mercaptopropionylglycine) is structurally related to D-penicillamine and has also been used as a second-line drug in rheumatoid arthritis. This compound also failed to suppress established arthritis in mice[98]. Sodium aurothiomalate administered intramuscularly at doses of 1–10 mg/kg either once per week or three times per week failed to suppress established arthritis. However, daily administration of the compound using the prophylactic schedule suppressed the synovitis (but not erosions) at doses of 1 and 3 mg/kg. Auranofin has variable activity in this model, suppression being seen with the prophylactic schedule on some occasions but not others. In contrast to the rabbit model, sulphasalazine at doses of 10–30 mg/kg daily reproducibly inhibits both synovitis and erosions in mouse arthritis using the therapeutic treatment schedule[97,98]. Investigation of the sulphapyridine moiety failed to reveal any activity, indicating that the whole molecule may be required for the expression of the activity of sulphasalazine.

The selective immunosuppressant cyclosporin A is currently on trial in rheumatoid arthritis in several centres. In the mouse model, suppression of established arthritis was observed with high doses of the drug (10–100 mg/kg daily); however this reached statistical significance only at 50 and 100 mg/kg, and evidence of toxicity was apparent at 100 mg/kg.

Despite the difficulties in injecting into mouse knee joint, Van den Berg et al.[99,100] have investigated the activity of locally injected catalase, amidated catalase, superoxide dismutase and peroxidase when administered 1 day prior to induction of arthritis. Native catalase and peroxidase showed some suppression of the inflammatory response (measured by [99m]Tc accumulation) at day 3 but not day 7. Cationic forms of these enzymes were prepared in order to increase the retention of the enzyme within the joint. Amidated catalase produced weak suppression of the inflammatory response at day 3, becoming more marked at day 7. Peroxidase-polylysine also produced a long-lasting suppression. In contrast, superoxide dismutase either in its native or amidated form had no suppressive effect on the arthritis, and at high doses produced some exacerbation. Interestingly, where suppression of the inflammatory response was observed with amidated catalase this effect was much less marked when assessed by histological means, implying that this effect is more palliative than disease-modifying.

So far, this model of arthritis has been used by only a few research groups. However, it is being adopted more widely within the pharmaceutical industry and consequently further information on novel compounds should appear before too long.

## VI. GLUCOSE OXIDASE-INDUCED ARTHRITIS IN MICE

The efficacy of cationic forms of peroxidase and catalase in the antigen-induced model of arthritis in mice suggests a role for hydrogen peroxide in the inflammatory processes and tissue damage in this model[99]. To investigate this further, Schalkwijk et al.[101] enzymatically generated hydrogen peroxide in the knee joints of mice by intra-articular injection of amidated glucose oxidase. This produced marked tissue damage as assessed histologically, inhibition of cartilage proteoglycan synthesis and increased vascular permeability as judged by $^{99m}$Tc uptake and $^{125}$I-albumin accumulation into the injected joint. This effect of glucose oxidase appeared to be dose-dependent, with high doses causing marked chondrocyte death and irreversible cartilage damage.

There are certain similarities between this model and the antigen-induced model in mice. High doses of amidated glucose oxidase produced joint swelling and $^{99m}$Tc accumulation in the joint comparable to a severe antigen-induced arthritis. Furthermore, histologically glucose oxidase produced marked cellular exudation, synovial cell hyperplasia, proteoglycan depletion from the surface of the articular cartilage and erosion by pannus-like tissue. However, the peri-articular lesions and chondrocyte death induced by amidated glucose oxidase appeared greater than those seen in antigen-induced arthritis[101].

Intra-articular injections of amidated catalase abolished the arthritogenic effect of the glucose oxidase when given simultaneously. The selenium-containing compound ebselen[102] which suppresses GSH peroxidase and also inhibits lipid peroxidation by a GSH-independent mechanism, given orally daily at a dose of 50 mg/kg commencing 1 day prior to the glucose oxidase injection, suppressed the arthritis, whereas indomethacin (10 mg/kg) or piroxicam (10 mg/kg) had no effect under the same conditions.

## VII. AUTOIMMUNE MOUSE MODELS

### (1) MRL/I mice

MRL-lpr/lpr (MRL/l) mice spontaneously develop a severe autoimmune disease which is characterized by massive generalized lymphadenopathy, arthritis, arteritis and immune complex-mediated glomerulonephritis. The serological abnormalities in these animals include antibodies against native DNA, rheumatoid factors and circulating immune complexes[103]. Thus this strain of mice may be regarded as a model of both human systemic lupus erythematosus (SLE) and rheumatoid arthritis. However, the incidence of arthropathy in these animals is much lower than the incidence of the SLE-like syndrome, and is much more variable in presentation. Consequently, this autoimmune syndrome should perhaps be regarded more as a model of SLE than of rheumatoid arthritis.

Since many of the novel antirheumatic drugs in development are immunomodulatory in their mechanism of action it is logical to investigate their potential activity in MRL/l mice, as well as in other spontaneous autoimmune disease models such as the NZB/W F1 hybrid mouse lupus model. One of the principal advantages of these two models is that, in contrast to the induced models of arthritis, they possess the serological features of the human diseases which can be used to monitor the progress of the disease and the efficacy of any treatment under investigation. However, these benefits are offset by the variable onset and severity of the disease which necessitates the use of large numbers of animals. Nevertheless, a considerable number of established and novel antirheumatic compounds have been investigated in MRL/l mice.

In this strain of mice, autoimmune manifestations begin to appear at the age of 8 weeks, and 12-week-old mice have histologically and serologically detectable signs of peripheral lymphoid hyperplasia and arthritis as well as functional renal disease. Consequently, two different treatment schedules have been employed: a prophylactic schedule with treatment commencing in the 4–8 week age range and therapeutic schedules where treatment commences in the 12–15 week age range. Both male and female mice express the disease, with females expressing slightly more severe disease than males. Both sexes have been used for pharmacological studies.

Dietary manipulation, sex hormones and prostaglandin $E_1$ have all been shown to modify the course of the autoimmune disease in MRL/l mice, but since these cannot be regarded as antirheumatic agents we consider these treatments as being outside the scope of this review.

Two cyclooxygenase inhibitors, aspirin and oxaprozin, have been evaluated in some detail in this model by Carlson et al.[104]. Daily treatment with these compounds at a dose of 100 mg/kg over a period of 3 months commencing at 8 weeks of age significantly reduced thymic hyperplasia. Aspirin, but not oxaprozin, also reduced total lymphocyte counts, spleen and lymph node hyperplasia and renal vasculitis. However, neither of these compounds had any effect on circulating anti-dsDNA levels or the glomerulonephritis. The effects of several NSAIDs on the production of acute phase reactants in this model have been investigated by other workers. Neither indomethacin (0.25–1 mg/kg) nor zomepirac sodium (0.5–2 mg/kg) had any effect on the elevation of ESR during the development of the disease[105]. Similarly, neither indomethacin nor piroxicam (both 0.5 mg/kg daily from 4 weeks of age to 24 weeks of age) had any effect on the rise in serum amyloid P-component (SAP), the anti-dsDNA antibody levels or the arthritis[106]. Tolfenamic acid (10 mg/kg daily) has also been shown to have no effect on serological parameters, the glomerulonephritis or survival of MRL/l mice using either prophylactic or therapeutic treatment schedules[107].

Two compounds which inhibit lipoxygenase as well as cyclooxygenase, namely BW 755C and benoxaprofen, have also been investigated in this model. BW 755C (50 mg/kg) suppressed the elevated ESR levels[105]; benoxaprofen (40 mg/kg daily) suppressed the rise in SAP and anti-dsDNA autoantibody levels without affecting the lymphoproliferation or the arthritis[105].

Corticosteroids and second-line antirheumatic agents have been investigated quite extensively in MRL/l mice. Rordorf-Adam et al.[106] found that prednisolone (0.6 and 6 mg/kg/day) reduced SAP levels and anti-dsDNA antibody levels but had no effect on the progression of the arthritis or the lymphoproliferation. Similarly, Stim et al.[105] showed that dexamethasone (0.5 mg/kg daily) reduced ESR levels, and Toivonen et al.[107] found that prednisolone (0.5 mg/kg daily) reduced lymph node enlargement without affecting anti-ssDNA levels, the development of the renal disease, or the survival of the mice.

Ackerman et al.[108] carried out a detailed study of the effect of therapeutic treatment with D-penicillamine (10, 30 and 100 mg/kg daily for 12 weeks commencing at 12 weeks of age) on the disease progression. Significant reductions in circulating IgG, IgM, rheumatoid factor, anti-DNA and anti-poly A antibodies were observed, particularly at the higher doses. However, the drug failed to have any effect on spleen weight or spleen cell number, or the responsiveness of the spleen cells to mitogens. Furthermore, there was no effect on the synovitis or the glomerulonephritis. Toivonen et al.[107] also found that low doses of D-penicillamine (5 mg/kg daily) given prophylactically failed to affect the renal disease, although there was some reduction in the lymph node enlargement. The effect of D-penicillamine on acute-phase reactants is equivocal. Stim et al.[105] reported suppression of the ESR with D-penicillamine at a dose of 25 mg/kg daily, whereas Rordorf-Adam et al.[106] found that 15 and 25 mg/kg/day D-penicillamine had no effect on either SAP levels or anti-dsDNA, and also failed to affect the arthritis.

Chloroquine and sodium aurothiomalate have also been investigated by Rordorf-Adam et al.[106]. Both compounds reduced the elevated levels of SAP in male mice, and sodium aurothiomalate also reduced the lymphoproliferation and arthritic changes. Fujitsu et al.[109] showed that aurothiomalate, and to a greater extent auranofin (10 mg gold/kg/day prophylactically) reduced anti-DNA antibody levels hypergammaglobulinaemia, polyclonal B-cell activation and the renal disease. However, in this case the lymphoproliferation was not prevented.

Cyclophosphamide is the only established drug to have shown a marked effect on the disease progression in MRL/l mice. Rordorf-Adam et al.[106] found that doses of 5 and 10 mg/kg/day i.p. given prophylactically completely suppressed the lymphoproliferation and SAP levels. The higher dose also significantly reduced the arthritic changes. Therapeutic treatment with cyclophosphamide at a dose of 100 mg/kg daily was also shown to reduce the lymphoproliferation, autoantibody levels, arthritic changes and renal lesions, as well as improving survival[110]. Similar results have been obtained by other workers using doses of 1.8 mg/mouse/week[111] and 25 mg/kg twice per week[112].

Although it cannot be truly classified as an established drug, lobenzarit (Carfenil) has recently entered the market in Japan as a second-line antirheumatic agent, although its efficacy needs to be confirmed through long-term use. Its efficacy in the MRL/l mouse model was investigated by Abe et al.[113]. They found that oral administration of the drug at a dose of 25 mg/kg three times per week commencing at 8 weeks of age produced a significant reduction in the arthritic changes, glomerulonephritis and lymphadenopathy.

Thus the responsiveness of this model to established drugs used in the treatment of rheumatoid arthritis is complex, with many of the drugs affecting one or more of the parameters measured. However, with the exception of cyclophophamide, none of the drugs has been shown to reproducibly retard the progression of the disease. Furthermore, the relationship between the serological parameters investigated and the lymphoproliferation and renal disease are unclear at present. Further controlled studies of this nature should clarify this point. In the meantime, several novel agents have been investigated in this autoimmune disease model.

The selective immunosuppressant cyclosporin A at very high doses (25 and 75 mg/kg/day) partially reduced the lymphoproliferation without affecting the SAP or anti-dsDNA antibody levels or the arthritis[106]. Mountz et al.[114] also demonstrated a reduction in lymphadenopathy by high-dose cyclosporin A treatment (40 mg/kg/day commencing at 2 weeks of age) without any effect on the anti-ssDNA levels. However, these workers also demonstrated suppression of the renal disease as evidenced by normal blood urea nitrogen and glomerular histology, as well as suppression of the synovitis and normalization of T cell responsiveness. Therefore these data suggest that the B cell hyperactivity can proceed without the T cell proliferative disease, and that the renal disease appears to be dependent on T cell responsiveness rather than the autoantibody response.

Suramin, a drug used for the treatment of African trypanosomiasis, had a suppressive effect on many parameters when given at doses of 20 and 50 mg/kg i.v. once per week[106]. Suramin treatment reduced the levels of SAP and anti-dsDNA as well as the arthritis, but had no effect on the lymphoproliferation[106]. These workers also showed that retinoic acid (2.5 and 12.5 mg/kg/day i.p) could partially inhibit the lymphoproliferation but had no effect on SAP or anti-dsDNA levels or the arthritis[106].

In view of the dependence of this disease model on aberrant immunological responses, several novel immunomodulatory compounds have been investigated in the model. The results of such studies should, as well as revealing information on the compounds themselves, shed light on the regulatory mechanisms contolling the aetiopathogenesis of the model.

The first of these compounds is DIAM 4, a cyclophosphazene derivative which inhibits polyclonal activation of lymphocytes and was originally developed as a potential antitumour drug. This compound was found to prevent the rise in anti-DNA antibody levels, the development of the renal disease, and the lymphoproliferation when administered at a dose of 10 mg/kg/day i.p. 5 days per week from 9 weeks of age[115].

SR 41 319 is a novel biphosphonate compound which is active in adjuvant arthritis in the rat and inhibits the production of collagenase and neutral proteases by chondrocytes and synoviocytes stimulated with interleukin-1-containing preparations[116]. Prophylactic treatment with this compound in MRL/1 mice delayed and reduced the onset of the clinical signs of disease, increased the lifespan and decreased the ESR. However, the compound only produced slight changes in the weight of some of the involved organs and this was apparent only in the first few weeks of treatment.

HWA 486 (leflunomide) is another immunomodulatory drug which shows activity in adjuvant arthritis in rats. In MRL/1 mice HWA 486, 20–30 mg/kg daily, increased the lifespan, prevented the development of proteinuria and arrested the development of splenomegaly. There was also an inhibition of anti-dsDNA antibody production[112].

Finally, the immunomodulatory compound LS 2616 was investigated in MRL/1 mice in comparison with cyclophosphamide[111]. Treatment was initiated either at 8 weeks (prophylactic) or 16 weeks (therapeutic) of age. Beneficial effects were seen with LS 2616 at doses as low as 1 mg/mouse/week i.p. given either prophylactically or therapeutically. These included suppression of the lymphadenopathy, splenomegaly, glomerulonephritis and vasculitis, as well as an increase in lifespan. Furthermore, the effects of LS 2616 at a dose of 32 mg/mouse/week were comparable to those of cyclophosphamide at 1.8 mg/mouse/week.

Thus there are several novel immunomodulatory compounds which appear to have marked suppressive effects on all the autoimmune manifestations in MRL/1 mice and increase the lifespan to a comparable extent to that seen with cyclophosphamide. These compounds appear to be much more selective in their effects on the immune system, and in some instances their immunomodulatory effects have still to be clearly delineated. The investigation of these compounds in the clinic should shed further light on the relevance of this animal model to rheumatoid arthritis and SLE.

## (2) NZB/W mice

New Zealand black x New Zealand white F1 hybrid (NZB/W) mice develop a spontaneous autoimmune disease similar to systemic lupus erythematosus (SLE). In female NZB/W mice the disease is characterized by the development of antinucleic acid antibodies, immune complex glomerulonephritis with proteinuria and uraemia, and a consequent shortened lifespan[117,118]. In general, proteinuria becomes apparent at 6–7 months of age and animals may die from 8 months of age. Males develop a less severe form of the disease. Although this spontaneous autoimmune disease model has been used for the investigation of antirheumatic drugs for many years, it has not been used as extensively as the MRL/l model, probably because the latter strain produces a more severe disease in a shorter period of time. This allows shorter treatment schedules to be used, and indications of compound efficacy to be obtained much more rapidly in MRL/l than NZB/W mice. Nevertheless, the latter model is still being used for evaluation of novel antirheumatic agents, although increasingly this is done after efficacy has been demonstrated in the MRL/1 model.

As with the MRL/l autoimmune model, the syndrome in NZB/W mice can be influenced by dietary manipulation and treatment with $PGE_1$ or sex steroids which are considered outside the scope of this review.

A number of studies have demonstrated the efficacy of immunosuppressive drugs in the treatment of glomerulonephritis in NZB/W mice. Hurd et al.[119] carried out a comparative study of the effects of daily i.p. treatment with cyclophosphamide (15 mg/kg) and 6-mercaptopurine (7.5 mg/kg) on the model. Treatment commenced at 1, 3, 5, 7 or 9 months of age and was continued for 4 months. Under these conditions, cyclophosphamide decreased antinuclear antibody production, immunoglobulin deposition in both skin and glomeruli, glomular cell proliferation and glomerulosclerosis. Similar results have been obtained with 12.5 mg/kg cyclophosphamide administered twice per week[120]. In contrast, 6-mercaptopurine treatment had no effect on antinuclear antibody production or immunoglobulin deposition in the glomeruli, although the glomerulosclerosis and glomerular cell proliferation were both reduced[119]. In this latter case, immunoglobulin deposition in skin was paradoxically increased.

Gelfand and Steinberg[121] compared the efficacy of azathioprine, cyclophosphamide and methylprednisolone at different doses and found that all three drugs reduced proteinuria, renal histology and anti-DNA antibody level and increased lifespan. At low doses (1.5 mg/kg/day) azathioprine appeared to be the most effective, whereas at high doses (4.5 mg/kg/day) cyclophosphamide was the most effective. Interestingly, the greatest effect was seen with a combination of methylprednisolone and cyclophosphamide (both at 1.5 mg/kg/day) which increased survival without increasing toxicity.

Thus this model of autoimmune disease is responsive to the classical immunosuppressant drugs such as corticosteroids and the cytotoxic agents. There have been very few investigations of the effects of NSAIDs in this model. Kelley et al.[122] have investigated the effect of ibuprofen treatment (8–9 mg/kg daily from 2 months of age) and found no effect on survival, the development of proteinuria or circulating levels of antibodies to DNA or retroviral gp70 immune complexes.

As seen in the MRL/l mice, cyclosporin A reduced some but not all of parameters of the autoimmune disease in NZB/W mice[123]. Treatment with the drug at a dose of 100 mg/kg five times per week commencing at 8 weeks of age increased lifespan and reduced proteinurea and glomerular proliferation. However, perivascular infiltration in the kidney, hypergammaglobulinaemia, circulating immune complex levels and the later development of auto-immune haemolytic anaemia were unaffected by the treatment. In parallel with the reduction in renal disease, there was a reduction in anti-dsDNA anti-body levels and T-cell function, although levels of rheumatoid factor were elevated. Gunn[124], also using cyclosporin A at 100 mg/kg five times per week, showed that the drug could reduce autoantibody levels when administered to mice commencing at either 12 or 36 weeks of age. In this study the novel cyclosporin derivative (Nva$^2$)-cyclosporin produced a similar effect to cyclosporin A.

Lobenzarit also produced a similar effect in NZB/W mice to that seen in MRL/l mice. Daily treatment with 5 and 50 mg/kg commencing at 9 weeks of age dose-dependently increased lifespan and reduced the proteinuria, glomerulonephritis, anti-DNA antibody levels and anti-thymocyte antibody levels, as well as the reduction in suppressor T-cell function which occurs with increasing age in these animals[125,126].

Mizoribine (bredinin) is an imidazole nucleoside immunosuppresant isolated from *Eupenicillium brefeldianum*, currently in use for renal trans-plantation in Japan because in this context it has comparable efficacy to aza-thioprine but produces fewer side effects[127]. In NZB/W mice mizoribine administered at a dose of 20 mg/kg on alternate days commencing at 14 weeks of age prolonged lifespan and suppressed both the anti-DNA antibody levels and the glomerulonephritis[128].

Frentizole was developed as a selective immunosuppressant since it was found to suppress immune responses without depressing peripheral blood granulocyte counts or predisposing animals or patients to infection. On the basis of this profile of activity, frentizole was evaluated in open-label and double-blind trials in patients with SLE. Although the drug appeared to be effective in suppressing the disease, it produced ischaemic bowel necrosis in approximately 10% of patients receiving the drug, and consequently the trials were abandoned[129]. During these studies frentizole was found to be effec-tive in treating autoimmune thrombocytpenia and the drug has subsequently been used to treat patients with life-threatening thrombocytopenia which is refractory to other therapies[129,130]. The efficacy of frentizole has been inves-tigated in NZB/W mice at two dose levels (8 and 80–84 mg/kg/day) under both prophylactic and therapeutic schedules (treatment commencing at 8 weeks or 24 weeks of age respectively)[131]. Prophylactic treatment with the higher dose effectively suppressed the anti-DNA antibody levels and in-creased lifespan, but had no effect on the progression of the renal disease. Under the therapeutic dosing schedule, high-dose frentizole produced some increase in lifespan but had no effect on either anti-DNA antibody levels or the renal disease. Low-dose frentizole treatment did not produce any benefi-cial effects under either schedule.

Several novel immunomodulatory compounds which have yet to be investigated in man have been studied in the NZB/W model. Two of these, LS-2616 and DIAM 4, have previously shown activity against the autoimmune syndrome in MRL/l mice. In NZB/W mice treatment with LS-2616 at doses of 1 and 8 mg/mouse/week commencing at either 4 weeks of age (early disease) or 7 weeks of age (established disease) increased lifespan and decreased splenomegaly and glomerulonephritis[113]. The results obtained with LS 2616 were comparable to those obtained with cyclophosphamide (1.8 mg/mouse/week). Similarly, DIAM 4 showed a comparable level of suppression of the disease in NZB/W mice to that obtained in MRL/1 mice under the same conditions, i.e. 10 mg/kg/day i.p. 5 days per week commencing at 20 weeks of age[115].

Zimet-3164 is a potent immunosuppressant belonging to the nitrogen mustard family. Doses of 20–40 mg/kg i.p. of Zimet-3164 given twice per week for up to 6 weeks were able to prevent the progression of the disease in NZB/W mice. The treatment was more effective in young adult animals with slight to moderate glomerular lesions than in older mice with advanced nephritis, and appeared to be more effective than treatment with cyclophosphamide[132]. The reduction in disease activity with Zimet-3164 treatment appeared to be due in part to diminished deposition of immune complexes within the glomeruli.

FUT-175 is a novel synthetic protease inhibitor which inhibits the C1r and C1 esterase of the complement system as well as thrombin, plasmin, kallikrein and trypsin. At the exceedingly high dose of 400 mg/kg six times per week the compound had a beneficial effect on the disease under both prophylactic and therapeutic regimes (treatment commencing at 16 and 32 weeks of age respectively[134]). The suppression of the disease was evidenced by a reduction in proteinuria, a decrease in blood urea nitrogen as well as a reduction in histological damage to the glomeruli. This effect was marginally superior to that observed with dexamethasone administered at a dose of 1–3 mg/kg under the same conditions. However, lower doses of FUT-175 appeared to be ineffective.

FCE 20696 is a synthetic immunomodulator which has been shown to induce suppressor cells after repeated administration to mice, and to reduce both adjuvant-induced arthritis and experimental allergic encephalitis in rats. In female NZB/W mice given FCE 20696 1.5 mg/kg biweekly commencing at 9 weeks of age, the drug prolonged lifespan and delayed the onset of proteinuria[135]. Subsequent studies with the compound in this model, employing a spleen cell transfer to syngeneic mice, revealed that the drug had induced a suppressor cell population in 21-week-old mice[136]. A similar induction of suppressor cells was observed with lobenzarit at a dose of 50 mg/kg.

In conclusion, there is a considerable degree of similarity in the effects of drugs on the autoimmune disease syndromes in NZB/W and MRL/l mice despite the differences in the autoimmune syndromes in the two strains, notably the increased disease severity, lymphadenopathy and arthritic manifestations in the latter. This similarity of responsiveness of the two strains coupled with the shorter disease duration in the MRL/l mice has led to the increasing popularity of the latter strain for investigation of novel com-

118

pounds. Consequently, in the future NZB/W mice may only be used once activity has been demonstrated in MRL/l mice. The activity of cytotoxic immunosuppressants and lack of activity of NSAIDs in these autoimmune disease models correlates well with their effects in SLE in man. Similarly, the efficacy of frentizole in both the clinic and the NZB/W model also indicates the usefulness of these spontaneous autoimmune disease models as predictors of efficacy in SLE. Several novel compounds covering a wide range of immunomodulatory activities have shown convincing activity in these models. Investigation of their activity in man should help to clarify this contention and determine the relevance of the models to other autoimmune diseases such as rheumatoid arthritis. Furthermore, many of these later compounds show greater efficacy than frentizole in the NZB/W model. It will be very interesting to see if they have a comparably greater level of efficacy in the clinical disease.

## VIII. EXPERIMENTAL ALLERGIC ENCEPHALOMYELITIS (EAE)

While not a model of arthritic disease *per se*, this is a model of cellular hypersensitivity that has been employed by some searching for disease-modifying agents acting on the T-lymphocyte arm of the immune system[137,138]. Various protocols are employed for the establishment of this disease in rats[137]. Essentially, crude spinal cord or preparations of myelin are admixed with suspending media and a Freund's-type adjuvant[137]. This is then injected intradermally at one or many sites, and after a period of about 2 weeks neurological manifestations of the disease ensue[137]. One such protocol which is relatively common and useful for reliably producing the disease involves i.d. injection into both hind paw foot pads of an 0.1 ml emulsion of 100 mg lyophilized and reconstituted spinal cord in Arlacel/Nujol/saline with 20 mg heat-killed mycobacteria[139].

The principal histopathological features in the central nervous system (CNS) which occur are perivascular injury and associated necrosis of the surrounding cells, with accompanying cellular infiltration, and degeneration of myelinated nerves[137]. The cellular-immune basis of this system has been investigated in some considerable detail[137,138]. Helper/inducer T-cells play a primary role in the induction of lesions[139]. It is suggested that upon infiltration of these cells they eleborate lymphokines which activate non-T cells to express Ia antigen, and this is followed by the ingress of suppressor/cytotoxic T-cells into the inflamed sites[139]. Clearly the specific cellular immune manifestations of this disease enable drug treatments to be applied at different stages of the induction thereof, and thus for drug effects to be identified as acting on $CD_4$ (helper), $CD_8$ (suppressor/cytotoxic) and macrophage-activating phases, even though there may be some degree of overlap.

Gold thiomalate and gold thioglucose were among the earlier agents shown to affect this disease in rats[140]. Other DMARDs and cytostats have been found to inhibit the progression of this disease, but NSAIDs are inef-

119

fective[139,141,142]. Cyclosporin and its analogues have been extensively investigated for their anti-arthritic effects, much of which probably originates from the actions on IL-2 receptors[139]. Cisplatin and related novel platinum compounds with anti-arthritic activity are very effective in EAE[143]. These observations suggest that EAE may at least be reasonably selective for detecting disease-modifying agents.

## IX. RELATIVE MERITS OF INDIVIDUAL MODELS

Table 1 summarizes the principal features of the animal models which have been discussed in this chapter. Also considered are the responses of the various classes of anti-arthritic agents, new and established. In some respects the responses to the different classes of drugs might be considered as a possible guide to the selectivity of a particular model for detection of disease-modifying compared with conventional controllers of soft tissue inflammation. Inspection of the table will reveal what many experimentalists regard as a depressing fact, i.e. one of chaos, for there is very little pharmacological basis for any basis for selection. While it is intuitively obvious to many working in the field of drug discovery that those animal models with predominant T-lymphocyte ($CD_4$) activation for their actions and specific disease manifestations resembling rheumatoid arthritis (e.g. adjuvant disease) or better still systemic lupus erythematosus (e.g. the MRL/l mouse) the great puzzle is to know why some of the established DMARDs enhance these diseases or have no effects in these models when they would be expected, classically, to have disease-remitting activity.

For the answer to these problems it is necessary to consider three possible aspects:

(1)     The DMARDs tested could be weak or ineffective when it comes to stringent testing.

(2)     These drugs could have biodisposition and modes of action in the rodent/lapine models employed such that their responses differ markedly from what are seen in the disease states in man.

(3)     The dosage regimes for the drugs employed in the animal studies could be out of relationship to the specific phases of the disease.

In essence all these points apply in particular to the comparative actions of the DMARDs. With the NSAIDs the actions are more or less clearcut, and in any case the point of interest with regard to selecting models or protocols for application with certain of these models is that they should enable the selection of disease-modifying or remitting actions. The question most often raised where NSAIDs are shown to have effects in an animal model (e.g. such as in adjuvant disease) is whether this of itself negates the applicability of such a model in the selection of drugs for disease-modifying actions. However, insight into the reactions at different phases of what is a disease of fast progression in most rat strains (though there is some considerable variation in the timing of different phases in different strains and responses of drugs therein - see refs 2 and 144), reveals that it is possible to select periods of both drug treatment and those for the observation(s) in order to discriminate out the actions of NSAID-like drugs from those with disease-remitting activity. In the experience of one of the authors (KDR, studies in preparation) combined with evidence from published studies[143,144] it is possible to achieve positive effects of most DMARDs, without NSAIDs having significant actions in adjuvant arthritic rats by dosing within a narrow time window shortly after establishment of the disease. Since this period is by far dominated by lymphocyte priming or activation it is not surprising that those drugs having effects only at the level of lymphocyte functions (the best example probably being cyclosporin A - see ref 143) will have quite selective actions on this phase of the disease.

It was considered during the past decade or so that this so-called period of prophylactic dosage was not one in which any degree of reliance would be placed for the identification of a drug with putative anti-arthritic effects (i.e. in a general sense). However, with futher insight in recent years into the development of the adjuvant disease, together with the above-mentioned observations on the narrow time frame for dosing to achieve selective effects, and improved methods for measuring the actions of the drugs, it has been possible to gain a greater degree of selectivity in screening for those drugs with disease-remitting actions in this model.

Even despite improvements in the application of the adjuvant arthritis model, there are still many points outlined in the three points above which are valid criticisms. Most especially, the relationship of drug pharmacokinetics in the diseased rats to their distribution in man, the responses of lymphocytes in arthritic rats to those in human subjects, and the timing of phases under treatment or those being analysed to the course of the rheumatoid disease in man, are all unsolved points.

The selection of various models is also a matter of much revelance, and often a point for intense debate among various pro- and anti-agonists. Thus many have regarded the Dumonde and Glynn model as being more appropriate to that of human rheumatoid disease based essentially on the joint pathology, compared with that of adjuvant disease in rats. This is in many respects true, especially in regard to local lymphoid nodular formation and the synovitis. One argument often stated is that the periostitis which is so dominant in adjuvant arthritis is not a major feature of human rheumatoid disease. This is in fact not true[145]. Also, it has been considered by many that the Dumonde and Glynn model is essentially a monoarticular arthropathy, and not a polyarthritis with attendant systemic manifestations (e.g. extensive alterations in the production of acute-phase proteins), which is in fact more indicative of the disease manifestations in human rheumatoid arthritis. Clearly the rational approach is to select the particular pathological responses in a select model to examine the drug actions. The key to the process of selection

Table 1 Summary of principal features of the main animal models used for the identification of anti-rheumatic activity

| Model inducing agent | Species | Joint pathology | Effects of | | | |
|---|---|---|---|---|---|---|
| | | | NSAIDs | DMARDs | CyA | Other newer agents |
| Mycobacterial Adjuvant (Freund's) | Rat | Autoimmune (?link protein Ag.) reaction, periostitis, new bone formation, cartilage erosion | ↓ (T)<br>↓ Some (P) | ↑ often (T)*<br>↓ (P) | ↓ (T)<br>↓ (P) | ↓ Ro-31,9848<br>bredinin<br>iobenzarit<br>BM41,3321<br>SA96 (T)<br>HWA 486<br>cyclophosphamide |
| CP20961 | Rat | as above (no evidence of Ag) | | | | |
| Collagen II | Rat | as above (Ag is collagen II) | ↓ (T) | ↑ (T) | ↑ (T)<br>↓ (P) | ↑ Retinoids |
| Collagen II | Mice | as above (Ag is collagen II) | ?NE<br>↓ INDO | ↑ Pn(P)<br>?Au NE | | ↓ Cyclophosphamide<br>cortico-oestrogenic steroids |
| Antigens + Freund's adjuvant | Rabbits | monoarticular local erosive arthropathy | NE except ↓ ketoprofen | NE Chloroquine<br>↓↑ D-Pen.<br>↓ ATM, ?AF<br>NE-SASP | | ↓ corticosteriods<br>azathioprine<br>cyclophosphamide<br>chlorambucil |

| | | | | | | |
|---|---|---|---|---|---|---|
| Antigen (e.g. BSA) (e.g. met-BSA) + Freund's adjuvant + Bordetella | Mice | as above | NE (P,T) | NE D-Pen. Tiopronin Chloroquine (P,T) ATM, ±AF(P) ↓SASP (T) | ?(T) | ↓ corticoids, azathioprine (T,P) ±methotroxate |
| Spontaneous autoimmune disease MRL/I | Mice | synovitis, erosive arthritis; variable disease | ↑, NE | NE, D-Pen, AF ↓ATM | NE | ±, NE corticoids ↓ cyclophosphamide lobenzarit biphosphonates |

*Abbreviations:* ↑ increase, ↓ decrease, or NE no effect on disease, ± variable effects, T = therapeutic, P = prophylactic dosing regimes, ATM = aurothiomalate, AF = auranofin, CyA = cyclosporin A, Pen = D-penicillamine, INDO = indomethacin, SASP = salicylsulphapyridine, Ag = antigen
*Depending on rat strain (see Haynes and Whitehouse, chapter 8, this volume, for details of effects of gold compounds, and see ref 144 for variable effects of D-penicillamine).

123

of the pathological responses to be monitored depends on the parameters being measured, and the methods of their measurement. This must still represent the greatest area for improvement in the application of the animal model(s) for drug development, especially in the automation and quantification of histopathological data.

## REFERENCES

1.  Hunneyball, IM, Stewart, GA and Stanworth, DR (1979). The effects of oral D-penicillamine on experimental arthritis and associated immune responses in rabbits. III. Reduction of the monoarticular arthritis. *Ann Rheum Dis*, **38**, 271–8

2.  Billingham, MEJ and Rushton, A (1985). Clozic. In *Anti-inflammatory and Anti-rheumatic Drugs*, Vol. III, ed. Rainsford, KD. CRC Press, Boca Raton, pp. 31–64

3.  Sporn, MB and Roberts, AB (1988). Peptide growth factors are multifunctional. *Nature*, **332**, 217–19

4.  Stoerk, HC, Bielinski, TC and Budzilovich, T (1954). Chronic polyarthritis in rats injected with spleen in adjuvants. *Am J Pathol*, **30**, 616

5.  Pearson, CM (1956). Development of arthritis, periarthritis and periostitis in rats given adjuvants. *Proc Soc Exp Biol (NY)*, **91**, 95–101

6.  Newbould, BB (1963). Chemotherapy of arthritis induced in rats by injection of mycobacterial adjuvant. *Br J Pharmacol*, **21**, 127–36

7.  Dumonde, DC and Glynn, LE (1962). The production of arthritis in rabbits by an immunological reaction to fibrin. *Br J Exp Pathol*, **43**, 373–83

8.  Brackertz, D, Mitchell, GF and Mackay, IR (1977). Antigen induced arthritis in mice. I. Induction of arthritis in various strains of mice. *Arth Rheum*, **20**, 841–50.

9.  Trentham, DE, Townes, AS and Kang, AH (1977). Autoimmunity to type II collagen: an experimental model of arthritis. *J Exp Med*, **146**, 857–68

10. Courtenay, JS, Dallman, MJ, Dayan, AD *et al.* (1980). Immunisation against heterologous type II collagen induces arthritis in mice. *Nature*, **238**, 666–8

11. Morgan, K, Evans, HB, Firth, SA *et al.* (1983). 1α2α3α collagen is arthritogenic. *Ann Rheum Dis,* **42**, 680–3

12. Glant, TT, Mikecz, K Arzoumanian, A and Poole, AR (1987). Proteoglycan-induced arthritis in Balb/C mice. Clinical features and histopathology. *Arth Rheum*, **30**, 201–12

13. Billingham, MEJ (1983). Models of arthritis and the search for anti-arthritic drugs. *Pharmacol Ther*, **21**, 389–428

14. Wright, V and Amos, R (1980). Do drugs change the course of rheumatoid arthritis. *Br Med J*, **280**, 964–6

15. Kohashi, O, Tanaka, A, Kotani, S *et al.* (1980). Arthritis-inducing ability of a synthetic adjuvant, N-acetyl muramyl peptides, and bacterial disaccharide, peptides related to different oil vehicles and their composition. *Infect Immun*, **29**, 70–5

16. Chang, YH, Pearson, CM and Abe, C (1980). Adjuvant polyarthritis, I.V. induction by a synthetic adjuvant: immunologic, histopathologic and other studies. *Arth Rheum*, **23**, 62–71

17. Kohashi, O, Aihara, K, Ozawa, A *et al.* (1982). New model of a synthetic adjuvant, N-acetyl muramyl-L-alanyl-D-isoglutamine-induced arthritis. Clinical and histological studies in athymic nude and euthymic rats. *Lab Invest*, **47**, 27–36

18. Taurog, JD, Sandberg, GP and Mahowald, ML (1983). The cellular basis of adjuvant arthritis. II. Characterisation of the cells mediating passive transfer. *Cell Immunol*, **80**, 198–204

19. Holoshitz, J, Naparstek, Y, Ben-Nun, A and Cohen, IR (1983). Lines of T-lymphocytes induce or vaccinate against autoimmune arthritis. *Science*, **219**, 56–8

20. Billingham, MEJ, Drayer, L, Fairchild, S et al. (1988). Monoclonal antibody therapy of experimental arthritis. Scand J Rheum (In press)

21. Van Eden, W, Thole, JER, Van Der Zee, R et al. (1988). Cloning of the mycobacterial epitope recognised by T lymphocytes in adjuvant arthritis. Nature, 331, 171–3

22. Janossy, G, Duke, O, Poulter, LW et al. (1981). Rheumatoid arthritis: a disease of T-lymphocyte/macrophage immunoregulation. Lancet, 2, 839–42

23. Trentham, DE, Belli, JA, Bloomer, WD et al. (1987). 2,000-centigray total lymphoid irradiation for refractory rheumatoid arthritis. Arth Rheum, 30, 980–7

24. Littler, TR (1982). Anti-rheumatic drugs. Pharmacol Ther, 15, 45–68

25. Koh, MS, Parente, L and Willoughby, DA (1978). The paradoxical effect of levamizole on different experimental models of inflammation. Eur J Rheum Inflam, 1, 254–60

26. Arrigoni-Martelli, E and Bramm, E (1975). Investigations of the influence of cyclophosphamide, gold sodium thiomaleate, and D-penicillamine on Nystatin oedema and adjuvant arthritis. Agents and Actions, 5, 264–7

27. Borel, JF, Feurer, C, Gubler, HV and Stahalin, H (19). Biological effects of cyclosporin A. A new antilymphocytic agent. Agents and Actions, 6, 468–75

28. Weinblatt, ME, Coblyn, JS, Fraser, PA et al. (1987). Cyclosporin A treatment of refractory rheumatoid arthritis. Arth Rheum, 30, 11–17

29. Dougados, M and Amor, B (1987). Cyclosporin A in rheumatoid arthritis: preliminary clinical results on an open trial. Arth Rheum, 30, 83–7

30. Iwata, H, Iwaki, H, Masukawa, T et al. (1987). Anti-arthritic activity of bredinin, an immunosuppressive agent. Experientia, 33, 502–3

31. Ohsugi, Y, Hata, S, Tanemura, M et al. (1977). N-(2-Carboxylphenyl)-4-chloroanthranilic acid disodium salt: a novel anti-arthritic agent without anti-inflammatory and immunosuppressive activities. J Pharm Pharmacol, 29, 636–7

32. Ohsugi, Y, Nakano, T and Hata, S (1983). A novel anti-arthritic agent, CCA (Lobenzarit disodium), and the role of thymus derived lymphocytes in the inhibition of rat adjuvant arthritis. Immunopharmacology, 6, 15–21

33. Shiokawa, Y, Horiuchi, Y, Mizushima, Y et al. (1984). A multicentre double-blind controlled study of Lobenzarit, a novel immunomodulator, in rheumatoid arthritis. J Rheumatol, 11, 615–23

34. Bicker, U (1982). Effect of the immunomodulant 2-cyanazinindine derivative BM41.332 on adjuvant arthritis in the rat. Arzneim Forsch, 32, 746–52

35. Komoriya, K, Tsuchimoto, M, Naruch, T et al. (1983). Immunopharmacological profile of TEI-3096: a new immunomodulator. J Immunopharm, 4, 285–301

36. Bender, PE, Hill, DT, Offen, PH et al. (1985). 5,6-Diaryl-2,3-dihydroimidazo[2,1-b]thizoles: a new class of immunoregulatory anti-inflammatory agents. J Med Chem, 28, 1169–77

37. Binderup, L (1985). Effects of isoprenozine in animals models of depressed T-cell function. Int J Immunopharmacol, 7, 93–101

38. Yamauchi, H, Hayashi, M, Kasamatsu, S et al. (1985). Pharmacological studies of N-(2-mercapto-2-methyl propanoyl)-L-cysteine (SA96). V. Effects of SA96 in combination with indomethacin or prednisolone on adjuvant arthritis in rats. Filio Pharmacol Japan, 85, 243–8

39. Bartlett, RR and Scleyerbach, R (1985). Immunopharmocological profile of a novel isoxazol derivative, HWA 486, with potential anti-rheumatic activity. I. Disease modifying action on adjuvant arthritis in the rat. Int J Immunopharmacol, 7, 7–18

40. Bartlett, RR (1986). Immunopharmacological profile of HWA486, a novel isoxazol derivative. II: In vivo immunomodulatory effects differ from those of cyclophosphamide prednisolone, or cyclosporin A. Int J Immunopharmacol, 8, 199–204

41. Rosenthale, ME, Santilli, AA, Scotese, AC et al. (1980). Immunopharmacologic properties of 1,6-bis[2-(diethylamino)ethoxy]xanthan-9-one dihydrochloride (WY-15297). J Immunopharmacol, 2, 257–64

42. Gilman, SC, Carlson, RP, Daniels, JF et al. (1987). Immunological abnormalities in rats with adjuvant-induced arthritis. II: Effect of antiarthritic therapy on immune function in relation to disease development. Int J Immunopharmacol, 9, 9–16

43. Rooney, TW, Rogers, SL, Maguire, R and Furst, DE (1986). Preliminary evaluation of the pharmacokinetics and pharmacodynamics of a potential immunomodulator, WY-18,251, in rheumatoid arthritis patients. Proc Ann Soc Exp Biol, 45, 332

44. Cohen, IR, Holoshitz, J, Van Eden, W and Frenkel, A (1985). T lymphocyte clones illuminate pathogenesis and effect therapy of experimental arthritis. Arth Rheum, 28, 841–5

45. Larsson, P, Holmdahl, R, Dencker, L and Klareskog, L (1985). In vivo treatment with W3/13 (anti-pan T) but not with OX8 (anti-suppressor/cytotoxic T) monoclonal antibodies impedes the development of adjuvant arthritis in rats. Immunology, 56, 383–91

46. Bloxham, DP, Bradshaw, D, Cashin, CH et al. (1987). RO31-3948, a potential disease modifying anti-rheumatoid drug (DMARD). Br J Rheumatol, 26, Abs. Suppl. 22

47. Hanifin, JW, Johnson, BD, Menschik, J et al. (1979). Potential anti-arthritic agents 1: benzolylacetonitriles. J Pharm Sci, 68, 535–6

48. Walker, GN (1981). Alpha-carbamoyl pyrrolepropionitriles and pharmaceutical preparations containing them. Eur Pat Appl, 21207

49. Bird, HA, Dixon, JS, Hill, J et al. (1987). A clinical and biochemical evaluation of the potential second-line activity of Primomide in the treatment of rheumatoid arthritis. Br J Rheumatol, 26, Abs. Suppl. 22

50. Cromartie, WJ, Craddock, JG, Schwab, JH et al. (1977). Arthritis in rats after systemic injection of streptococcal cell walls. J Exp Med, 146, 1485–1602

51. Wilder, RL, Allen, JB and Hansen, C (1987). Thymus-dependent and independent regulation of Ia antigen expression in situ by cells in the synovium of rats with streptococcal cell wall-induced arthritis. J Clin Invest, 79, 1160–71

52. Yocum, DE, Allen, JB, Wahl, SM et al. (1986). Inhibition by cyclosporin A of streptococcal cell wall-induced arthritis and hepatic granulomas in rats. Arth Rheum, 29, 262–73

53. Haraori, B, Wilder, RL, Allen, JB et al. (1985). Dose dependent suppression by the synthetic retinoid, 4-hydroxyphenyl retinamide, of streptococcal cell wall-induced arthritis in rats. Int J Immunopharmacol, 7, 903–16

54. Ridge, SC, Rath, N, Galivan, J et al. (1986). Studies on the effect of D-penicillamine, gold thioglucose and methotrexate on streptococcal cell wall arthritis. J Rheumatol, 13, 895–8

55. Trentham, DE, Dynesius, RA and David, JR (1978). Passive transfer by cells of type II collagen-induced arthritis in rats. J Clin Invest, 62, 359–66

56. Sloboda, AE, Birnbaum, JE, Oronsky, AL and Kerwar, SS (1981). Studies on type II collagen-induced polyarthritis in rats. Effect of anti-inflammatory and anti-rheumatic agents. Arth Rheum, 24, 616–24

57. Billingham, MEJ, Clague, RB, Morgan, K and Smith, MN (1981). Effect of ICI 55897 (Clozic) and inodmethacin on type II collagen-induced arthritis in the rat. Br J Pharmacol, 72, 551P

58. Phadke, K and Nanda, S (1982). Effects of benoxaprofen on the inflammatory, humoral and cellular components of type II collagen–induced arthritis in rats. Eur J Rheum Inflam, 5, 170–4

59. Gilbertsen, RB (1986). Rat haptoglobin: Method of quantitation and response to antiarthritic therapy in collagen arthritis. Immunopharmacology, 11, 69–77

60. Stuart, JM, Myers, LK, Townes, AS and Kang, AH (1981). Effect of cyclophosphamide, hydrocortisone, and levamisole on collagen-induced arthritis in rats. Arth Rheum, 24, 790–4

61. McCure, WJ, Trentham, DE and David, JR (1980). Gold does not alter the arthritic,

humoral or cellular responses in rats with type II collagen arthritis. *Arth Rheum*, **23**, 932–6

62. Henderson, B, Staines, NA, Burrai, I and Cox, JH (1984). The anti-arthritic and immunosuppressive effects of cyclosporine on arthritis induced in the rat by type II collagen. *Clin Exp Immunol*, **57**, 51–6

63. Kaibara, N, Hotokebuchi, T, Takagishi, K and Katsuki, I (1983). Paradoxical effects of cyclosporin A on collagen arthritis in rats. *J Exp Med*, **158**, 2007–15

64. Trentham, DE and Brinckerhoff, CE (1982). Augmatation of collagen arthritis by synthetic analogues or retinoic acid. *J Immunol*, **129**, 2668–72

65. Larsson, P and Holmdahl, R (1987). Oestrogen-induced suppression of collagen arthritis. II. Treatment of rats suppresses development of arthritis but does not affect the anti-type II collagen humoral responses. *Scand J Immunol*, **26**, 579–83

66. Burrai, I, Henderson, B, Knight, SC and Staines, NA (1985). Suppression of collagen type II-induced arthritis by transfer of lymphoid cells from rats immunised with collagen. *Clin Exp Immunol*, **61**, 368–72

67. Brahn, E and Trentham, DE (1987). Attenuation of collagen arthritis and modulation of delayed type hypersensitivity by type II collagen reactive T-cell lines. *Cell Immunol*, **109**, 139–47

68. Arita, C, Kaibara, N, Jingushi, S *et al*. (1987). Suppression of collagen arthritis in rats by heterologous anti-idiotypic antisera against anticollagen antibodies. *Clin Immunol Immunopathol*, **43**, 354–61

69. Thompson, HSG, and Staines, NA (1986). Gastric administration of type II collagen delays the onset and severity of collagen induced arthritis in rats. *Clin Exp Immunol*, **64**, 581–6

70. Watson, WC, Brown, PS, Pitcock, JA and Townes, AS (1987). Passive transfer studies with type II collagen antibodies in B10.D2/old and new line and C57BL/6 normal and beige strains: evidence for important roles for C5 and multiple inflammatory cell types in development of erosive arthritis. *Arth Rheum*, **30**, 460–5

71. Holmdahl, R, Klareskog, L, Robin, K *et al*. (1986). Role of T-lymphocytes in murine collagen induced arthritis. *Agents and Actions*, **19**, 295–305

72. Ranges, GE, Sriram, S and Cooper, SM (1986). Prevention of type II collagen-induced arthritis by in vivo treatment with anti–L3T4. *J Exp Med*, **162**, 1105–10

73. Hom, JT, Butler, LD, Riedl, PE and Bendele, AM (1988). Evidence for a role of T cells in perpetuating the chronicity of the inflammation in established collagen-induced arthritis of mice. *J Immunol* (In press)

74. Phadke, K, Fouts, RL, Parrish, JE and Butler, LD (1985). Evaluation of the effects of various anti-arthritic drugs on type II collagen-induced mouse arthritis model. *Immunopharmacology*, **10**, 51–60

75. Paska, W, McDonald, KJ and Croft, M (1986). Studies on type II collagen induced arthritis in mice. *Agents and Actions*, **18**, 413–20

76. Wooley, PH, Whalen, JD, Zimmerman, JL and Champion, TM (1987). The effect of etodolac on type II collagen-induced arthritis in mice. *Agents and Actions*, **21**, 244–6

77. Takagishi, K, Kaibara, N, Hotokebuchi, T *et al*. (1986). Effects of cyclosporin on collagen induced arthritis in mice. *Ann Rheum Dis*, **45**, 339–44

78. Holmdahl, R, Jansson, L, Meyerson, B and Klareskog, L (1987). Oestrogen induced suppression of collagen arthritis: I. Long term oestradiol treatment of DBA/1 mice reduces severity and incidence of arthritis and decreases the anti type II collagen immune response. *Clin Exp Immunol*, **70**, 372–8

79. Waites, GT and Whyte, A (1987). Effect of pregnancy on collagen-induced arthritis in mice. *Clin Exp Immunol*, **67**, 467–76

80. Hunneyball, IM, (1984). Use of experimental arthritis in the rabbit for the development of antiarthritic drugs. In Otterness, I, Capetola, R and Wong, S (eds), *Advances in Inflammation Research*, pp. 249–262. (New York: Raven Press)

81. Blackham, A and Radziwonik, H (1977). The effect of drugs on established rabbit

monoarticular arthritis. *Agents and Actions*, **7**, 473–80

82. Goldlust, MB and Rich, LC (1981). Chronic immune synovitis in rabbits II. Modulation by anti-inflammatory and anti-rheumatic agents. *Agents and Actions*, **11**, 729–35

83. Blackham, A, Farmer, JB, Radziwonik, H and Westwick, J (1974). The role of prostaglandins in rabbit monoarticular arthritis. *Br J Pharmacol*, **51**, 35–44

84. Hunneyball, IM (1981). Some further effects of prednisolone and triamcinolone hexacetonide on experimental arthritis in rabbits. *Agents and Actions*, **11**, 490–8

85. Lewis, AJ (1980). The local antiinflammatory activity of rimexolone (ORG 6216) in fibrin-induced monoarticular arthritis and adjuvant-induced arthritis. *Agents and Actions*, **10**, 258–65

86. Wright, JM, Knight, CG and Hunneyball, IM (1986). The effect of side chain structure on the biochemical and therapeutic properties of intraarticular dexamethasone 21-esters. *Clin Exp Rheumatol*, **4**, 331–9

87. Reimann, I and Rasmussen, GG (1975). Questionable effects of myocrisin in experimental arthritis in rabbits. *Scand J Rheumatol*, **4**, 221–4

88. Dingle, JT, Gordon, JL, Hazleman, BL *et al*. (1978). Novel treatment for joint inflammation. *Nature*, **271**, 372–3

89. Bard, DR, Knight, CG and Page Thomas, DP (1983). The retention and distribution in the rabbit knee of a radionuclide complexed with a lipophilic chelator in liposomes. *Clin Exp Rheumatol*, **1**, 113–17

90. Bard, DR, Knight, CG and Page Thomas, DP (1985). Effect of the intra-articular injection of lutetium-177 in chelator liposomes on the progress of an experimental arthritis in rabbits. *Clin Exp Rheumatol*, **3**, 237–42

91. Foong, WC and Green, KL (1982). The retention of free and liposome-entrapped methotrexate in arthritic joints. *Br J Pharmacol*, **77**, Suppl, 553P

92. Foong, WC, Green, KL, Patterson, LT *et al*. (1985). Treatment of arthritis in the rabbit with intra-articular daunorubicin linked to protein. *J Pharm Pharmacol*, **37**, Suppl, 98P

93. Foong, WC and Green, KL (1985). Effect of intra-articular yttrium 90 or chlorambucil on an experimental arthritis. *Br J Pharmacol*, **86**, Suppl, 522P

94. Meier-Ruge, W, Muller, W and Pavelka, K (1976). Effect of yttrium 90 on experimental allergic arthritis in rabbits. *Ann Rheum Dis*, **35**, 60–6

95. Brackertz, D, Mitchell, GF and Mackay, IR (1977). Antigen-induced arthritis in mice. I. Induction of arthritis in various strains of mice. *Arthr Rheum*, **20**, 841–50

96. Hunneyball, IM, Crossley, MJ and Spowage, M (1986). Pharmacological studies of antigen-induced arthritis in BALB/c mice I. Characterisation of the arthritis and the effects of steroidal and non-steroidal anti-inflammatory agents. *Agents and Actions*, **18**, 384–93

97. Hunneyball, IM, Crossley, MJ and Spowage, M (1986). Pharmacological studies of antigen-induced arthritis in BALB/c mice II. The effects of second-line antirheumatic drugs and cytotoxic agents on the histopathological changes. *Agents and Actions*, **18**, 394–400

98. Crossley, MJ, Spowage, M and Hunneyball, IM (1987). Studies on the effects of pharmacological agents on antigen-induced arthritis in BALB/c mice. *Drugs Exp Clin Res*, **13**, 273–8

99. Schalkwijk, J, Van Den Berg, WB, Van De Putte, LBA *et al*. (1985). Cationisation of catalase, peroxidase and superoxide dismutase: effect of improved intra-articular retention on experimental arthritis in mice. *J Clin Invest*, **76**, 198–205

100. Van Den Berg, WB, Schalkwijk, J, Joosten, LAB and Van De Putte, LBA (1986). Experimental allergic arthritis in mice: effects of local enzyme therapy with native and cationic derivatives. *Agents and Actions*, **17**, 350-1

101. Schalkwijk, J, Van Den Berg, WB, Van De Putte, LBA and Joosten, LAB (1986). An experimental model for hydrogen peroxide-induced tissue damage. Effects of a single

inflammatory mediator on (peri) articular tissues. *Arthr Rheum*, **29**, 532–8

102.  Müller, A, Cadenas, E, Graf, P and Sies, H (1984). A novel biologically active sele-
no-organic compound. I. Glutathione peroxidase-like activity in vitro and antioxidant
capacity of PZ51 (ebselen). *Biochem Pharmacol*, **33**, 3235–9

103.  Hang, L, Theofilopoulos, AN and Dixon, FJ (1982). A spontaneous rheumatoid arthritis–like disease in MRL/1 mice. *J Exp Med*, **155**, 1690–1701

104.  Carlson, RP, Gilman, SC, Hodge, TG *et al.* (1984). Effects of oral aspirin and oxaprozin on the development of lupus-like disease in MRL/1 mice. *J Immunopharmacol*, **6**, 69–78

105.  Stim, TB, Garrabrant, TA and Persico, FJ (1985). Erythrocyte sedimentation rate as
a parameter for drug evaluation in the MRL/1 autoimmune mouse. *Agents and Actions*, **16**, 603–4

106.  Rordorf-Adam, C, Rordorf, B, Serban, D and Pataki, A (1986). The effects of anti-
inflammatory agents on the serology and arthritis of the MRL 1pr/1pr mouse. *Agents
and Actions*, **19**, 309–11

107.  Toivonen, M-L, Linden, I-B, Gripenberg, M and Vapaatalo, H (1984). The usability
of the MRL/1 mouse strain in detection of anti-rheumatic drugs. *Agents and Actions*,
**15**, 578–83

108.  Ackerman, NR, Trimble, B, Kowalski, WJ *et al.* (1984). The effects of D-penicillamine in the MRL/1 mouse. In Otternesss, I, Capetola R and Wong, S (eds), *Advances in Ifflammation Research*, pp. 249–262. (New York: Raven Press)

109.  Fujitsu, T, Sakuma, S, Seki, N *et al.* (1986). Effect of auranofin on autoimmune disease in a mouse model. *Int J Immunopharmacol*, **8**, 897–910

110.  Smith, HR, Chused, TM and Steinberg, AD (1984). Cyclophosphamide-induced
changes in the MRL-1pr/1pr mouse: effects upon cellular composition, immune
function and disease. *Clin Immunol Immunopathol*, **30**, 51–61

111.  Tarkowski, A, Gunnarsson, K, Nilsson, L-A *et al.* (1986). Successful treatment of
autoimmunity in MRL/1 mice with LS-2616, a new immunomodulator. *Arthr Rheum*,
**29**, 1405–9

112.  Popovic, S and Bartlett, RR (1986). Disease modifying activity of HWA 486 on the
development of SLE in MRL/1-mice. *Agents and Actions*, **19**, 313–15

113.  Abe, C, Shiokawa, Y, Ohishi, T *et al.* (1982). Effect of CCA on spontaneous joint lesions in MRL/1 mice. *Int Congr Ser – Excerpta Med*, **563**, 511–14

114.  Mountz, JD, Smith, HR, Wilder, RL *et al.* (1987). CS-A therapy in MRL-1pr/1pr
mice: amelioration of immunopathology despite autoantibody production. *J Immunol*, **138**, 157–63

115.  Dueymes, M, Fournié, GJ, Mignon-Conté, M *et al.* (1986). Prevention of lupus disease in MRL/1, NZB x NZW, and BXSB mice treated with a cyclophosphazene
derived drug. *Clin Immunol Immunopathol*, **41**, 193–205

116.  Barbier, A, Planchenault, C and Breliere, JC (1986). Effect of (chloro-4-phenyl)-
thiomethylene bisphosphonic acid (SR 41319) on the autoimmune disease activity in
MRL/1 mice. *Agents and Actions*, **19**, 311–12

117.  Howie, JB and Helyer, BJ (1968). The immunology and pathology of NZB mice. *Adv
Immunol*, **9**, 215–66

118.  Theofilopoulos, AN and Dixon, FJ (1981). Etiopathogenesis of murine SLE. *Immunol Rev*, **55**, 179–216

119.  Hurd, ER, Gilliam, JN and Ziff, M (1976). The differential effects of cyclophosphamide and 6-mercaptopurine on the renal disease and skin immunoglobulin deposits
of the NZB-NZW F1 hybrid mice. *Agent and Actions*, **6**, 364–8

120.  Klassen, LW, Williams, GW, Reinertsen, JL *et al.* (1979). Ribavirin treatment in
murine autoimmune disease I. Therapeutic efficacy and effect on the immune response. *Arthr Rheum*, **22**, 145–54

121.  Gelfand, MC and Steinberg, AD (1972). Therapeutic studies in NZB/W mice II.
Relative efficacy of azathioprine, cyclophosphamide and methylprednisolone. *Arthr*

*Rheum*, **15**, 247–52

122.  Kelley, VE, Izui, S and Halushka, PV (1982). Effect of ibuprofen, a fatty acid cyclooxygenease inhibitor on murine lupus. *Clin Immunol Immunopathol*, **25**, 223–31

123.  Jones, MG and Harris, G (1985). Prolongation of life in female NZB/NZW (F1) hybrid mice by cyclosporin A. *Clin Exp Immunol*, **59**, 1–9

124.  Gunn, HC (1986). Successful treatment of autoimmunity in (NZB x NZW) F1 mice with cyclosporin and (Nva$^2$-cyclosporin: I. Reduction of autoantibodies. *Clin Exp Immunol*, **64**, 225–33

125.  Ohsugi, Y, Nakano, T, Hata, S et al. (1978). N-(2-carboxyphenyl)-4-chloroanthranilic acid disodium salt: prevention of autoimmune kidney disease in NZB/NZW F1 hybrid mice. *J Pharm Pharmacol*, **30**, 126–8

126.  Nakano, T, Yamashita, Y, Ohsugi, Y et al. (1983). The effect of CCA (Lobenzarit disodium) on the suppressor T cell function and the production of autoantibodies in NZ black and NZ white F1 mice. *Immunopharmacology*, **5**, 293–302

127.  Tsukagoshi, S (1985). Mizoribine (Bredinin): an immunosuppressive agent. *Drugs of Today*, **21**, 173–6

128.  Kamata, K, Okubo, M, Uchiyama, T et al. (1984). Effect of mizoribine on lupus nephropathy of New Zealand black/white hybrid mice. *Clin Immunol Immunopathol*, **33**, 31–8

129.  Bang, NU (1980). Frentizole in systemic lupus erythematosus: current status (editorial). *Arthr Rheum*, **23**, 1388–90

130.  O'Duffy, JD, Colgan, JP, Phyliky, RL and Ferguson, RH (1980). Frentizole therapy of thrombocytopenia in systemic lupus erythematosus and refractory idiopathic thrombocytopenic purpura. *Mayo Clin Proc*, **55**, 601–5

131.  Walker, SE, Solsky, M and Schnitzer, B (1982). Prolonged lifespans in female NZB/NZW mice treated with the experimental immunoregulatory drug frentizole. *Arthr Rheum*, **25**, 1291–7

132.  Guttner, J (1979). Therapeutic effect of β-[1-pheny-5-bis(β-chloroethyl)aminobenzimidazolyl-(2)-DL-alanin (Zimet-3164) on immune complex nephritis of NZB hybrid mice. *Agents and Actions*, **9**, 527–33

133.  Tarkowski, A, Gunnarsson, K and Stalhandske, T (1986). Effects of LS2616 administration upon the autoimmune disease of (NZB x NZW) F1 hybrid mice. *Immunology*, **59**, 589–94

134.  Ikehara, S, Shimamura, K, Aoyama, T et al. (1985). Effect of FUT-175, a new synthetic protease inhibitor, on the development of lupus nephritis in (NZB x NZW) F1 mice. *Immunology*, **55**, 595–600

135.  Isetta, AM, Fornasiero, MC, Ferrari, M and Trizio, D (1985). Activity of the immunomodulator FCE 20696 in experimental models of autoimmunity. *Int J Immunopharmacol*, **7**, 390

136.  Fornasiero, MC, Isetta, AM, Ferrari, M and Trizio, D (1986). Antigen specific, suppressor cells induced by the immunomodulator FCE 20696 in aged NZB/W F1 mice. *Agents and Actions*, **19**, 315–17

137.  Paterson, PY (1982). Molecular and cellular determinants of neuroimmunologic inflammatory disease. *Fed Proc*, **41**, 2569–76

138.  Lassmann, H, Vass, K, Brunner, CH and Seitelberger, F (1986). Characterization of inflammatory infiltrates in experimental allergic encephalomyelitis. In Zimmerman, HM (ed), *Progress in Neurobiology*, pp. 33–62 (New York: Raven Press)

139.  Borel, JF, Gubler, HU, Hiestand, PC and Wenger, RM (1986). Immunopharmacological properties of cyclosporine (Sanimmune®) and (rat$^2$)-dihydrocyclosporine and their prospect in chronic inflammation. In Otterness, I, Lewis, A and Capetola, R (eds), *Therapeutic Control of Inflammatory Diseases; Advances in Inflammation Research*, vol. II, pp. 277–291 (New York: Raven Press)

140.  Waltz, DT, Di Martino, MJ and Sutton, BM (1974). Design and laboratory evaluation of gold compounds as anti-inflammatory agents. In Scherrer, RA and White-

house, MW (eds), *Anti-inflammatory Agents, Chemistry and Pharmacology*, vol. I, pp. 209–244 (New York: Academic Press)

141.    Rosenthale, ME, Datko, LJ, Kassarich, J and Schneider, F (1969). Chemotherapy of experimental allergic encephalo-myelites (EAE). *Arch Int Pharmacodyn*, 179, 251–75

142.    Rosenthale, ME, Begany, AJ, Dervinis, A *et al.* (1974). Anti-inflammatory properties of 4,5-diphenyl-2-oxazolepropionic acid (oxaprozin). *Agents and Actions*, 4, 151–9

143.    Fairlie, DP, and Whitehouse, MW (1981). Cis-platinum (II) amines: toxicities and immunosuppressant/anti-arthritic activities. In Rainsford, KD, Brune, K and Whitehouse, MW (eds), *Trace Elements in the Pathogenesis and Treatment of Inflammation, Agents and Actions*, Suppl. 8, pp. 399–434 (Basel: Birkhaeuser)

144.    Nakaike, S, Takeshita, K, Shiono, M *et al.* (1985). Studies of D-penicillamine on strain variability and lymphnode cellularity in adjuvant arthritis. *Agents and Actions*, 16, 514–20

145.    Harris, ED (1981). Pathogenesis of rheumatoid arthritis. In Kelley, WN, Harris, ED Jr, Ruddy, S and Sledge, CB (eds), *Textbook of Rheumatology*, chap. 59, pp. 896–927 (Philadelphia: Saunders)

# 5
# Novel eicosanoid inhibitors

**Lisa A. Marshall and Joseph Chang**
Immunopharmacology Subdivision, Wyeth-Ayerst Research Inc.
CN 8000, Princeton, NJ 08543-8000, USA

## I. INTRODUCTION

Our understanding of arachidonic acid (AA) metabolism and its role in inflammation has increased significantly since the discovery of prostaglandins over 50 years ago. We now know that AA can be transformed into not just prostaglandins (PGs) and thromboxanes (TxB2) but also 5-lipoxygenase (5-LO) products collectively termed leukotrienes (LTs). Whether all the metabolites of AA have been identified is uncertain and the recent discovery of lipoxins[1], which are trihydroxy AA metabolites, underscores this view.

Present knowledge suggests that PGs and LTs are major contributors to the inflammatory process[2-4]. Indeed, non-steroidal anti-inflammatory drugs (NSAIDs) by inhibiting cyclo-oxygenase (CO) are major drugs in the treatment of inflammation associated with various rheumatic disorders. However, NSAIDs do not inhibit 5-LO-catalysed reactions that generate LTs, leaving a potentially important proinflammatory pathway unaffected. Thus, drugs that can reduce LT synthesis or their actions, as well as the formation of PGs, may be more effective than NSAIDs as anti-inflammatory drugs. In this chapter we review the evidence for this proposal and consider approaches designed to achieve this result. These approaches fall principally into two categories: (1) inhibition of LT formation and (2) antagonism of LT action. Discussion will initially focus on inhibitors of key enzymes of the AA cascade, followed by a review on the development of LT receptor antagonists.

## II. AA METABOLISM

The pathways of AA metabolism are illustrated in Figure 1. The principal source of AA is phospholipids, structural components of cell membranes and activation of a phospholipase or phospholipases leads to the release of free AA from phopholipid stores[5-7]. Unlike preformed mediators, both PGs and

*New Developments in Antirheumatic Therapy.* Rainsford, KD and Velo, GP(eds), Inflammation and Drug Therapy Series, Volume III.

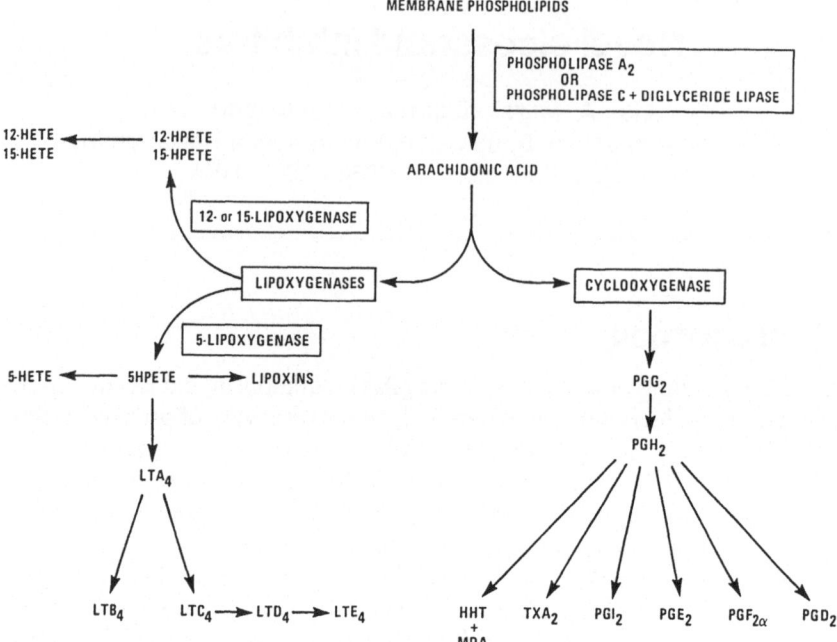

**Figure 1** Pathway of arachidonic acid metabolism

LTs are not stored and require *de novo* synthesis, suggesting that availability of free AA is the first rate-limiting step in eicosanoid synthesis. The phospholipase which releases free AA from the sn-2 position of membrane phospholipids in several tissues is phospholipase $A_2$ (PLA2)[5-7]. However, AA release is also possible through the sequential actions of a phosphatidyl inositol-specific phospholipase C and diglyceride lipase[8-10]. The relative contribution of this pathway to overall substrate availability is still unclear, although the release of AA from diacylglycerol, at least in certain cells, appears to correspond with the rate of synthesis of AA metabolites[9].

Following the release of AA, CO catalyzes the addition of molecular oxygen to AA and cyclizes it to the unstable intermediate, $PGG_2$. This is then converted to $PGH_2$, which in turn isomerizes enzymatically or non-enzymatically to various PGs ($PGE_2$, $PGF_{2\alpha}$ and $PGD_2$). In certain tissues the endoperoxides are also transformed to unstable $TxA_2$ and prostacyclin (PGI2) which are rapidly degraded to TxB2 and 6-keto-$PGF_{1\alpha}$, respectively. Concurrently, malondialdehyde and 12-hydroxy-5,8,10-heptadecatrienoic acid (HHT) are formed.

Oxidative metabolism of AA also occurs through the action of lipoxygenases (LO) such as 5-, 12- and 15-LO, and such enzymes have been found in inflammatory cells[11-13]. Among these the 5-LO has attracted the most attention because its activation catalyzes the conversion of AA into 5-hydroperoxyeicosatetraenoic acid (5-HPETE) that is the precursor of 5-hydroxyeicosatetraenoic acid (5-HETE), LTB4 and the peptidoleukotrienes LTC4, LTD4 and LTE4. Depending on the cell type, one or more of these products are formed. For example, whereas neutrophils[13-15] synthesize predominantly 5-HETE and LTB4, eosinophils[16] and mast cells[17] are major producers of LTC4. There are even subtle differences within the same cell type depending on its anatomical location. Whereas human peritoneal macrophages are capable of producing both LTB4 and LTC4 [18], human alveolar macrophages synthesize only LTB4[19].

The 5-LO enzyme has been isolated from rat basophilic leukaemia cells (RBL-1)[20], MC-9 mast cells[21], guinea pig[22] and rat peritoneal exudate cells[23] and human leukocytes[13]. Its amino acid structure is not known, although efforts to purify and sequence the enzyme are underway in several laboratories. Evidence suggests that 5-LO and LTA4 synthase activities reside in the same protein; both have the same co-factor requirements and sensitivity to inhibitors[24]. The enzyme requires $Ca^{2+}$ for activity and is stimulated by several nucleotides, of which ATP is the most potent. It is unstable and loses activity upon purification; therefore stabilizers such as gelatin, ethylene glycol or glycerol are usually added during purification to preserve enzyme integrity, particularly if the enzyme is frozen. Sulphur-containing compounds, such as dithiothreitol (DTT) or glutathione (GSH), protect enzyme longevity and are included in enzyme reactions. Initial enzyme velocity is characterized by a lag phase which is not observed in the presence of fatty acid hydroperoxides[25]. This suggests that hydroperoxides activate enzyme activity and may be important endogenous factors in the regulation of leukotriene synthesis.

Utilization of the purified 5-LO enzyme for identifying 5-LO inhibitors is in its infancy. Such studies are undoubtedly useful since they provide in-depth information on mechanism of drug action on the enzyme. However, until the enzyme is available in a purified state a complete understanding of its physical characteristics and co-factor requirements is lacking. Direct enzyme analysis of 5-LO inhibitors should, therefore, be interpreted cautiously.

## III.  BIOLOGICAL ACTIONS OF LTS

The chemical synthesis and availability of synthetic LTs has facilitated the characterization of the biological actions of these metabolites[26–28]. In general, the LTs may be classified under two groups: (a) the peptidoleukotrienes (LTC4, LTD4 and LTE4) whose actions are primarily on smooth muscle and (b) the hydroxylated metabolites of AA (LTB4 and 5-HETE) which exert cellular actions such as chemotaxis and degranulation.

The peptidoleukotrienes are potent constrictors of several smooth muscle preparations and specific LT receptor sites have been identified on these tissues[29,30]. Airway smooth muscle, gastrointestinal smooth muscle and coronary smooth muscle are all responsive to peptidoleukotrienes, although there is considerable species variation, making it difficult to generalize about the absolute potency of these mediators. *In vivo*, the smooth muscle contractile activity of LTs is further complicated by the fact that LTs can act directly or indirectly via the release of CO products (e.g. $TxA_2$ and $PGE_2$), depending on the route of administration and the rapid conversion of $LTC_4$ to $LTD_4$ [31,32]. Nonetheless, human and guinea pig lungs are exquisitely sensitive to $LTC_4$ and $LTD_4$ which have been shown to be several orders of magnitude more potent than histamine as bronchoconstrictors[29].

In the cardiovascular system LTs cause a marked arterial constriction when injected intradermally or applied directly to the microcirculation[33,34]. When given intravenously to guinea-pigs, LTs cause an initial hypertensive response followed by long-lasting hypotension, whereas intra-arterial injection produces a less marked hypertensive effect but a more prolonged hypotensive effect. These actions are species-dependent; in cats $LTC_4$ given into the right atrium causes a rise in mean arterial pressure without observable hypertension[29]. An additional vascular effect produced by peptidoleukotrienes is the augmentation of vascular permeability. Intradermal injection of nmol amounts of LTs produces a local wheal-and-flare reaction in human and guinea-pig skin which is potentiated by co-administration of PGs[35]. In the hamster cheek pouch, $LTC_4$ causes an extravasation of macromolecules from post-capillary venules at doses which do not exert vasoconstrictor effects. Notably, LTs (especially $LTC_4$) are as potent as angiotension II in this respect[36].

Unlike peptidoleukotrienes, $LTB_4$ and 5-HETE exert their main actions on inflammatory cells. Both are known to be chemokinetic and chemotactic for human polymorphonuclear leucocytes (PMN) with $LTB_4$ being the most potent endogenous chemotactic factor known[37–39]. $LTB_4$'s *in vitro* actions on PMN are stereospecific; not shared by other leukotrienes and distinct from the actions of $C_{5a}$ or f-met-leu-phe (FMLP). $LTB_4$-induced chemotactic activity is observed *in vitro* with isolated preparations of neutrophils, eosinophils and monocytes and in a variety of *in vivo* models such as the hamster cheek pouch[40], guinea-pig peritoneal cavity[41], rabbit eye[42] and human skin[43]. However, $LTB_4$ is virtually inert as a chemoattractant in rats and dogs, and in our laboratory, intra-articular injection of $LTB_4$ does not cause an influx of neutrophils into the dog synovial joint[44,45].

$LTB_4$ may also modulate other aspects of inflammatory cell function. Enhancement of lysosomal enzyme release, superoxide generation, $C3_b$ receptor site expression and T-cell function have all been reported[46] with $LTB_4$. Leukotriene $B_4$ augments lymphocyte activation as suggested by the suppression of concanavalin A (Con-A)-stimulated murine spleen cell proliferation and the reduction in interleukin IL-1 and IL-2 formation after administration of 5-LO inhibitors such as esculetin and caffeic acid[47]. This appears to be the case with natural killer and lymphokine-activated cytotoxic lymphocytes since inhibition of LTB$_4$ in these systems results in reduced cytotoxic activity of human peripheral blood leucocytes against chromium labelled-K562 tumor cells[48]. Monocyte IL-1 and PG production are moderately increased[49] when incubated in the presence of LTB$_4$. On the other hand, LTB$_4$ induces the appearance of suppressor T lymphocytes, suggesting that it exerts an indirect inhibitory action on lymphocyte proliferation[49]. LTB$_4$ binds to certain T cell subclasses exerting a suppression of T$_4$ cell (helper) proliferation and an enhancement of the T$_8$ (suppressor) cell response which results in immunosuppression[50].

The ability of LTs to regulate inflammatory and immune cell function suggests that these mediators may potentiate the inflammatory response in disease such as rheumatoid arthritis (RA). However, the relative importance of LTs in relation to other potential inflammatory mediators such as histamine, kinins, interferon or the interleukins remains to be established. Furthermore, inhibition of 5-LO metabolism may be deleterious, considering that some immune functions require LTB$_4$ for optimal activity. Nonetheless, LTB$_4$ produces biologically diverse effects which may impact on immune and inflammatory processes.

## IV. LT INVOLVEMENT IN HUMAN DISEASES

Based on the evidence as described above, LTs have been implicated in the pathophysiology of several diseases including RA, gout, asthma, endotoxin shock, myocardial ischaemia and psoriasis. LTB$_4$ has been identified in lesional skin from psoriatic patients[51] and a putative 5-LO/CO inhibitor, lonapalene, is reportedly an effective topical antipsoriatic agent[52]. Synovial fluid of RA patients[53] contain elevated levels of LTB$_4$, suggesting that it may act as a chemotactic agent for infiltrating neutrophils. Similarly, the immune actions of LTB$_4$ may explain, in part, the immune abnormalities observed in RA patients. Exacerbation of the pain response in arthritis is another aspect of potential LT involvement[54,55].

Perhaps the putative role of LTs in disease is best exemplified in asthma. Certain, but not all, features of an asthmatic response can be reproduced by exogenous application of LTs, especially LTD$_4$. Antigen challenge of human asthmatic lung tissue causes both LT release and mucus secretion. Eosinophil infiltration, a prominent feature of asthma, may be due to the generation of chemotactic LTB$_4$ in the lung. Indeed, cells infiltrating the asthmatic lung, such as neutrophils, basophils and eosinophils, have all been shown to produce substantial amounts of LTs in response to antigen challenge[56]. However, it is prudent to point out that unequivocal evidence for the *in vivo* role of LTs as proinflammatory mediators is lacking. Classically, to attain mediator status in chronic inflammation the following criteria must be met: (1) the compound must be active at physiological levels ($10^{-9}$–$10^{-7}$ mol/l), (2) it must be recovered *in vivo* at the sites of inflammation and (3) the symptoms characterizing chronic inflammation must be attenuated by inhibition of mediator synthesis or function. The first two criteria have been met fairly successfully, even though it is yet unclear whether enhanced LT is the cause of or the result of the inflammatory process. The third criterion is more difficult to satisfy, due primarily to the lack of a clinically effective drug that is a potent and specific 5-LO inhibitor. The problem is further compounded by the difficulty of *in vivo* LT measurement which would enable an *in vivo* correlation between LT inhibition and a therapeutic effect. Clinical evaluation of a bioavailable 5-LO inhibitor is therefore essential for defining the role of LTs as mediators of human inflammatory disease.

## V. AGENTS THAT MODIFY AA METABOLISM

The pathway leading to LT synthesis is regulated by several key enzymes, providing several approaches to drug design, which will now be considered.

### (1) PLA₂ inhibitors

Modulation of $PLA_2$ activity results in the attenuation of AA availability and subsequent conversion to products of both the CO and 5-LO pathways. The ability to interfere with the enzyme is shared by many structurally unrelated compounds. However, not all compounds reported to inhibit $PLA_2$ are direct enzyme inhibitors. Any agent that disturbs the architecture of the lipid–water interface would physically prevent $PLA_2$ from hydrolysing phospholipid substrate. For example, compounds that make cell membranes more fluid (e.g. halothane) or those which make the membranes more rigid (e.g. cholesterol) indirectly affect $PLA_2$ activity[57]. Complex formation between the phospholipid substrate and drug also prevents enzyme attack of the substrate. For example, local anaesthetics (cincaine, butacaine and lidocaine), antimalarial agents (chloroquine, mepacrine), polyamines (spermine, spermidine and putrescine), antipsychotic agents (chlorpromazine, promethazine, and fluphenazine), n-alkanols (methanol, n-tetradecanol and ethanol), antibiotics (streptomycin and gentamicin), and calcium antagonists have all been reported to interfere with the substrate/enzyme interface[58–60].

NSAIDs are believed to owe their therapeutic efficacy to inhibition of CO. However, at high concentrations sulindac sulphide, tiaramide, indomethacin, sodium meclofenate and sodium flufenamate also inhibit $PLA_2$ activity[61–63]. Franson and co-workers[63] have further shown that this inhibition is sensitive to calcium concentrations; the $PLA_2$ inhibitory activity of indomethacin and sodium meclofenamate is greatly diminished in the presence of high calcium concentrations (5 mmol/l). More recently, LO inhibitors such as quercetin, 4,8,11,14-eicosatetraenoic acid (ETYA) and nordihydroguaiaretic acid (NDGA) have also demonstrated[64] inhibition of $PLA_2$. Again, it should be emphasized that inhibition of $PLA_2$ by these agents can only be observed at concentrations which may not be easily attainable under *in vivo* conditions.

5,6-dehydroarachidonic acid

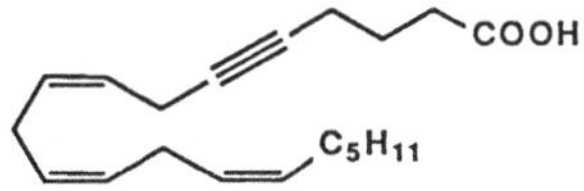

Piriprost (U-60,257)

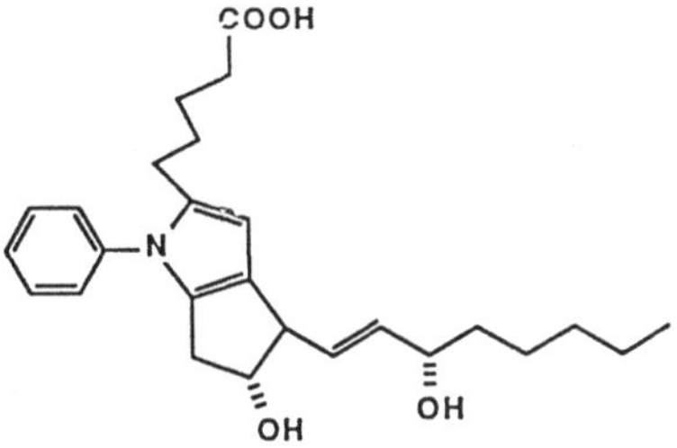

AA-861

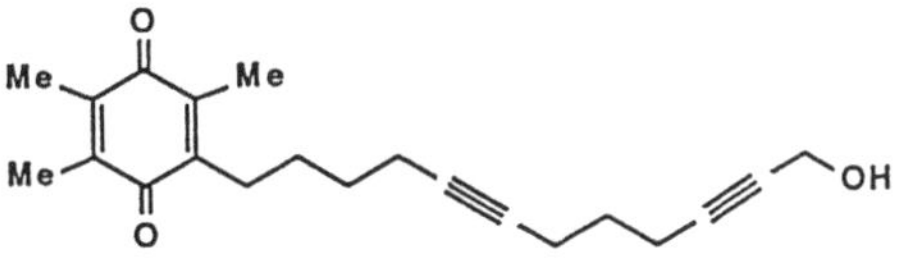

REV-5,901

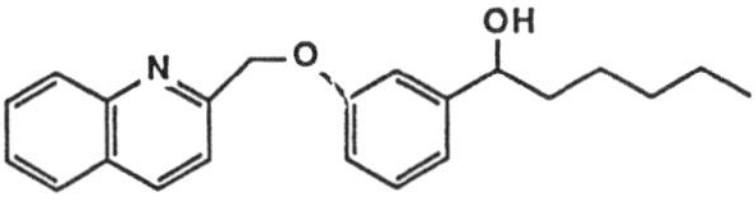

L-651,392

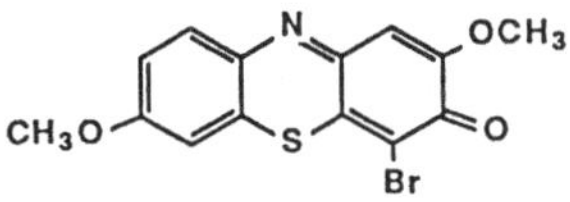

**Figure 2** Specific 5-LO inhibitors

The first systematic description of novel $PLA_2$ inhibitors was reported by Wallach and Brown[65], where a series of butyrophenone derivatives were shown to inhibit hog pancreas, cobra venom and bee venom $PLA_2$. The butyrophenone analogue, U-3, 585 (Figure 2), a non-competitive $PLA_2$ inhibitor, also inhibited collagen-induced platelet aggregation, prostanoid synthesis by isolated perfused guinea-pig lung and UV-induced skin erythema. More recently, KF-4939 and CGP 35,949B have also been reported[66,67] to inhibit $PLA_2$. However, neither compound is specific because of its ability to inhibit phospholipase C and antagonize leukotriene receptors, respectively.

Anti-inflammatory steroids are believed to act primarily by reducing $PLA_2$ activity. Indeed, the rank order of potency of steroids as anti-inflammatory agents correlates with their $PLA_2$ inhibitory activity[68]. In recent years several laboratories have proposed that steroids induce the synthesis of an endogenous $PLA_2$ inhibitory protein called lipocortin, which interacts directly with $PLA_2$ resulting in an anti-inflammatory effect[69]. Lipocortin has been sequenced and cloned, but its therapeutic potential is severely limited by its peptidic nature[70]. It may be possible, however, to design traditional organic molecules as lipocortin mimics, provided a small active fragment (molecular weight < 2000) can be identified. Whether the side-effects of steroids may also be duplicated by such inhibitors is not known.

Recently, a natural product, manoalide, has been described as a $PLA_2$ inhibitor[71]. This sesterterpenoid, isolated from the sponge *Luffanella variabilis*, inhibits $PLA_2$ at low concentrations and has demonstrated *in vivo* anti-inflammatory activity. Manoalide reacts with several lysine residues on $PLA_2$ which reduces the *in vitro* hydrolysis of phosphatidylcholine but not phosphatidylethanolamine[72] by $PLA_2$; in fact, phosphatidylethanolamine hydrolysis is enhanced. This differential effect suggests that at least one of the lysine residues is at or near the substrate binding site of $PLA_2$. Manoalide forms a covalent complex with $PLA_2$, suggesting that it is an irreversible enzyme inhibitor. Its use an an oral or topical anti-inflammatory agent remains to be determined.

Although several types of compounds exist, a specific $PLA_2$ inhibitor has not reached the stage of clinical development. Because of the attractiveness of this approach such inhibitors will probably be evaluated in the clinic in the near future.


## (2)  5-LO inhibitors

An LO inhibitor is defined as a compound which directly or indirectly reduces LO metabolite formation. The 5-LO enzyme system is composed of several enzymes which contribute to the formation of LTs. Therefore, pharmacological approaches to achieve inhibition of synthesis include direct interference with one or more of the enzymes listed in Table 1. To date, the design of inhibitors has focused on 5-LO, since this allows all 5-LO metabolites to be reduced.

**Table 1 Enzymes leading to LT formation**

| Enzyme | Inhibitory drugs |
|---|---|
| 5-lipoxygenase | 5,6 DHA, Rev 5901, piriprost, AA 861 |
| LTA$_4$ synthase (5-HPETE dehydrase | Piriprost |
| LTA$_4$ hydrolase (LTB$_4$ synthetase) | None |
| Glutathione s-transferase | |
| ($\alpha$-glutamyltranspeptidase, LTC$_4$ synthetase | Piriprost |
| Peptidase (cysteinyl-glycinase) | None |

Novel compounds are initially assessed for 5-LO activity *in vitro* either by using broken cell preparations or by monitoring eicosanoid release from whole-cell cultures. Immunocompetent cell populations such as rat PMNs, human blood neutrophils, murine and/or guinea-pig peritoneal macrophages or representative cell lines (e.g. RBL-1, mastocytoma cells, HL-60 leukaemia cells) have all been used to assess drug activity[73].

5-LO inhibitors are usually assessed in animal models of acute and chronic inflammation. These models and their predictive clinical efficacy have been reviewed in depth[74]. In brief, traditional models such as pleurisy, sponge implantation, Arthus reaction, adjuvant-induced arthritis and type II collagen arthritis in the rat and spontaneous autoimmunity in the MRL/1 mouse have all been used. These models are NSAID-sensitive and it is not known whether they are appropriate to detect the anti-inflammatory activity of 5-LO inhibitors.

The current emphasis is to profile 5-LO inhibitors in a variety of models that span the course of the inflammatory process. Examination of *in vivo* eicosanoid changes through assays such as A23187-induced rat peripheral blood leucocyte eicosanoid production[75] or the zymosan-induced mouse peritonitis model[76] establishes 5-LO inhibitor oral biochemical efficacy which can then be correlated with oral anti-inflammatory activity. Pulmonary and cutaneous models, where 5-LO metabolites are thought to be important mediators, are often utilized to lend support to the 5-LO inhibitory activity of the drug.

Many compounds have been reported to exhibit 5-LO metabolite inhibitory activity[77]. In general, 5-LO inhibitors can be classified as selective inhibitors such as NDGA[78], dual CO and 5-LO inhibitors such as phenidone, BW 755c[79], SKF 86002[80], lonapalene[52], flavonoids such as cirsiliol, quercetin or baicalein[81], sulfasalazine[82] (a compound used in treatment of inflammatory bowel disease), nafazatrom[83] (a free radical scavenger), AA analogues such as ETYA[84], AA metabolites such as 15-HPETE or 15-HETE[85], benoxaprofen[86] and various natural products such as eicosapentaenoic acid (EPA)[87], caffeic acid, epupatilin, and esculetin[88]. These compounds demonstrate reasonable 5-LO inhibitory activity but also exert other activities which could contribute to their anti-inflammatory properties. For example, ETYA,

BW 755c, phenidone, lonapalene, SKF 86002 and EPA all inhibit CO. Benoxaprofen, initially reported to be a selective 5-LO inhibitor, was later found to directly affect A23187 rather than exerting an action on 5-LO[89]. Nafazatrom is a reducing co-factor for peroxidase and is thought to inhibit 5-LO activity by increasing levels of the 5-LO inhibitor, 15-HETE.

Compounds demonstrating a greater degree of specificity include 5,6-dehydroarachidonic acids (DHA)[90], piriprost (U 60, 257)[91], AA 861[92], Rev 5901[93] and L 651,392[94] (Figure 1). These compounds inhibit 5-LO at concentrations which do not affect other enzyme systems. For example, L 651,392 (4-mono-2,7-dimethoxy-3H-phenothiazine-3-one) a phenothiazinone, effectively reduces LTB$_4$ production by both stimulated human and rat PMN and LTC$_4$ by rat basophilic leukaemic cells (IC$_{50}$ 6–9 x 10$^{-8}$ mol/l)[95]. By contrast, this compound does not affect sheep seminal vesicle CO or soybean 15-LO at these concentrations. Furthermore, L 651, 392 reduces zymosan-induced mouse macrophage LTC$_4$ by 50% at 4 x 10$^{-7}$ mol/l but does not affect PGE$_2$ or PGI$_2$ release. Oral activity of L 651,392 has been demonstrated by its inhibition of rat antigen-induced bronchoconstriction[95], a model where LTs are thought to mediate the bronchoconstriction process. In squirrel monkeys sensitized against ascaris, oral administration of L 651,392 (1 and 5 mg/kg) suppresses antigen-induced changes in airway resistance and dynamic compliance[94]. The *in vivo* anti-inflammatory activity of L 651,392 remains to be established.

AA 861 (2-(12-hydroxydodeca-5,10-dinyl)-3,5,6-trimethyl-1,4-benzoquinone) is one of the most potent 5-LO inhibitors yet described. It selectively reduces rat peritoneal macrophage A 23187-induced 5-HETE and LTB$_4$ release (IC$_{50}$; 3 x 10$^{-8}$ and 8 x 10$^{-8}$ mol/l respectively)[92]. SRS-A generation as measured by the contractile response of the guinea-pig ileum is inhibited 50% by 1.8 x 10$^{-6}$ mol/l which is several-fold more potent than ETYA, NDGA or BW 755c. When tested for activity against guinea-pig peritoneal PMN cell free 5-LO, AA 861 is a substrate competitive, reversible inhibitor (IC$_{50}$ = 0.8 $\mu$mol/l). Concentrations of 10 $\mu$mol/l or greater are required to express other activities such as inhibition of 12-LO or CO enzyme activity in other cell-free preparations[92].

Oral administration of AA 861 reduced carrageenan-induced rat paw oedema in a dose-dependent manner, but is significantly less potent than indomethacin[92]. Exudate volume, but not cell infiltration, is reduced by AA 861 in the carrageenan pleurisy model. In the rat reverse passive Arthus pleurisy model, AA 861 administered intrapleurally, effectively reduces vascular permeability, oedema, cell migration and LTs in exudate fluids[96]. Despite the failure of AA 861 to affect 12-LO enzyme activity[92], this compound significantly reduces 12-HETE production in mouse epidermis, which suggests that potency and selectivity of AA 861 may vary with the species of animal or type of cell used[97].

Piriprost, a prostacyclin (PGI$_2$) analogue, 6,9-de-epoxy-6,9-(phenyl-imino-6,8-prostaglandin I, (U 60,257)) inhibits LT release from A 23187-

challenged rat peritoneal mononuclear cells but fails to affect human platelet 12-LO or human PMN cell-free 15-LO[91,98]. Conversely, release of $PGD_2$ by human lung mast cells is potentiated, while $TxB_2$ is inhibited by exposure to piroprost[99]. Piriprost is reported to selectively inhibit RBL-1 glutathione-s-transferase, suggesting that this compound is more selective that the aforementioned drugs[100]. However, experiments examining the interaction of piriprost with diethyl carbamazine (DEC), an inhibitor of glutathione-s-transferase, reveal that low levels of piriprost augment DEC inhibition. This is thought to be due to a reduction of $LTA_4$ levels and inhibition of 5-LO by piriprost[101]. Additionally, piriprost has since been reported to inhibit 5-HETE and 5,12 diHETE formation by A 23187-stimulated human lung cells in the presence of exogenous [$^{14}$C]AA94. The mode of action, therefore, appears to be more complex than originally thought.

Piriprost has demonstrated anti-inflammatory activity in various animal models. Leucocyte accumulation during glycolate-induced acute inflammation in rats is effectively reduced by oral administration of 5 mg/kg piriprost[102]. Intradermal injections of various jellyfish venoms in rats results in rapid cutaneous capillary leakage and oedema formation which is significantly reduced by administration of piriprost 5 min prior to challenge[103]. Piriprost has also been shown to ameliorate symptomatology in animal models of asthma. Hydrogen peroxide-induced pulmonary vasoconstriction is effectively inhibited by aerosol pretreatment with 10 $\mu$mol/l piriprost[104]. Guinea-pigs sensitized against ovalbumin and pretreated with an antihistamine, atropine and indomethacin exhibit a dose-dependent reduction in antigen-induced insufflation pressure when given piriprost (0.1-10 mg/kg, i.v.)[105]. Again, similar results were obtained when piriprost was administered by aerosol (0.01% solution for 180 s). Dynamic lung and pulmonary resistance in ascaris-sensitized monkeys are also inhibited by piriprost[106].

Finally, Rev 5901 (2-[3-(1-hydroxyhexyl1)phenomethyl]quinoline hydrochloride) irreversibly inhibits A 23187-induced 5-HETE production by rat and human PMN[107]. When tested in the cell free RBL-1 5-LO enzyme assay, Rev 5901 is a direct enzyme inhibitor, and preliminary kinetic analysis suggests that it acts through substrate competition[108]. When tested against a semi-purified guinea pig PMN 5-LO preparation, Rev 5901 reversibly inhibits 5-HETE formation in a concentration-dependent but time-independent manner[24]. Marginal activity against rat platelet 12-LO or sheep seminal vesicle cyclo-oxygenase is observed[108].

The *in vivo* effects of Rev 5901 have been extensively evaluated in models of asthma. Guinea-pig airway resistance and dynamic lung compliance are inhibited 91% and 48%, respectively, when the drug is administered intraduodenally (0.1–100 mg/kg)[108]. Higher doses are required when administered orally to reduce resistance and compliance with no notable effects on ventilation or bronchomotor tone. The topical anti-inflammatory activity of Rev 5901 in the AA-induced mouse ear inflammation model was compared to that of phenidone. Both Rev 5901 and phenidone (2 mg/ear)

143

significantly reduce the acute inflammatory oedema, but Rev 5901 has a longer duration of action. Both compounds decrease neutrophil infiltration into the inflammatory site as measured by myeloperoxidase activity[107]. Finally, a recent report documented the anti-inflammatory activity of Rev 5901 against lens protein-induced ocular inflammation in rabbits (both i.v. and topically administered)[109]. Rev 5901 therefore demonstrates a good topical anti-inflammatory profile, but its usefulness as an orally active agent may be limited.

### (3)  Clinical status of 5-LO inhibitors

The above 5-LO inhibitors, except for L 651,392, have undergone preliminary clinical evaluation. Rev 5901, AA 861 and piriprost are in phase II clinical trials primarily as antiallergic/antiasthmatic agents. Lonapalene and L 651,343, dual 5-LO/CO inhibitors, are currently being evaluated as topical anti-inflammatory drugs. To the best of our knowledge an orally effective 5-LO inhibitor has not been evaluated in RA. The lack of a suitable animal model hampers the developmental progress of compounds in this area. It may be necessary ultimately to determine the therapeutic value of these inhibitors without establishing anti-inflammatory activity in animal models.

### VI.  ANTAGONISTS

In addition to inhibiting the synthesis of LTs, an alternative approach to developing 'anti-LT' drugs is to antagonize the actions of LTs. This approach offers the attraction of specificity and obviates the need for a drug to penetrate cells. Furthermore, it may also avoid any possible shunting that may occur with enzyme inhibition, leading to increased synthesis of other lipid mediators. The development of an LT antagonist is, however, proceeding despite our lack of knowledge concerning the geometric and electronic characteristics of the LT receptor site.

Specific $LTD_4$ antagonists are now available. An orally active $LTD_4$ antagonist, LY 171,883, has been reported to be a clinical candidate for asthma therapy[110]. Subsequently, other $LTD_4$ antagonists including L 649,923[111], ICI 198,615[112,113], SKF 104,353[114] and Wy 48,252[115] have also been announced as anti-asthmatic candidates.

It should be stressed, however, that despite their potential as anti-asthmatic agents, the anti-inflammatory actions of these antagonists remain to be established. For example, although effective against antigen-induced bronchoconstriction in the guinea-pig, such compounds have not demonstrated efficacy against traditional models of inflammation.

The LT that is believed to play a major role in inflammation is $LTB_4$. Unlike antagonists to $LTD_4$, there are very few reports of compounds that are selective $LTB_4$ antagonists. In view of its biological actions that were pre-

144

viously described, it would appear that a LTB$_4$ antagonist holds the most promise as an anti-inflammatory agent.

## VII. SUMMARY

There is now sufficient evidence to suggest that LTs are potent biological entities. LTs appear to induce changes in biological processes that resemble certain facets of inflammatory diseases, and these observations have led to the notion that LTs play an important role in mediating the inflammatory process. While elevated levels of LTs have been found in various human diseases, a causative relationship is yet to be established. The availability of specific inhibitors or antagonists will provide answers to this question.

## ACKNOWLEDGEMENTS

We would like to thank Bernadette Reczek for preparing this manuscript and Pearl Stark for her bibliographic assistance.

## REFERENCES

1.      Serhan, CN, Hambery, M and Samuelsson, B (1984). Lipoxins: novel series of biologically active compounds formed from arachidonic acid in human leukocytes. *Proc Natl Acad Sci USA*, **81**, 5335-9
2.      Malsten, CL (1982). Leukotrienes: mediators of inflammation and immediate hypersensitivity reactions. *CRC Rev Immunol*, **4**, 307-34
3.      Higgins, AJ (1985). The biology, pathophysiology and control of eicosanoids in inflammation. *J Vet Pharmacol Ther*, **8**, 1-18
4.      Salmon, JA and Higgs, GA (1987). Prostaglandins and leukotrienes as inflammatory mediators. *Br Med Bull*, **43**, 285-96
5.      Bills, TK, Smith, JB and Silver, MJ (1976). Metabolism of [$^{14}$C]arachidonic acid by human platelets. *Biochim Biophys Acta*, **424**, 303-14
6.      Blackwell, GJ, Duncombe, WG, Flower, RJ *et al.* (1977). The importance of phospholipase A$_2$ in prostaglandin biosynthesis. *Br J Pharmacol*, **59**, 353-66
7.      Kunze, H and Vogt, W (1971). Significance of phospholipase A for prostaglandin formation. *Ann NY Acad Sci*, **180**, 123-5
8.      Kennerly, DA, Sullivan, TJ, Sylvester, P and Parker, CW (1979). Diacylglycerol metabolism in mast cells: A potential role in membrane fusion and arachidonic acid release. *J Exp Med*, **150**, 1039-44
9.      Rittenhouse, S (1980). Indomethacin-induced accumulation of diglyceride in activated human platelets. The role of diglyceride lipase. *J Biol Chem*, **255**, 2259-62
10.     Bell, RL, Kennerly,. DA, Stanford, N and Majerus, PW (1979). Diglyceride lipase: a pathway for arachidonate release from human platelets. *Proc Natl Acad Sci USA*, **76**, 3238-41
11.     Nugteren, H (1975). Arachidonate lipoxygenase in blood platelets. *Biochim Biophys Acta*, **380**, 299-307
12.     Wong, PY-K, Westland, P, Hamberg, M *et al.* (1985). 15-lipoxygenase in human platelets. *J Biol Chem*, **260**, 9162-5
13.     Rouzer, CA and Samuelsson, B (1985). On the nature of the 5-lipoxygenase reaction in human leukocytes: enzyme purification and requirement for multiple stimulating factors. *Proc Natl Acad Sci USA*, **82**, 6040-4

14.	Borgeat, P and Samuelsson, B (1979). Arachidonic acid metabolism in polymorpho-nuclear leukocytes: effects of ionophore A23187. *Proc Natl Acad Sci USA*, **76**, 2148-52

15.	Borgeat, P and Samuelsson, B (1979). Arachidonic acid metabolism in polymorpho-nuclear leukocytes: unstable intermediate in formation of dihydroxy acids. *Proc Natl Acad Sci USA*, **76**, 3213-17

16.	Shaw, RJ, Cromwell, O and Kay, AB (1984). Preferential generation of leukotriene $C_4$ by human eosinophils. *Clin Exp Immunol*, **56**, 716-22

17.	Peters, SP, MacGlashan Jr, DW, Schleimer, RP *et al*. (1984). IgE-mediated release of inflammatory mediators from human basophils and mast cells *in vitro* and *in vivo*. *Adv Inflamm Res*, **8**, 227-41

18.	Du, JT, Foegh, M, Maddox, Y and Ramwell, PW (1983). Human peritoneal macrophages synthesize leukotrienes $B_4$ and $C_4$. *Biochim Biophys Acta*, **753**, 159-63

19.	Fuller, RW, Kelsey, CR, Cole, PJ *et al*. (1984). Dexamethasone inhibits the production of thromboxane $B_2$ and leukotriene $B_4$ by human alveolar and peritoneal macrophages in culture. *Clin Sci*, **67**, 653-6

20.	Jakshik, BA, Sun, FF, Lee, L and Steinhoff, MM (1987). Calcium stimulation of a novel lipoxygenase. *Biochem Biophys Res Commun*, **95**, 103-10

21.	Bryant, RW, She, HS, Ng, KJ and Siegal, MI (1986). Modulation of the 5-lipoxyge-nase activity of MC-9 mast cells: activation by hydroperoxides. *Prostaglandins*, **32**, 615-27

22.	Ochi, K, Yoshimoto, T, Yamamoto, S *et al*. (1982). Arachidonate 5-lipoxygenase of guinea pig peritoneal polymorphonuclear leukocytes. *J Biol Chem*, **258**, 5754-8

23.	Evans, JF, Dupius, P and Ford-Hutchinson, AW (1985). Purification and characterization of leukotriene $D_4$ hydrolase from rat neutrophils. *Biochim Biophys Acta*, **840**, 43-50

24.	Hogaboom, GK, Cook, M, Varrichio, A *et al*. (1986). $LTA_4$ synthetase. Leukotriene $A_4$ formation from 5-hydroperoxyeicosatetraenoic acid by purified 5-lipoxygenase of rat basophilic leukemia (RBL-1) cells. *Pharmacologist*, **28**, 186, Abstract 513

25.	Riendeau, D and Leblanc Y (1986). Modulation of rat polymorphonuclear leukocyte 5-lipoxygenase activity by 5-HPETE and NADH-dependent flavin inhibition. *Biochem Biophys Res Commun*, **141**, 534-40

26.	Lewis, RA, Austen, KF, Drazen, JM *et al*. (1980). Slow reacting substances of anphy-laxis: Identification of leukotrienes C-1 and D from human and rat sources. *Proc Natl Acad Sci USA*, **77**, 3710-14

27.	Morris, HR, Taylow, GW, Piper, PJ and Tippins, JR (1980). Structure of slow reacting substances of anaphylaxis from guinea pig lung. *Nature*, **285**, 104-6

28.	Murphy, RC, Hammerstom, S and Samuelsson, B (1979). Leukotriene C: a slow-reacting substance from murine mastocytomas cells. *Proc Natl Acad Sci, USA*, **76**, 4275-9

29.	Piper, PJ (1984). Formation and actions of leukotrienes. *Physiol Rev*, **64**, 744-61

30.	Fleisch, JH, Rinkema, L and Marshall, WS (1984). Pharmacologic receptors for the leukotrienes. *Biochem Pharmacol*, **33**, 2919-3922

31.	Engineer, DM, Morris, HR, Piper, PJ and Sirois, P (1978). The release of prosta-glandins and thromboxanes from guinea pig lung by slow reacting substance of an-aphylaxis, and its inhibition. *Br J Pharmacol*, **64**, 211-18

32.	Folco, G, Hansson, G and Granstom, E (1981). Leukotriene $C_4$ stimulates $TxA_2$ formation in isolated sensitized guinea pig lungs. *Biochem Pharmacol*, **30**, 2491-3

33.	Dahlen, S-E, Bjork, J, Hedqvist, P *et al*. (1981). Leukotrienes promote plasma leak-age and leukocyte adhesion in postcapillary venules: *in vivo* effects with relevance to the acute inflammatory response. *Proc Natl Acad Sci, USA*, **78**, 3887-91

34.	Bjork, J, Dahlen, S-E, Hadqvist, P and Arfors, K-E (1983). Leukotrienes $B_4$ and $C_4$ have distinct microcirculatory actions *in vivo*. In Samuellson, B, Paoletti, R and Ramwell, P (eds) *Advances in Prostaglandin, Thromboxane and Leukotriene Research*, vol 12, pp. 1-6. (New York: Raven Press)

35. Lindbom, L, Hedqvist, P, Dahlen, S-E, Lindgren, JA and Arfors, K-E (1982). Leukotriene B4 induces extravasation and migration of polymorphonuclear leukocytes *in vivo*. *Acta Physiol Scand*, **116**, 105-8

36. Peck, MJ, Piper, PJ and Williams, TJ (1981). The effect of leukotrienes C4 and D4 on the microvasculature of guinea pig skin. *Prostaglandin*, **21**, 315-21

37. Goetzl, EJ and Sun, FF (1979). Generation of unique mono-hydroxyeicosatetraenoic acids from arachidonic acid by human neutrophils. *J Exp Med*, **150**, 406-11

38. Palmer, RMJ, Stepney, RJ, Higgs, GA and Eakins, KE (1980). Chemokinetic activity of arachidonic acid lipoxygenase products on leukocytes from different species. *Prostaglandins*, **20**, 411-18

39. Goldman, DW and Goetzl, EJ (1982). Specific binding of leukotriene B4 to receptors on human polymorphonuclear leukocytes. *J Immunol*, **129**, 1600-4

40. Bray, MA, Ford-Hutchinson, AW and Smith, MJH (1981). Leukotriene B4: an inflammatory mediator *in vivo*. *Prostaglandins*, **22**, 213-22

41. Smith, MJH, Ford-Hutchinson, AW and Bray, MA (1980). Leukotriene B: a potential mediator of inflammation. *J Pharm Pharmacol*, **32**, 517-18

42. Bhattacherjee, P, Hammond, B, Salmon, JA *et al.* (1981). Chemotactic response to some arachidonic acid lipoxygenase products in the rabbit eye. *Eur J Pharmacol*, **73**, 21-7

43. Camp, RDR, Coutts, AA, Greaves, MW *et al.* (1982). Responses on human skin to intradermal injection of leukotrienes C4, D4 and B4. *Br J Pharmacol*, **85**, 168P

44. Carlson, RP, Chang, J, Datko, L and Lewis, AJ (1986). Questionable role of LTB4 in MSU-induced synovitis in the dog. *Prostaglandins*, **32**, 579-85

45. Palmer, RMJ, Stepney, RJ, Higgs, GA and Eakins, KE (1980). Chemokinetic activity of arachidonic acid lipoxygenase products on leukocytes of different species. *Prostaglandins*, **20**, 411-18

46. Davies, P, Bailey, PJ and Goldenberg, MM (1984). The role of arachidonic acid oxygenation products in pain and inflammation. *Ann Rev Immunol*, **2**, 335-57

47. Kato, K, Koshihara, Y and Murata, S (1986). Contribution of lipoxygenase metabolites to IL 2 production in the early phase of lymphocyte activation. *Prostaglandins, Leukotrienes Med*, **22**, 301-11

48. Sibbitt Jr, WL, Imir, T and Bankhurst, AD (1986). Reversible inhibition of lymphokine-activated killer cell activity by lipoxygenase-pathway inhibitors. *Int J Cancer*, **38**, 517-21

49. Rola-Pleszczynski, M (1985). Immunoregulation by leukotrienes and other lipoxygenase metabolites. *Immunol Today*, **6**, 302-7

50. Payan, DG, Missirian-Bastian, A and Goetzle, J (1984). Human T-lymphocyte subset specificity of the regulatory effects of leukotriene B4. *Proc Natl Acad Sci, USA*, **81**, 1-5

51. Brain, W, Camp, R, Dowd, P *et al.* (1984). The release of leukotriene B4-like material in biologically active amounts from the lesional skin of patients with psoriasis. *J Invest Dermatol*, **83**, 70-3

52. Lassus, A and Forsstrom, S (1985). A dimethoxynaphthalene derivative (RS-43179 gel) compared with 0.025% fluocinolone acetonide gel in the treatment of psoriasis. *Br J Dermatol*, **113**, 103-6

53. Klickstein, LB, Shapleigh, C and Goetzl, EJ (1980). Lipoxygenation of arachidonic acid as a source of polymorphonuclear leukocyte chemotactic factors in synovial fluid and tissue in rheumatoid arthritis and spondyloarthritis. *J Clin Invest*, **66**, 1166-70

54. Bisgaard, H and Kristensen, JK (1985). Leukotriene B4 products hyperalgesia in humans. *Prostaglandins*, **30**, 791-7

55. Levine, JD, Lau, W, Kwiat, G and Goetzl, EJ (1984). Leukotriene B4 produces hyperalgesia that is dependent on polymorphonuclear leukocytes. *Science*, **225**, 743-5

56. Kay, AB, Austen, KF and Lichenstein, LM (1984). *Asthma (New York: Academic Press)*

57. Vigo, C, Lewis, GP and Piper, PJ (1980). Mechanisms of inhibition of phospholipase A$_2$. *Biochem Pharmacol*, **29**, 623-7

58. Loffler, BM, Bohn, E, Hesse, B and Kunze, H (1985). Effects of antimalarial drugs on phospholipase A and lysophospholipase activities in plasma membrane, mitochondrial, microsomal and cytosolic subcellular fractions of rat liver. *Biochim Biophys Acta*, **31**, 448-55

59. Sechi, AM, Cabrini, L, Landi, L *et al.* (1978). Inhibition of phospholipase A$_2$ and phospholipase C by polyamines. *Arch Biochem Biophys*, **186**, 248-54

60. Jain, MK and Jahagirdar, DV (1985). Action of phospholipase A$_2$ on bilayers. Effect of inhibitors. *Biochim Biophys Acta*, **11**, 319-26

61. Franson, RC (1981). From physical structure to therapeutic applications. In Knight, K (ed.) *Liposomes*, pp. 349-379. (Amsterdam: Elsevier/North Holland)

62. Takano, S (1985). Inhibition of phospholipase A$_2$ by tiaramide in rabbit platelets. *Jpn J Pharmacol*, **39**, 302-16

63. Franson, RC, Eisen, D, Jesse, R and Lanni, C (1980). Inhibition of highly purified mammalian phospholipase A$_2$ by nonsteroidal antiinflammatory agents. *Biochem J*, **186**, 633-6

64. Lanni, C and Becker, EL (1985). Inhibition of neutrophil phospholipase A$_2$ by p-bromophenylacyl bromide, nordihydroguaiaretic acid, 5,8,11,14-eicosatetraenoic acid and quercetin. *Int Arch Allergy Appl Immunol*, **76**, 214-17

65. Wallach, DP and Brown, VJR (1981). Studies on the arachidonic acid cascade-I. Inhibition of phospholipase A$_2$ *in vitro* and *in vivo* by several novel series of inhibitor compounds. *Biochem Pharmacol*, **30**, 1315-24

66. Yamada, K, Kumada, Y and Kubo, K (1985). KF4939, a new antiplatelet agent, inhibits activation of phospholipase C and A$_2$ in rabbit platelets. *Jpn J Pharmacol*, **39**, 108-11

67. Bray, MA, Beck, A, Wenk, P *et al.* (1987). CGP-35949: potent leukotriene antagonist and inhibitor of phospholipase A$_2$ biological profile. In Samuelsson, B, Paoletti, R and Ramwell, PW (eds) *Advances in Prostaglandin, Thromboxane and Leukotriene Research*, (New York: Raven Press)

68. Flower, RJ, Blackwell, GJ, DiRosa, M and Parenti, L (1981). Mechanism of steroid-induced inhibition of arachidonate oxygenation. In Lewis, GP and Grusberg, M (eds) *Mechanism of Steroid Action*, pp. 97-114. (New York: Macmillan Press)

69. Flower, RJ (1984). Macrocortin and the antiphospholipase proteins. In Weissmann, G (ed.) *Advances in Inflammation Research*, pp. 1-34. (New York: Raven Press)

70. Wallner, BP, Mattaliano, RJ, Hession, C *et al.* (1986). Cloning and expression of human lipocortin, a phospholipase A$_2$ inhibitor with potential antiinflammatory activity. *Nature*, **320**, 77-81

71. Deems, RA, Lombardo, D, Morgan, BP *et al.* (1987). The inhibition of phospholipase A$_2$ by manoalide and manoalide analogues. *Biochim Biophys Acta*, **917**, 258-68

72. Lombardo, D and Dennis, EA (1985). Cobra venom phospholipase A$_2$ inhibition by manoalide: a novel type of phospholipase inhibitor. *J Biol Chem*, **260**, 7234-40

73. Salmon, JA (1986). Inhibition of prostaglandin, thromboxane and leukotriene biosynthesis. *Adv Drug Res*, **15**, 112-67

74. Lewis, AJ, Carlson, RP and Chang, J (1985). Experimental models of inflammation. In Bonta, IL, Bray, MA and Parnham, MJ (eds) *The Pharmacology of Inflammation*, pp. 371-397. (Amsterdam: Elsevier Science Publishers, BV)

75. Patrignani, P and Canete-Soler, R (1987). Biosynthesis, characterization and inhibition of leukotriene B$_4$ in human whole blood. *Prostaglandins*, **33**, 539-51

76. Doherty, NA, Peubelle, P, Borgeat, P *et al.*. (1985). Intraperitoneal injection of zymosan in mice induces pain, inflammation and the synthesis of peptidoleukotrienes and prostaglandin E$_2$. *Prostaglandins*, **30**, 769-90

77. Bach, MK (1984). Inhibitors of leukotriene synthesis and action. In Chakrinard, LW and Bailey, DM (eds) *The Leukotrienes: Chemistry and Biology*, pp. 163-194. (New York: Academic Press)

78. Salari, H, Braquet, P and Borgeat, P (1984). Comparative effects of indomethacin, acetylenic acids, 15-HTE, nordihydro-guaiaretic acid and BW 755c on the metabolism of arachidonic acid in human leukocytes and platelets. *Prostaglandin, Leukotrienes Med*, 13, 53-68

79. Blackwell, GJ and Flower, RJ (1978). 1-phenyl-3-pyrazolidine: An inhibitor of cyclooxygenase and lipoxygenase pathways in lung and platelets. *Prostaglandins*, 16, 417-25

80. DiMartino, MJ, Griswold, DE, Berkowitz, BA *et al.* (1987). Pharmacologic characterization of the antiinflammatory properties of a new dual inhibitor of lipoxygenase and cyclooxygenase. *Agents and Actions*, 20, 113-23

81. Yoshimoto, T, Furukawa, M, Yamamoto, S *et al.* (1983). Flavonoids: Potent inhibitors of arachidonic 5-lipoxygenase. *Biochem Biophys Res Commun*, 116, 612-19

82. Stenson, WF and Labs, E (1982). Sulfasalazine inhibits the synthesis of chemotactic lipids by neutrophils. *J Clin Invest*, 69, 494-6

83. Busser, WD, Mardin, M, Gruetzmann, R *et al.* (1982). Nafazatrom (Bay g 6575) an inhibitor of cellular lipoxygenase activity. *Fed Proc Am Soc Exp Biol*, 41, 1717, Abstr 8464

84. Bach, MK, Brashler, JR and Gorman, RR (1977). The structure of slow reacting substances of anaphylaxis: evidence of biosynthesis from arachidonic acid. *Prostaglandins*, 14, 21-8

85. Chang, J, Skowronek, MD and Lewis, AJ (1985). Differential effects of monohetes (monohydroxyeicosatetraenoic acids) on arachidonic acid metabolites in glycogen-elicited rat polymorphonuclear leukocytes. *Inflammation*, 9, 395-405

86. Walker, JR, Boot, JR, Cox, B and Dawsen, W (1980). Inhibition of the release of slow-reacting substance oof anaphylaxis by inhibitors of lipoxygenase activity. *J Pharm Pharmacol*, 32, 866-7

87. Terano, T, Salmon, J, Higgs, GA and Moncada, S (1986). Eicosapentaenoic acid as a modulator of inflammation: Effect of prostaglandin and leukotriene synthesis. *Biochem Pharmacol*, 779-85

88. Neichi, T, Koshihara, Y and Murota, S (1983). Inhibitory effect of esculetin on 5-lipoxygenase and leukotriene biosynthesis. *Biochem Biophys Acta*, 753, 130-2

89. Salmon, JA, Tilling, LC and Moncada, S (1985). Evaluation of inhibitors of eicosanoid synthesis in leukocytes: Possible pitfall of using the calcium ionophore A23187 to stimulate 5-lipoxygenase. *Prostaglandins*, 29, 377-85

90. Corey, EJ and Munroe, JE (1982). Irreversible inhibition of prostaglandin and leukotriene biosynthesis from arachidonic acid by 11,12 dehydro- and 5,6 dehydroarachidonic acids, respectively. *J Am Chem Soc*, 104, 1752-4

91. Bach, MK, Bowman, BJ, Brashler, JR *et al.*. (1985). Piriprost, a selective inhibitor of leukotriene synthesis. In Hayaishi, O and Yamamoto, S (eds) *Advances in Prostaglandin, Thromboxane and Leukotriene Research*, pp. 225-227. (New York: Raven Press)

92. Ashida, Y, Saigo, T, Kuriki, H *et al.* (1983). Pharmacological profile of AA 861, a 5-lipoxygenase inhibitor. *Prostaglandins*, 26, 955-72

93. Robinson, C and Holgate, ST (1986). Ionophore-dependent generation of eicosanoids in human dispensed lung cells. *Biochem Pharmacol*, 35, 1903-8

94. Letts, LG, McFarland, C, Pietchuta, H and Ford-Hutchinson, AW (1986). The effects of a 5-lipoxygenase inhibitor (L-651-392) and leukotriene D4 antagonist (L-649,923) in two animal models of immediate hypersensitivity reactions. *6th International Conference on PG and related compounds*, Abstract 418, Florence, Italy

95. Guindon, Y, Girard, Y, Maycock, A *et al.* (1986). L-651-392, A novel, potent and selective 5-LO inhibitor. *6th International Conference on PG and related compounds*, pp. 256, Florence, Italy

96.     Makino, H, Ashida, Y, Saigo, T *et al.* (1986). Role of leukotrienes in rat reversed passive arthus pleurisy and the effect of AA-861, a 5-lipoxygenase inhibitor. *Int Arch Allergy Appl Immunol*, **79**, 38-44

97.     Nakadate, T, Yamamoto, S, Aizu, E and Kato, R (1985). Inhibition of mouse epidermal 12-lipoxygenase by 2,3,4-trimethyl-6-(12-hydroxy-5,10-dodecadienyl)-1,4-benzoquinone (AA-861). *Pharm Pharmacol*, **37**, 71-3

98.     Bach, MK, Brashler, JR, Smith, HW *et al.* (1982). 6,9-deepoxy-6,9-(phenylimino)-6,8-prostaglandin I, (U-60,257), a new inhibitor of leukotriene C and D synthesis: *in vitro* studies. *Prostaglandins*, **23**, 759-71

99.     Holgate, ST and Robinson, C (1984). 6,9-deepoxy-6,9-(phenylimino)-6,8-prostaglandin I, (U-60,257) stimulates prostaglandin $D_2$ and inhibits thromboxane $B_2$ release from ionophore challenged human dispersed lung cells. *Br J Pharmacol*, **83**, 603-5

100.    Bach, MK, Brashler, JR, Peck, PE and Morton, DR (1984). Leukotriene C synthetase, a special glutathione S-transferase: Properties of the enzyme and inhibitor studies with special reference to the mode of action of U-60,257, a selective inhibitor of leukotriene synthesis. *J Allergy Clin Immunol*, **74**, 353-7

101.    Bach, MK and Brashler, JR (1986). Inhibition of the leukotriene synthetase of rat basophil leukemia cells by diethylcarbanazine, and synergism between diethylcarbanazine and piriprost a 5-lipoxygenase inhibitor. *Biochem Pharmacol*, **35**, 425-33

102.    Lawsen, CF, Smith, HW and Fitzpatrick, FA (1986). Effect of piriprost, a 5-lipoxygenase inhibitor on leukocyte accumulation during thioglycollate-induced acute inflammation. *Wien Klin Wochenschr*, **98**, 110-13

103.    Burnett, JW and Calton, GJ (1986). Pharmacological effects of various venoms on cutaneous capillary leakage. *Toxicon*, **24**, 614-17

104.    Burghuber, OC, Strife, R, Kirolli, J *et al.* (1986). Hydrogen peroxide induced pulmonary vasoconstriction in isolated rat lungs is attenuated by U-60,257, a leukotriene synthesis blocker. *Wien Klin Wochenschr*, **98**, 117-19

105.    Ritchie, DM, Sierchio, JN, Capetola, RJ and Rosenthale, ME (1981). SRSA-mediated bronchospasm by pharmacologic modification of lung anaphylaxis *in vivo*. *Agents and Actions*, **11**, 396-401

106.    Johnson, HG, McNee, MC, Bach, MK and Smith, HW (1983). The activity of a new novel inhibitor of leukotriene synthesis in rhesus monkey ascaris reactions. *Int Arch Allergy Appl Immunol*, **70**, 169-73

107.    Sonnino-Goldman, P, DonigiRuzza, D, Hujman, S *et al.* (1985). Comparative effects of topically applied Rev 5901, phenidone (PHEN) and indomethacin (INDO) on arachidonic acid (AA)-induced ear inflammatin in DBA/25 mice. *Agents and Actions*, **16**, 598-9

108.    Coutts, S, Khandwala, A, Van Invegen, R *et al.* (1984). Arylmethyl phenyl ethers: A new class of specific inhibitors of 5-lipoxygenase. *4th International Symposium on Prostaglandins and Leukotrienes*, Abstract 70, Washington

109.    Chlou, LY and Chrom, GCY (1985). Ocular antiinflammatory action of a lipoxygenase inhibitor in the rabbit. *J Ocul Pharmacol*, **1**, 383-90

110.    Fleisch, JH, Rinkema, LE, Haisch, KD *et al* (1985). LY-171,883,1-[2-hydroxy-3-propyl-4-[4-(1H-tetrazol-5-yl)butoxy]phenyl]ethanone, an orally active leukotriene $D_4$ antagonist. *J Pharmacol Exp Ther*, **222**, 148-57

111.    Jones, TR, Young, R, Champion, E *et al.* (1986). L-649-923 sodium ($\beta S^*$. $\gamma R^*$)-4-(3-(4-acetyl-3-hydroxy-2-propylphenoxy)-propylthio)-$\gamma$-hydroxy-$\beta$-methylbenzine-butanoate, a selective, orally active leukotriene receptor antagonist. *Can J Physiol Pharmacol*, **64**, 1068-75

112.    Krell, RD, Snyder, DW, Giles, RE *et al* (1986). ICI-198,615, a novel peptidoleukotriene (LT) receptor antagonist: *in vivo* pharmacology. Joint meeting - American Society for Pharmacology and Experimental Therapeutics and Society of Toxicology, August *Pharmacologist*, **28**, 185, Abstr 506

113.    Snyder, DW, Krell, RD, Keith, RA *et al.* (1986). ICI-198,615, a novel peptidoleuko-triene (LT) receptor antagonist: *In vitro* pharmacology. Joint meeting - American Society for Pharmacology and Experimental Therapeutics and Society for Toxico-logy, August *Pharmacologist*, **28**, 185 Abstr 505

114.    Vickery, L, Gleason, JG and Wasserman, MA (1986). Comparison of the effects of SKF-104,353, salbutamol and FPL-55,712 sa. $LTD_4$-induced bronchoconstriction in guinea pigs (GPs). Joint meeting - American Society for Pharmacology and Ex-perimental Therapeutics and Society of Toxicology, August *Pharmacologist*, **28**, 142, Abstr 278

115.    Hand, JM, Musser, JH, Kreft, AF *et al.* (1987). Wy-48,252 (1,1,1-trifluoro-N-[3-(2-quinolinylmethoxy)phenyl]methane sulfonamide): a selective orally active leuko-triene antagonist. Conference on the Biology of the Leukotrienes, New York Academy of Sciences

# 6
# New steroidal anti-inflammatory drugs

**Henry J. Lee, Ann S. Heiman and Irach B. Taraporewala**
Center for Anti-inflammatory Research
College of Pharmacy
Florida A&M University
Tallahassee, Florida 32307, USA

## I. INTRODUCTION

It has become increasingly evident that new anti-inflammatory steroids introduced in the 1980s are a consequence of focused efforts towards the development of local corticosteroids. Two synthetic approaches have been dominant: a traditional means of increasing lipophilicity of potent corticosteroids by masking the hydroxyl group and synthesis of non-systemic steroids by introducing metabolically labile functional groups. The slow increase in the number of chemically distinct steroids in the post-dexamethasone era is indicative of the difficulty in synthesizing effective steroids with new functional groups at non-conventional positions or modifying the 3-one-4-ene, 11-hydroxy and 17-ketol groups which have been regarded as essential for glucocorticoid activities. The impact of new local anti-inflammatory steroids, a few of whose structures are quite distinct from conventional corticosteroids, as anti-arthritis agents has been minimal due to insufficient research in pharmacotherapeutic evaluations and drug delivery systems.

This review gives a brief account of the evolution of anti-inflammatory steroids from 1951 to 1979, a survey of new steroids in the 1980s and progress in the pharmacology of steroids. Regrettably, it has not been a feasible task to include relative efficacies of the new products.

Chemical names of the anti-inflammatory steroids which have appeared in the 1980s are listed in Table 1. Roman numerals correspond to the steroids in the text and figures.

*New Developments in Antirheumatic Therapy.* Rainsford, KD and Velo, GP (eds), Inflammation and Drug Therapy Series, Volume III.

**Table 1 Chemical names of anti-inflammatory steroids in the 1980s**

| | |
|---|---|
| Alclometasone (XIa) | 7α-Chloro-11β,17α,21-trihydroxy-16α-methyl-1,4-pregnadiene-3,20-dione. |
| Budesonide (I) | 16,17-(22R,S)-Propylmethylene-pregna-1,4-diene-11β,21-diol-3,20-dione |
| Cloprednol (XIII) | 6-Chloro-11β,17α,21-trihydroxypregna-1,4,6-triene-3,20-dione |
| Cortivazole (XXXVIII) | 11β,21-Dihydroxy-6α,16α-dimethyl-2,3(phenyl[3,2-c]pyrazolo)-pregna-2,4,6-triene-20-one |
| Deflazacort (III) | 11β,21-Dihydroxy-2'-methyl-5'H-pregna-1,4-dieno[16α,17β-d]oxazolin-3,20-dione-21-acetate |
| Domoprednate (XLII) | 11β-Hydroxy-17α-(1-oxobutoxy)-D-homopregna-1,4-diene-3,20-dione |
| Halometasone (XIV) | 2-Chloro-6α,9α-difluoro-11β,17α,21-trihydroxy-16α-methyl-pregna-1,4-diene-3,20-dione |
| Halopredone (XIIb) diacetate | 17α,21-Diacetoxy-2-bromo-6β,9α-difluoro-11β-hydroxy-pregna-1,4-diene-3,20-dione |
| Hydrocortisone-17-butyrate-21-propionate (VIII) | 11β-Hydroxy-pregna-4-ene-3,20-dione-17α-butyrate-21-proprionate |
| Nivazol (XXI) | (17α)2'-(4-fluorophenyl)-2'H-pregna-2,4-dien-20-yno-[3.2-c]pyrazol-17-ol |
| Prednicarbate (V) | 11β-Hydroxy-17α-ethylcarbonyloxy-21-propionyloxy-pregna-1,4-diene-3,20-dione |
| Rimexolone (XVIII) | 11β-Hydroxyl-16α,17β,21-trimethyl-pregna-1,4-diene-3-one |
| Tipredane (XVII) | 17α(ethylthio)-9α-fluoro-11β-hydroxy-17β-(methylthio)androsta-1,4-dien-3-one |
| Tixocortol pivalate (XV) | 11β,17α-Dihydroxy-21-tert-pentanoylthiopregna-4-ene-3,20-dione |
| RS-35909 (XVI) | 6β,9α-Difluoro-11β-hydroxy-16α-methyl-17β-methylthio-carbonyl-androsta-1,4-dien-3-one 17α-propionate |
| Sch 22219 (IX) | 7α-Chloro-11β-hydroxy-16α-methyl-pregna-1,4-diene-3,20-dione-17,21-diproprionate |
| Sch 23409 (X) | 21-Acetoxy-17α-benzoyloxy-7α-bromo-11β-hydroxy-16α-methyl-pregna-1,4-diene-3,20-dione |
| SQ 26,490 (IV) | (11β,16α)-9-fluoro-1',2',3',4'-tetrahydro-11,21-dihydroxypregna-1,4-dieno[16,17-b]naphthalene-3,20-dione |

| | |
|---|---|
| P8 (XXII) | Methyl 11β,17α-dihydroxy-3,20-dioxo-1,4-pregnadiene-21-oate |
| DeoxyP8 (XXVII) | Methyl 11β-hydroxy-3,20-dioxo-1,4-pregnadiene-21-oate |
| P4Al (XXIII) | Methyl 11β,17,20α-trihydroxy-3-oxo-1,4-pregnadiene-21-oate |
| P4Be (XXIV) | Methyl 11β,17,20β-trihydroxy-3-oxo-1,4-pregnadiene-21-oate |
| P4AlAc (XXV) | Methyl 11β-hydroxy-17α,20α-isopropylidenedioxy-3-oxo-1,4-pregnadiene-21-oate |
| P4BeAc (XXVI) | Methyl 11β-hydroxy-17α,20β-isopropylidenedioxy-3-oxo-1,4-pregnadiene-21-oate |
| P4AlNPr (XXXc) | 11β,17,20α-trihydroxy-3-oxo-1,4-pregnadiene-21-N-(n-propyl)-carboxamide |
| P4BeNPr (XXXIc) | 11β,17,20β-trihydroxy-3-oxo-1,4-pregnadiene-21-N-(n-propyl)-carboxamide |
| P16CM (XXXIV) | Methyl 11β,17α,21-trihydroxy-3,20-dioxo-1,4-pregnadiene-16-carboxylate |
| DeoxyP16CM (XXXIII) | Methyl 11β,21-dihydroxy-3,20-dioxo-1,4-pregnadiene-16-carboxylate |
| TAMe (XXVIII) | Methyl 9α-fluoro-11β-hydroxy-16,17α-isopropylidenedioxy-1,4-pregnadiene-21-oate |

## II. EVOLUTION OF CORTICOSTEROID DRUGS

Three very important observations were reported by Hench and his co-workers following the first cortisone therapy of a rheumatoid arthritis patient[1]. First, doses less than 100 mg/day were not therapeutically effective. Second, beneficial effects of cortisone were limited to the duration of treatment while the natural progression of the disease was not altered. Third, a number of adverse effects, cushingoid symptoms, appeared after about 3 weeks of cortisone administration.

The awesome potential of cortisone, as well as its adverse effects, were thus recognized by the early 1950s before general use of steroids. The early task of the steroid chemist was to synthesize corticosteroids which were more potent anti-inflammatory agents but had reduced incidences of side-effects. As a result of this research effort, very potent semi-synthetic corticoids with virtually no salt-retaining activity have been produced.

Figure 1 depicts the structure of hydrocortisone, with arrows indicating the four favourite positions at which medicinal chemists introduce modifications: a double bond between carbons 1 and 2 and a halogen atom, methyl or hydroxyl group at carbons 6, 9 and 16.

155

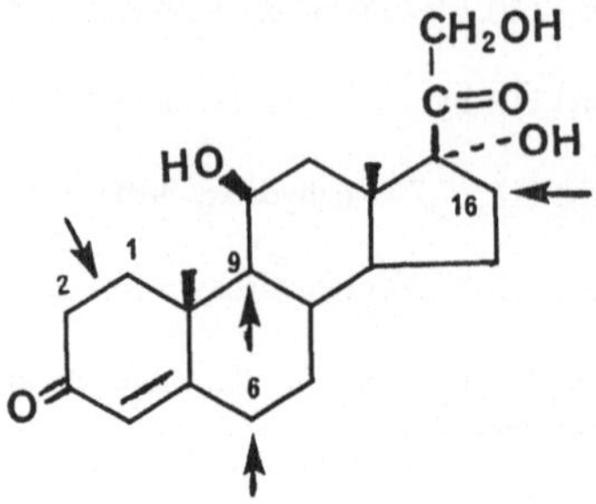

**Figure 1** Structure of hydrocortisone. Arrows indicate four favourite positions for functional group introduction

Significant structural modifications of hydrocortisone which enhance glucocorticoid potency and were introduced prior to 1980 are chronologically listed below:

1.  Introduction of fluorine at the $9\alpha$-position for the protection of the proximal 11-hydroxy group was one of the earliest modifications and resulted in agents such as fluorocortisone (1954).

2.  Placement of a double bond between carbon 1 and 2, as in prednisolone (1955), led to increased potency with reduced salt-retaining activity. This structural feature has endured in most subsequent corticosteroid drugs.

3.  The incorporation of a C-6 methyl to prevent hydroxylation at the position as in methyl prednisolone (1956). led to the synthesis of more potent agents with longer durations of action.

4.  The introduction of C-16 hydroxy groups as in triamcinolone (1956) or methyl groups as in dexamethasone (1958) and betamethasone (1958), resulted in drugs with 30 times the potency of hydrocortisone.

5.  Formation of C-16, C-17 acetonides and esterification at C-17 and/or C-21 hydroxy groups have resulted in compounds with greater lipophilicity and consequently higher local activity. Examples include triamcinolone acetonide (1957) and betamethasone-17-valerate and betamethasone-17,21-diproprionate (1959).

Other chemical changes, more significant from the chemistry viewpoint than the pharmacotherapeutic viewpoint, include the replacement of the hydroxyl group at C-21 with chlorine (Halcinonide, 1962), incorporation of a fused phenylpyrazole ring at C-2 and C-3 ($9\alpha$-fluoro-$11\beta$,$17\alpha$,21-trihydroxy-6,16$\alpha$-dimethyl-4,6-prednadieno[3,2-C]-2'-phenylpyrazole, (1963), substitution of the 11-hydroxy group with chlorine (Meclorisone Dibutyrate, 1967), incorporation of a fused oxazole ring at C-16 and C-17 (Azacort, 1967), and the ester of steroid-21-oate (Fluocortin Butyl, 1977)[2].

156

Three therapeutic approaches have been employed to reduce the systemic adverse effects of potent steroids. First, various dosage forms have been developed for local administration such as topical preparations for treatment of skin disorders, drops for treatment of ophthalmic disorders, aerosols for asthmatic conditions and preparations for intra-articular injections for joint diseases. Second, alternate-day therapeutic regimens have been used to minimize the effect on the hypothalamic-pituitary adrenal (HPA) axis. A 48-hour regimen of administering intermediate-acting steroids is preferred for maintenance, and has proven particularly effective in asthma, systemic lupus erythematosus, uveitis and nephrotic syndrome. The third strategy has been to use a concomitant "protective" therapy such as the administration of antihypertensive agents, potassium replacement agents, immunizations to prevent chronic infection or administration of vitamin D or its metabolites to reduce bone loss.

Advances in the therapeutic strategy and proliferation of corticosteroid products in the 1950s and 1960s have not been entirely successful, since therapy with powerful corticosteroids is routinely beset with undesirable and toxic side-effects which can be debilitating. Until recently many investigators have been resigned to accepting the relatively poor therapeutic indices associated with chronic use of corticosteroids. This gloomy attitude has been reflected in a general discontinuance of corticosteroid research by several manufacturing firms, and has created a state of inertia in terms of new corticosteroids. Now, out of the efforts of a few laboratories, new concepts and new compounds have evolved. Three important new concepts which were introduced in the late 1970s are: (1) a rational approach to improve the physicochemical properties of corticosteroids for local use, (2) development of steroidal or non-steroidal anti-glucocorticoids, and (3) drug design within the "antedrug" concept.

Examples of rational approaches for the improvement of physicochemical properties of corticosteroids for local use appear in the next section as extensions of traditional modifications or novel alterations. Steroidal or non-steroidal anti-glucocorticoids, discussed later with steroid binding studies, have been useful as probes for determining agonist, partial agonist or antagonist activity for given steroid-receptor complexes. Drug design within the antedrug concept is applicable to many of the new corticosteroids whose descriptions follow.

Somewhat in contrast to the term prodrug, which is used to describe compounds which undergo biotransformation prior to exhibiting their pharmacological effects, is the antedrug concept. In developing the new antedrug concept, the following considerations have served as guidelines: (1) corticosteroid pharmacotherapy appears to offer an abundance of agents, but no truly safe drug; (2) systemic manifestations of steroids are unnecessary complications which accompany treatment of many inflammatory conditions; (3) an intact ketol side-chain is not an absolute requirement for the anti-inflammatory activity of corticosteroids; and (4) steroid acid esters with intact ring structures of potent glucocorticoids retain anti-inflammatory activity of the parent compound but upon entry into the circulatory system from the site of administration are hydrolyzed to steroid acids which are inactive and readily excreted[3]. The term antedrug can be applied to an active synthetic derivative which is inactivated by the first metabolic step upon entry into the circulation. Thus, a true antedrug acts only locally, and undergoes only one predictable metabolic step to an inactive metabolite. Compounds which have at least one active intermediary metabolite can be considered as partial antedhe former might include the esters of steroid acids, and the latter might include cortisone acetate and budesonide. As a logical extension of the prototype ester and amide derivatives of steroid-21-oates, steroids with carboxy ester and amide groups at other strategic positions of the steroid nucleus are under investigation[4].

## III.  NEW ANTI-INFLAMMATORY CORTICOSTEROIDS IN THE 1980s

The recent research activities in developing anti-inflammatory steroids have been to increase the therapeutic index of potent corticosteroids by reducing their systemic side-effects. While many of the new steroids have been obtained by the extension of traditional chemical manipulations, new corticoid molecules with significant structural changes have also been developed. The novel structural modifications include the alteration of the essential functional groups and the introduction of new functional groups in the glucocorticoid molecules.

The new compounds are discussed according to the following chemical modifications:

1.  Steroids developed from traditional modifications:
    (a)  C-16, C-17 acetals and acetonides.
    (b)  C-16, C-17 fused ring compounds.
    (c)  C-17 esters and C-21 diesters of steroidal alcohols.
    (d)  Halogenated steroids.

2.  Steroids developed from novel modifications:
    (a)  Side-chain modified compounds.
    (b)  Esters and amides of steroidal carboxylates.
    (c)  Miscellaneous compounds.

## (1)  Steroids developed from traditional modifications

### (a)  C-16, C-17 acetals and acetonides

One of the earliest approaches employed to improve the potency of anti-inflammatory steroids for local use was to prepare acetonides at the C-16, C-17 positions. Extensive work in this line of structure modification was prompted when triamcinolone acetonide was found to be ten times more active topically than triamcinolone, but having similar systemic effects. Recently, new types of acetal and acetonides having reportedly high local to systemic activity ratios have been prepared.

*Budesonide* (I), introduced by Brattsand *et al.*, is a newer non-halogenated steroid with a unique asymmetric acetal group at the C-16, C-17 positions[5]. It is a mixture of two epimers with [22R] and [22S] configurations. The [22R] isomer has the higher local anti-inflammatory potency[6]. Low systemic effects are attributed to its rapid biotransformation in the liver. Negligible metabolism was noted in skin homogenates, but rapid biodegradation occurred in liver homogenates from rats and mice[7]. In human liver the [22R] isomer was found to be more prone to biotransformation than the [22S] isomer. Budesonide metabolism is considerably faster than that of triamcinolone acetonide, which contains a 9α-fluoro substituent[8]. In clinical studies on severe steroid-dependent asthmatics, adrenal function was not suppressed by budesonide[9,10].

An asymmetric acetal substitution at the 16α,17α positions markedly enhanced the topical anti-inflammatory potency when compared to the conventional symmetric acetonide substitution. The halogenation of the steroid molecule by 9α-fluoro or 6α-,9α-difluoro substitution increases the systemic activity of 16α,17α substituted acetals and acetonides.

*Flunisolide* (II) is a topical corticosteroid containing 6α-fluoro and a 16α,17α-acetonide group. Rapid oxidation of the 11-hydroxy group in the absence of a 9α-fluoro substituent, in contrast to triamcinolone acetonide, accounts for reduced systemic effects. Current therapeutic applications of flunisolide are limited to bronchial asthma and allergic rhinitis[11,12].

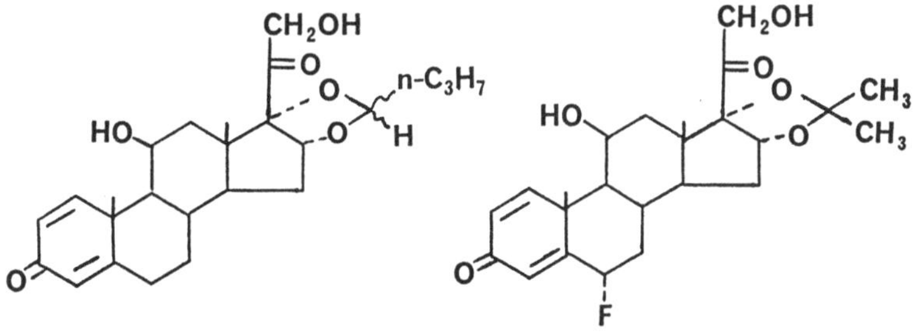

I    II

**Figure 2** C-16, C-17 acetonides and acetals

## (b) C-16,C-17 fused ring compounds

As an outcome of the favourable pharmacological evaluation of C-16,C-17 acetals and acetonides as local anti-inflammatory agents, attempts have been

made to bridge these positions of the D-ring with other heterocyclic structures.

*Deflazacort* (III) has a fused 2-methyloxazoline ring at the 16α,17α-po-
sitions of ring D in the steroid nucleus. In a clinical study deflazacort has a
comparable anti-inflammatory potency but a lower hyperglycaemic effect in
comparison to prednisone[13]. Pretreatment with deflazacort partially inhibited serum cortisol secretion but did not alter basal or thyrotropin-releas-
ing hormone (TRH) stimulated secretion of prolactin when compared with
dexamethasone or placebo[14].

*Compound SQ 26,490* (IV), a 9α-fluorinated compound contains a te-
trahydronaphthalene ring fused at the 16β,17α positions of the D ring[15]. The
reported activity of this agent was 5.5 times greater than that of hydrocortisone in the croton-oil induced rat ear oedema bioassay. After extended topical applications, SQ 26,490 continuously suppressed oedema with much less
dermal atrophy compared to several reference steroids. A low plateau level
of dermal atrophy was maintained with SQ 26,490 at doses considerably
higher than the dose necessary to achieve a significant anti-inflammatory effect.

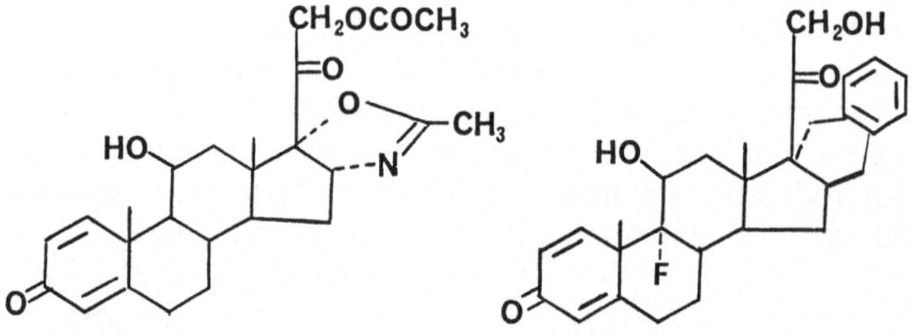

**Figure 3** C-16, C-17 fused ring steroids

## (c) C-17 esters and C-17,C-21 diesters of steroidal alcohols

Esterification of hydroxyl groups at the C-17 and C-21 positions has been a
classical means to increase lipophilicity. A necessary compromise between
the lipophilicity and the steric size of the ester groups has been studied recently. Esterification of the 17α-hydroxyl group in particular has been shown
to increase the affinity of steroids for their cytosolic receptors, which correlates well with anti-inflammatory activity[17,18].

Steroids with longer alkyl ester groups incorporated at either the C-
17 or C-21 positions have higher binding affinities. However, diesterification
at both positions with bulky groups such as valerate reduces the binding affinity[19]. This is evident from the order of binding affinities of betamethasone-

derived esters: betamethasone 17-valerate > betamethasone 17α,21-divalerate > betamethasone-21-valerate. Various C-17 esters and C-17,C-21 diesters with favourable therapeutic indices as anti-inflammatory agents have appeared recently.

*Prednicarbate* (V), the 17-ethylcarbonate-21-propionate diester of prednisolone is reported to have topical anti-inflammatory activity comparable to that of desoximethasone but exhibits reduced systemic effects measured as thymus involution, glycogen deposition and dermal atrophy[20,21].

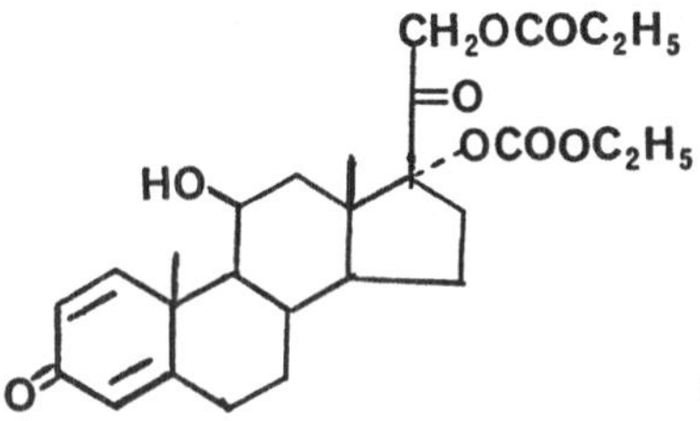


V

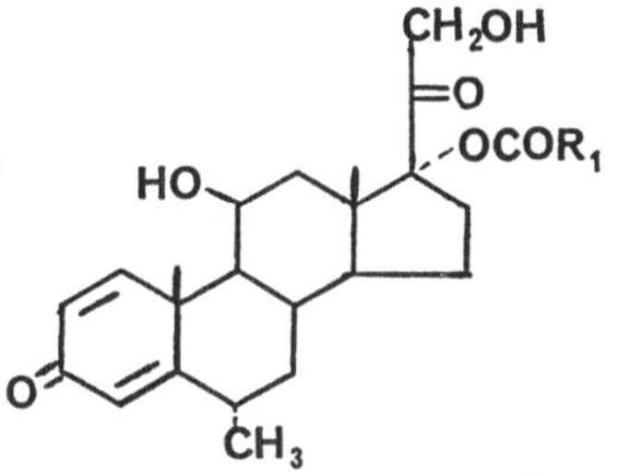


VI a, $R_1 = CH(CH_3)_2$

b, $R_1 = CH_2CH(CH_3)_2$

c, $R_1 = CH_2OCH_3$

d, $R_1 = CH_2SCH_3$

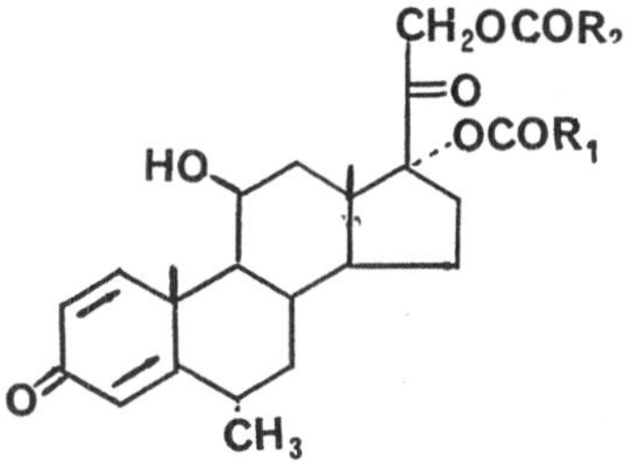


VII a, $R_1, R_2$ = n-$C_4H_9$

b, $R_1, R_2 = CH_2OCOCH_3$

c, $R_1, R_2 = CH_2SCOCH_3, CH_2OCOCH_3$

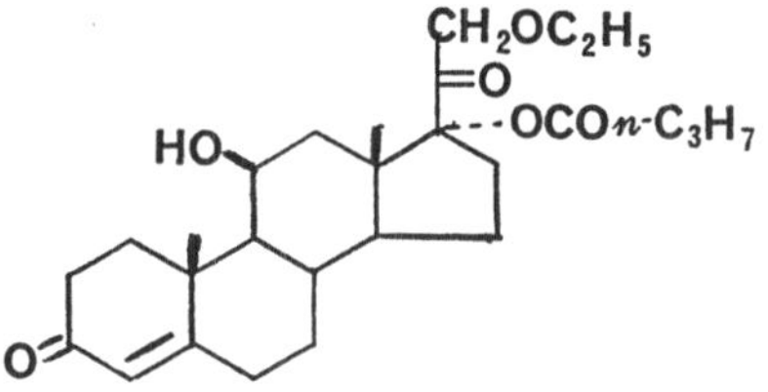


VIII

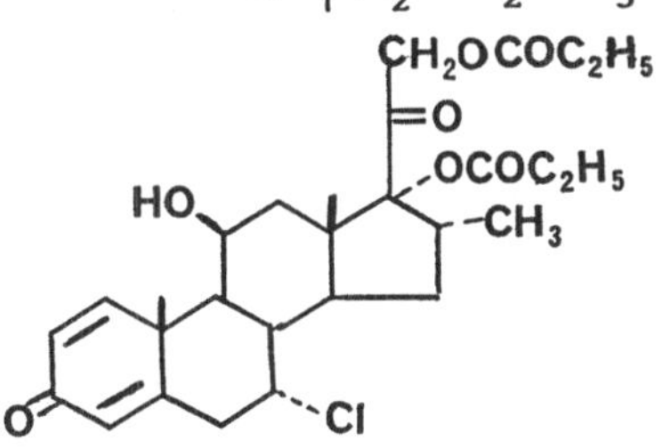


IX

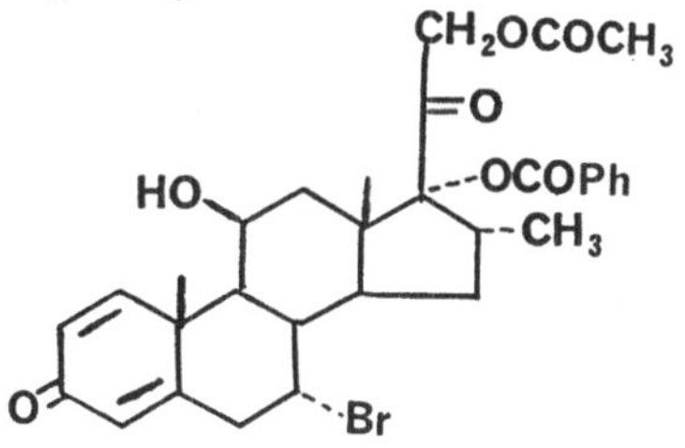


X

**Figure 4** C-17 esters and C-17, C-21 diesters derived from steroid alcohols

The 17-monoesters (VI) and 17,21-diesters (VII) derived from $6\alpha$-methyl prednisolone were investigated as anti-inflammatory agents using the skin vasoconstriction test[22]. The highest activities in the series were observed with C-17 mono substituted branched-chain alkyl esters such as the isopropylcarbonyl (VIa) and isobutylcarbonyl (VIb). However, compounds having bulky ester groups at both C-17 and C-21 positions such as the 17,21-di-n-butyl ester (VIIa) had low anti-inflammatory activity.

The 17,21-diester (VIIb,c) and 17-esters (VIc,d) which have methoxyacetate ($R_1 = CH_2OCH_3$) and methylthioacetate ($R_1 = CH_2SCH_3$) groups were prepared from 6-methylprednisolone. All the monoesters, and 17,21-diesters studied were as active or more potent than the parent molecule. Since the 17-substituted methylthioacetyl derivatives were more potent than the corresponding methoxyacetates, the higher lipophilicity of the sulphur atom compared to the corresponding oxygen atom was suggested by Sugai *et al.* to be responsible for the enhanced activity[23].

*Hydrocortisone-17-butyrate-21-proprionate (HBP)* (VIII), a diester derived from hydrocortisone, has been introduced in Japan as an anti-inflammatory agent for dermal application[24]. In a comparative study, HBP produced less adverse effects than other steroids as measured by body weight gain, serum cholesterol and triglyceride levels and the atrophy of lymphatic tissues and skin[25]. HBP is rapidly metabolized to hydrocortisone 17-butyrate by cultured human keratinocytes. Non-enzymatic transacylation of the butyrate moiety from C-17 to C-21 produces hydrocortisone-21-butyrate, which is eventually hydrolysed to hydrocortisone[26]. The rapid hydrolysis of the diester in the skin before the drug enters the systemic circulation is believed to be responsbile for its favourable therapeutic index.

*Compounds Sch 22219* (IX) and *Sch 23409* (X) are two new C-17,C-21 diesters with low systemic activities[27]. These compounds have a $7\alpha$ and $16\alpha$-methyl substituent in addition to moderately bulky C-17 and C-21 ester group substitutions. The role of the $7\alpha$-halo substitution is discussed in the next section.

### (d) Halogenated corticosteroids

Increased topical anti-inflammatory activity has been reported for compounds having halogen substitution at the C-2 and C-7 positions.

*Alclometasone* (XIa, R = H), a $16\alpha$-methylprednisolone derivative with a $7\alpha$-chloro substituent, has a relatively high topical therapeutic index[29]. Esterification of the 17,21 positions of alclometasone increases the topical anti-inflammatory activity. The 17,21-diproprionate derivative of alclometasone also exhibitied enhanced topical potency when compared with the parent drug[30,31].

*Halopredone* (XIIa, R = H) and its diacetate ester derivative THS-201 (XIIb, R = COCH$_3$) are trihalogenated derivatives with fluorine atoms at the

162

6β and 9α positions and a bromo substituent at the new C-2 position of ring A. These steroids are claimed to act exclusively at the site of administration and exert a prolonged therapeutic effect[32]. In antigen-induced bilaterally arthritic rabbits an intra-articularly administered single dose of THS-201 at 2mg per joint decreased the swelling of the treated knee joint for more than 24 days, but no such effect was seen in the untreated knee joint[33]. In the carrageenan-induced oedema test, THS-201 showed greater potency than triamcinolone acetonide, methylprednisolone acetate or hydrocortisone acetate[33].

*Cloprednol* (XIII), a 6-chloro substituted derivative of 6,7-dehydroprednisolone, is another topical halogenated steroid with low systemic activity as evidenced by reduced effects upon the HPA axis[34].

*Halometasone* (XIV) is a topical steroid with a 2-chloro substituent useful in a variety of acute and chronic eczematous dermatoses and psoriatic conditions and is reportedly devoid of skin toxicity and systemic side-effects[35-37].

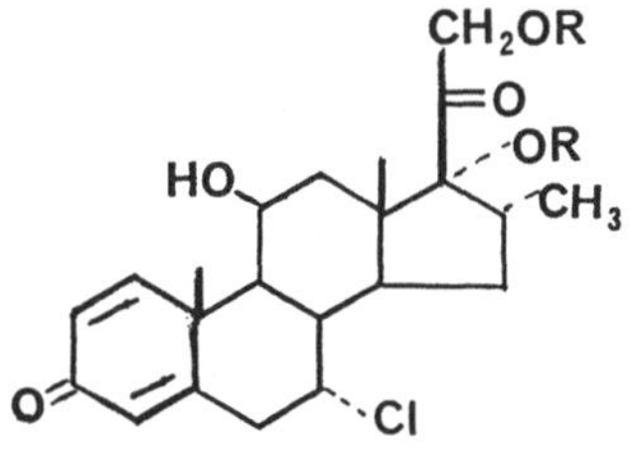


XI a, R = H
b, R = $COC_2H_5$

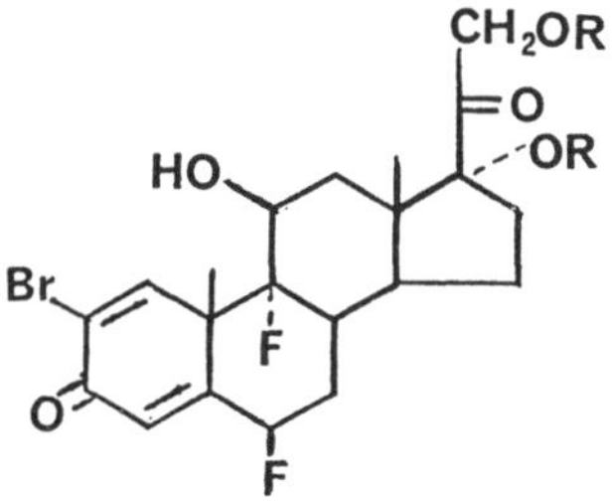


XII a, R = H
b, R = $COCH_3$

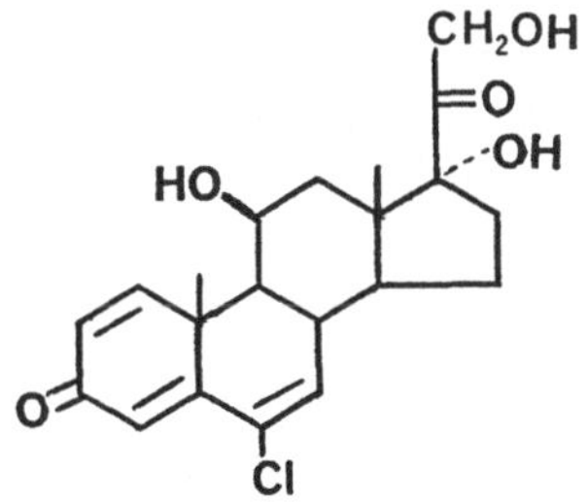


XIII

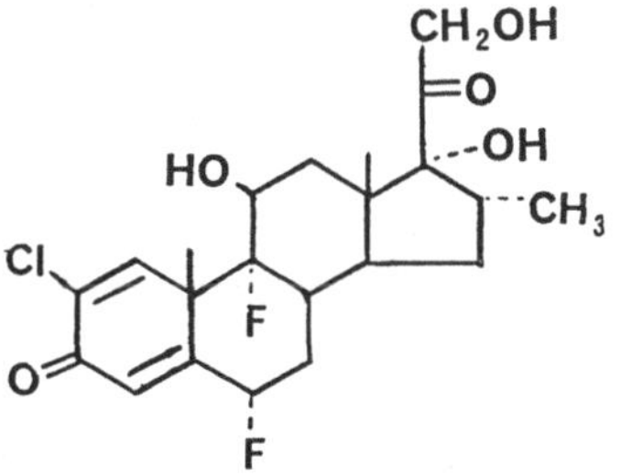


XIV

**Figure 5** Halogenated corticosteroids

## (2) Steroids developed from novel modifications

### (a) Side-chain modified compounds

Improved local to systemic activity ratios have been achieved by various chemical modifications of the 17-ketol side-chain which has been regarded as being an essential functional group for anti-inflammatory activity. This new class of steroids in which radical modifications have been made suggests that a greater degree of latitude is available in modifying the 17-ketol group, a unique structural moiety of adrenal steroids.

Tixocortol pivalate (XV) is a pivalyl thiolester compound derived from hydrocortisone and introduced by Juvenal Laboratories in France. This drug exhibits anti-inflammatory activity equal or less than that of hydrocortisone acetate when applied locally or topically, but possesses very little systemic activity. The lack of glucocorticoid or anti-inflammatory effects following oral or subcutaneous doses of tixocortol pivalate is ascribed to its rapid biotransformation to inactive metabolites[38]. Following single oral or intrarectal doses or short-term intranasal applications, tixocortol pivalate did not suppress plasma cortisol levels, leucocyte counts, blood glucose levels and 24-hour urinary excretion of sodium[39]. Tixocortol pivalate also demonstrates a lack of immunosuppressive activity on lymphocytes in vivo in comparison to hydrocortisone acetate or beclomethasone diproprionate[40,41]. Tixocortol pivalate, which is currently licensed to very limited applications, is a potentially superior, albeit relatively weaker, local anti-inflammatory agent.

RS-35909 (XVI), in which a 17β-methylthiocarbonyl group replaces the ketol side-chain, also contains two fluorine substituents at C-6 and C-9 of Ring B and a 17α-butyrate ester function[42]. RS-35909 is rapidly metabolized in vivo to the inactive C-20 carboxylic acid and has a plasma half-life of 34 minutes after intravenous administration. The low systemic activity of RS-35909 in comparison to its topical activity is attributable to the metabolically labile methyl thiolester group which provides a site for the rapid biotransformation of the steroid to an inactive metabolite.

Tipredane (XVII) is a structurally unique 17α,β-bisthioalkyl 9α-fluoro steroid. The 17β side-chain and the 17α hydrogen atom are both replaced by thioalkyl substituents[43]. It has been shown to possess moderate anti-inflammatory activity in the carrageenan oedema test. When tipredane is applied to the skin of psoriatic patients, no decreases in plasma cortisol or urinary 17-hydroxy corticoid levels were observed. Tipredane appears to undergo complete metabolism before excretion, since no unchanged drug could be detected in urine. The compound is metabolized 5-30 times faster than hydrocortisone in liver homogenates of rats and mice.

Rimexolone (XVIII) represents a novel corticosteroid having a 17β-propionyl side-chain in place of the ketol group. The 17α-hydroxy group is also replaced by a methyl group. It is reported to have local anti-inflammatory activity comparable to that of betamethasone valerate, but has low systemic effects when administered either locally or systemically[44].

Rimexolone exhibits no significant atrophogenic activity in the skin when administered topically or intravenvously in animals. The reduction of joint swelling in rabbit adjuvant-induced arthritis was comparable to triamcinolone hexacetonide and prednisolone t-butyl acetate in an intra-articular injection test. The drug showed no significant thymolytic or adrenolytic effects, but had a relatively long duration of action[45].

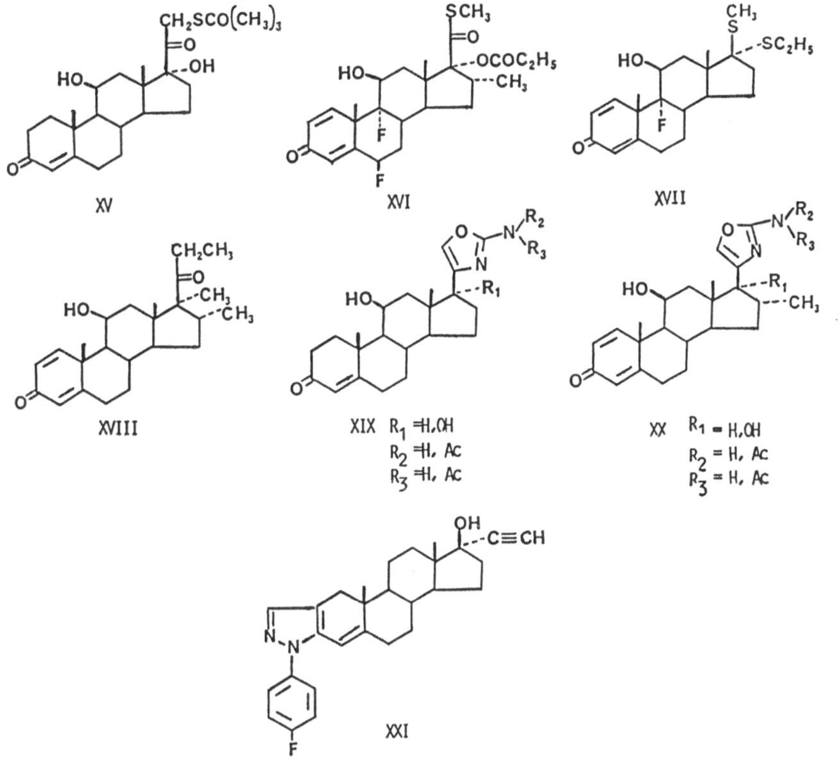

**Figure 6** Steroids with modified side-chains

*Amino-oxazolyl-17β-corticosteroids* (XIX and XX), derived from hydrocortisone and dexamethasone respectively, represent a more drastic side-chain modification involving the replacement of the 17-ketol side-chain by a heterocyclic amino-oxazole substituent[46]. A series of 15 compounds with these structural elements was evaluated in the cotton pellet granuloma and the carrageenan paw oedema bioassay in rats. All the amino-oxazolyl steroids showed local anti-inflammatory activity. Those compounds derived from dexamethasone (XX, $R_2,R_3$ = H,H; $R_2,R_3$ = H,Ac; $R_2,R_3$ = Ac,Ac) were the most potent in the cotton pellet granuloma assay but did not have inhibitory effects upon the thymus or adrenal glands, or influence alterations in body weights. The 17β-amino-oxazolyl steroids failed to inhibit prostaglandin synthesis[47], which suggested that these new steroids exert their anti-inflammatory action by an alternative mechansism to the inhibition of phospholipase-induced release of arachidonic acid from membrane phospholipids. Their mechanism of action has been attributed to the heterocyclic 2-amino-oxazolyl side-chain which interacts with possible cytotoxic oxidant species such as peroxides and peroxy radical scavengers[47].

*Nivazol* (XXI) is a steroid whose structure is an even further departure from conventional corticosteroids. Not only is the ketol group replaced by a 17β-hydroxy-17α-ethynyl group, but the 1,4-dien-3-one system is replaced by a 1-(4-fluorophenyl)pyrazole ring system fused at the 2,3 positions of ring A[48]. Although nivazol lacks three of the essential groups traditionally considered important for glucocorticoid activity (the 3-keto, 11-hydroxy and 20-keto groups), it nevertheless exhibits a complete spectrum of glucocorticoid activities in the rat, including suppression of the hypothalamic–pituitary–adrenal axis, thymolytic action and hepatic glycogen deposition[49].

In the rhesus monkey, however, nivazol displays the HPA-inhibitory activity, but lacks peripheral glucocorticoid actions[50]. The selectivity of action is brought about by drastic structural changes of the steroid structure. This warrants further investigation and re-evaluation of the structure–activity relationships of anti-inflammatory corticosteroids[51].

### (b) Esters and amides derived from steroidal carboxylic acids

A new class of anti-inflammatory steroids, the derivaties of steroid acids, has been synthesized by modifying the 17β-ketol side-chain of potent corticosteroids. The rationale for the modification was that the esters and amides derived from corticosteroid-21-oic acids might retain local activity but would be hydrolysed to the inactive steroid acids and hence cause minimal systemic side-effects.

Thus the ester derivatives would have a different spectrum of activity dependent upon the route of adminstration. In accord with this hypothesis, the local anti-inflammatory activity of methyl prednisolonate (XXII) and the two epimers of methyl 20ξ-dihydroprednisolonate, the 20α-hydroxy (XXIII) and the 20β-epimer (XXIV) was comparable to that of the parent drug prednisolone, but their systemic effects were greatly reduced[52]. Moreover, steroid acid esters did not have suppressive effects on relative adrenal weights or plasma corticosterone levels[53], or inhibit skin collagen synthesis or dermal thickness[54]. These derivatives also stabilized lysosomal membranes and competed with [³H]dexamethasone for rat liver receptors[55]. The metabolite of the steroid acid esters, 20-dihydroprednisolonic acid, was inactive in pharmacological tests and had no affinity for cytosol glucocorticoid receptors. Results obtained with the two epimers of methyl 20-dihydroprednisolonate (XXIII and XXIV) reveal the necessary orientation of the 20-hydroxyl group for anti-inflammatory potency. For example, the 20β-isomer was 2-3 times more potent than the 20α-epimer (Table 2). Typically, the C-20 carbonyl function has been considered essential for anti-inflammatory activity. No glucocorticoid currently in clinical use has a reduced keto group, that is, a hydroxy group, at the C-20 position as is present in methyl 20-dihydroprednisolonate. It is therefore significant that the corresponding C-20β hydroxy compound is not only an active local anti-inflammatory agent but also is as potent as the C-20 keto compound.

The corresponding acetonides (XXV) and (XXVI) derived from the epimers were also prepared and evaluated. In the cotton pellet granuloma assay these derivatives showed local anti-inflammatory activities comparable to prednisolone, but had reduced systemic effects. The topical anti-inflammatory activities of the steroidal 21-oate esters and acetonides were measured in the croton oil-induced ear oedema bioassay in rats[56]. The order of anti-inflammatory potency in this assay was prednisolone > XXV > XXVI > XXIII > XXIV. This order was paralleled by their 1-octanol:water partition coefficients.

The effects of these new anti-inflammatory steroids on leucocyte migration and prostanoid liberation in rats was studied by subcutaneous implantation of saline-soaked polyester sponges impregnated with the steroids[58]. The methyl 20α- and 20β-dihydroprednisolonates XXIII and XXIV had no effect on cell migration but depressed the levels of 6-keto $PGF_{1\alpha}$, $PGE_2$ and elastase. On the other hand, the acetonides XXV and XXVI inhibited the liberation of these inflammatory mediators and also inhibited neutrophil migration.

The effect of a 17α-hydroxy group of steroidal 21-oate esters upon the electrolyte balance was studied on methyl prednisolonate (XXII) and methyl 17-deoxyprednisolonate (XXVII). The latter compound, which lack the 17α-hydroxyl group, has significant mineralocorticoid activity, while the former had no effect upon the electroylte balance[59].

Encouraged by the activity profiles of steroid acid esters, a fluorinated analogue (XXVIII), the methyl 16,17-acetonide-2-oate derived from triamcinolone acetonide, was prepared by Gorsline et al. [60]. The binding affinity of XXVIII was found to be comparable to that of triamcinolone acetonide, and the ester was rapidly hydrolyzed upon incubation with serum at 37°C. The ester lacks the adverse side-effects such as suppression thymic weight or plasma corticosterone levels, and shows local activity comparable with that of triamcinolone acetonide in the cotton pellet granuloma bioassay.

Various steroidal 20-carboxamides as topical agents have also been investigated[61]. While the 17β-carboxamides derived from hydrocortisone or dexamethasone (XXIX) have been shown to be glucocorticoid antagonists[62] in rat HTC cells, the 20-carboxamides were glucocorticoid agonists in vivo. A series of steroidal carboxamides (XXX) and (XXXI) (Figure 8) shows anti-inflammatory activity in the cotton pellet granuloma bioassay (Table 3). The binding affinities for the 20α-hydroxy carboxamide compounds (XXX) are higher than those for the 20β-hydroxy compounds (XXXI), as in the case of the 21-oate esters. However, the amide derivatives exhibit systemic activities as evidenced by suppressed plasma corticosterone levels. It appears, therefore, that these carboxamide derivatives, while retaining the anti-inflammatory activity seen in the esters, are probably not hydrolyzed as readily *in vivo*. Continuing comparative studies of the metabolism and pharmacokinetics of the derivatives should indicate whether these agents act as true antedrugs. Also under investigation currently are the 20-keto carboxamides (XXXII).

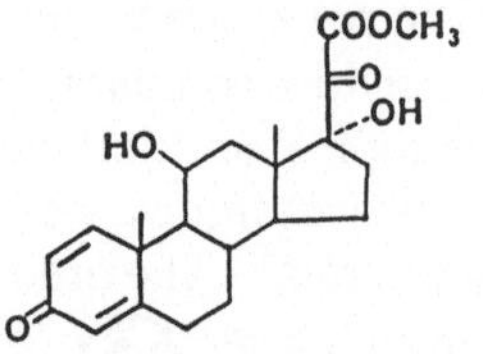


XXII

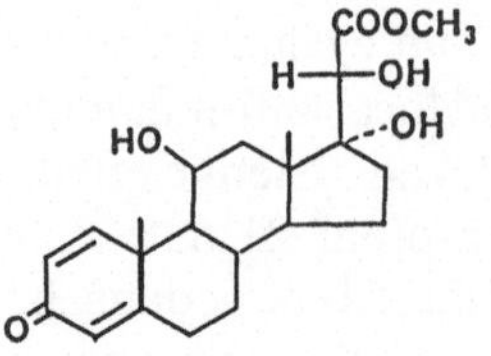


XXIII

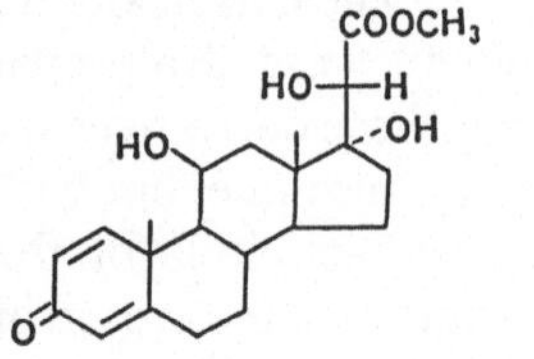


XXIV

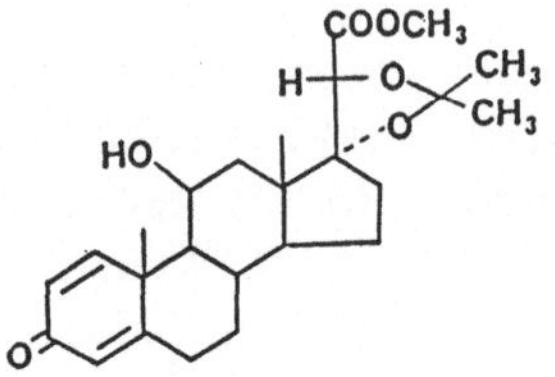


XXV

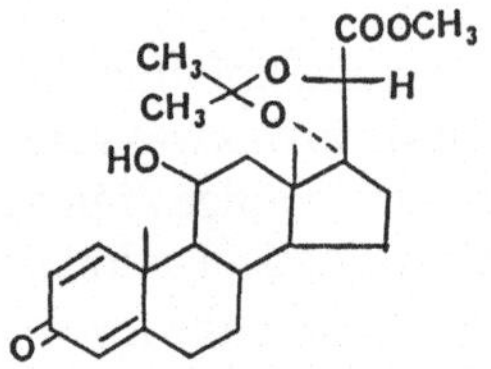


XXVI

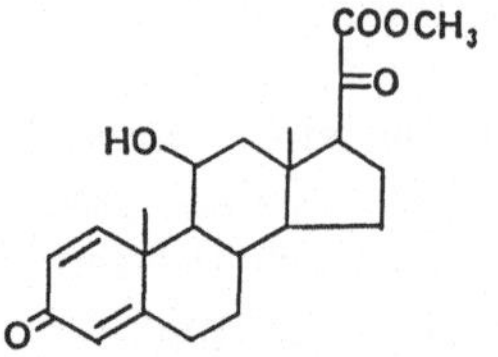


XXVII

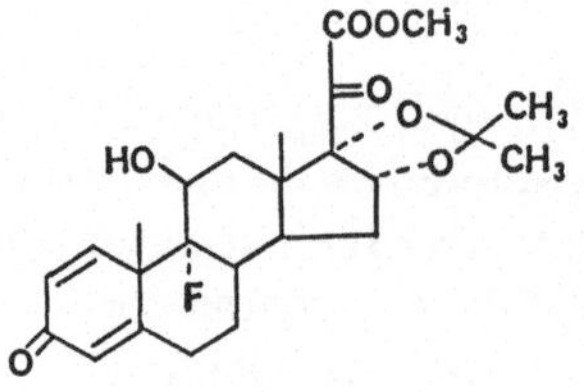


XXVIII

**Figure 7** Steroid 21-oate esters

As a logical extension of the protoypes of esters and amides of steroidal 21-oates, a new generation of derivatives of steroidal acids, i.e. steroids with various carboxylic acid groups at the strategic positions of 6α, 9α and 9β and 16α and 16β are under investigation[4]. The anti-inflammatory activity of some of these derivatives (Figure 9) is shown in Table 4. Of the 16-substituted derivatives tested to date, the methyl 16α-carboxylate 17-hydroxy derivative (XXXIV) shows the highest anti-inflammatory activity in the cotton pellet granuloma bioassay. Compared to prednisolone in full dose-response granuloma inhibition experiments, the estimated $ID_{50}$ for XXXIV was 0.4 mg/rat while the estimated prednisolone $ID_{50}$ was 2.2 mg/rat. Similarly, estimated $ID_{50}$ values for the systemic effect, thymic involution, have been calculated and are 1.5 mg/rat for both XXXIV and prednisolone. Thus, while the derivative XXXIV shows 5.5 times the local anti-inflammatory activity of prednisolone, there was no increased effect on relative thymic weights. The corresponding deoxy compound XXXIII showed lower local anti-inflammatory activity, and has an estimated $ID_{50}$ of 4 mg/rat for granuloma inhibition, but shows no significant thymic involution.

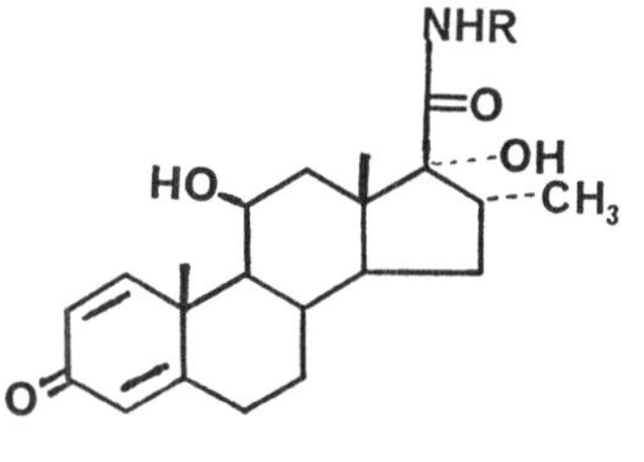

XXIX

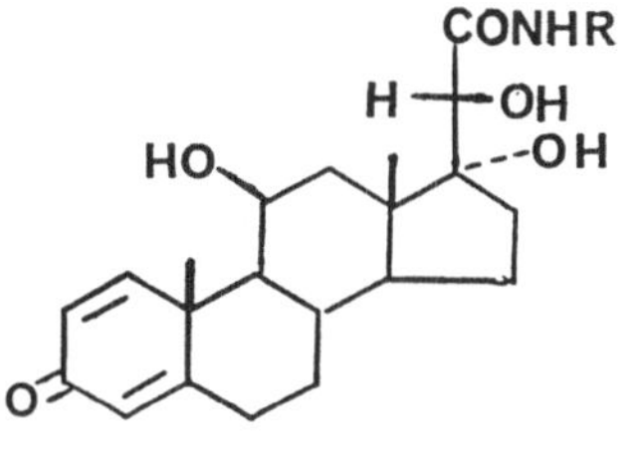

XXX a , R = $CH_3$
b , R = $C_2H_5$
c , R = $n\text{-}C_3H_7$
d , R = $CH_2Ph$

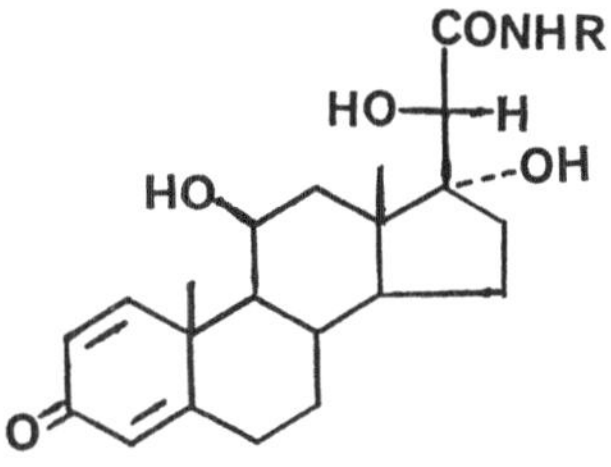

XXXI a, R = $CH_3$
b, R = $C_2H_5$
c, R = $n\text{-}C_3H_7$
d, R = $CH_2Ph$

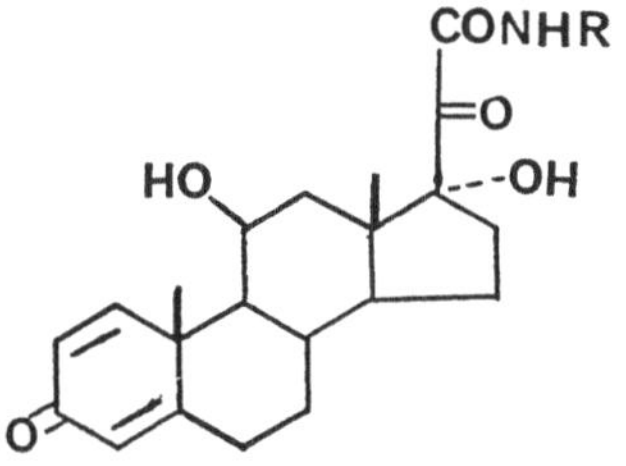

XXXII a, R = $CH_3$
b, R = $C_2H_5$
c, R = $n\text{-}C_3H_7$
d, R = $CH_2Ph$

**Figure 8** Steroidal carboxamides

Introduction of the bulkier malonate ester group at C-16, as in XXXV and XXXVI, essentially abolished the activity. Likewise, the methyl carboxymethyl ester XXXVII showed low anti-inflammatory activity but retained some thymic involution properties. This suggests that there is a steric size restriction for ester substituents at C-16. Various C-16 carboxamide derivatives are also currently under investigation.

**Table 2. Anti-inflammatory activity of methyl 20ξ-dihydroprednisolonate and its epimers**

| Test compound | Dose (mg/cotton pellet) | Dry weight of granuloma (mg) | Percentage granuloma inhibition | Relative weight of thymus (mg/100 g of body weight) | Relative weight of adrenals (mg/100 g of body weight) | Plasma corticosterone (μg/100 mg) |
|---|---|---|---|---|---|---|
| Control | 0.0 | 48.3 ± 2.6 | ---- | 217.8 ± 12.4 | 14.4 ± 0.4 | 25.8 ± 4.1 |
| Prednisolone | 2.5 | 16.6 ± 0.5** | 65.7 | 91.1 ± 8.0** | 11.9 ± 0.6 | 16.2 ± 6.9** |
| XXIII + XXIV | 2.5 | 18.9 ± 0.6** | 61.0 | 231.9 ± 10.5 | 13.8 ± 0.3 | 28.1 ± 5.5 |
| XXIII | 2.5 | 35.5 ± 1.3** | 26.5 | 217.6 ± 35.8 | 17.8 ± 0.3 | 25.4 ± 4.1 |
| XXIV | 2.5 | 18.3 ± 1.3** | 62.1 | 188.0 ± 28.1 | 13.1 ± 0.1 | 23.5 ± 8.1 |

Values are expressed as the mean ± SEM for six animals in each group. For steroid nomenclature refer to Figure 7. The Student's t-test was used to determine significant differences from the controls at $p < 0.01$ (**).

**Table 3  Effect of locally administered steroidal 20-carboxamides on cotton pellet-induced granuloma formation**

| Treatment | Treated pellet | | Untreated pellet | |
|---|---|---|---|---|
| | Dry weight (mg) | Percentage inhibition | Net dry weight (mg) | Percentage inhibition |
| Vehicle | 77.9 ± 2.6 | | 79.2 ± 3.9 | |
| Prednisole | 30.7 ± 5.2*** | 60.6 | 58.2 ± 6.8* | 26.6 |
| XXXa | 18.9 ± 1.3*** | 75.5 | 40.8 ± 5.4*** | 48.6 |
| XXXIa | 61.6 ± 9.9 | 21.1 | 82.8 ± 4.4 | − 4.5 |
| XXXb | 36.4 ± 5.0*** | 53.3 | 58.1 ± 5.0*** | 26.7 |
| XXXIb | 59.9 ± 5.3** | 23.1 | 83.1 ± 5.6 | − 4.9 |
| XXXc | 23.9 ± 5.6*** | 69.3 | 46.6 ± 9.6** | 41.2 |
| XXXIc | 33.4 ± 5.2*** | 57.1 | 48.3 ± 4.5*** | 39.1 |
| XXXd | 24.0 ± 4.7*** | 69.3 | 48.4 ± 6.9*** | 38.9 |
| XXXId | 61.6 ± 4.2** | 20.9 | 75.2 ± 5.9 | 5.2 |

Table values are the mean ± SEM for six animals. Treated pellets received 2.0 mg steroid. For steroid nomenclature, refer to Figure 8. The student's t-test was used to determine significant differences from the vehicle-treated controls at $p < 0.05$ (*), $p < 0.01$ (**) and $p < 0.005$ (***).

**Table 4  Anti-inflammatory activity and systemic effects of 16-carboxylate derivatives of prednisolone**

| Compound | Percent granuloma inhibition | | | Percenage control relative weights | |
|---|---|---|---|---|---|
| | Dose (mg/pellet) | Local | Systemic | Thymus | Adrenals |
| Prednisolone | 2.5 | 51.3*** | 24.7* | 45.2*** | 97.5 |
| XXXIII | 2.5 | 26.3* | 1.4 | 108.2 | 112.4 |
| XXXIV | 2.5 | 76.9*** | 39.7* | 24.3*** | 86.7* |
| | 0.25 | 34.1** | 1.7 | 100.6 | 111.6 |
| XXXV | 2.5 | −6.8 | 3.1 | 103.0 | 65.2* |
| XXXVI | 2.5 | 14.0 | 12.3 | 88.9 | 76.3 |
| XXXVII | 2.5 | 19.0* | 13.7 | 47.3*** | 81.3 |

Values indicate the average percentage inhibition or percentage of control with six animal per group. Indicated amounts of steroid were impregnated in one pellet which is used to determine local anti-inflammatory activity while the contralateral pellet received only vehicle (acetone) and is used to determine systemic anti-inflammatory activity. Student's t-test was used to determine values significantly different from controls at $p < 0.05$ (*), $p < 0.01$ (**) and $p < 0.005$(***). For steroid nomenclature refer to Figure 9.

171

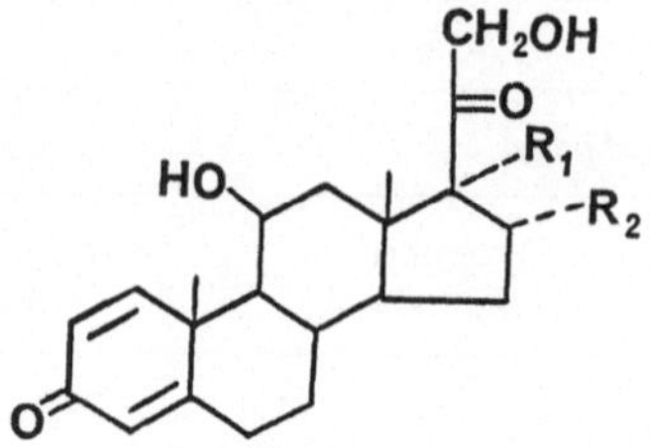

| XXXIII | $R_1 = H$, $R_2 = COOCH_3$ |
| XXXIV | $R_1 = OH$, $R_2 = COOCH_3$ |
| XXXV | $R_1 = H$, $R_2 = CH(COOCH_3)_2$ |
| XXXVI | $R_1 = OH$, $R_2 = CH(COOCH_3)_2$ |
| XXXVII | $R_1 = H$, $R_2 = CH_2COOCH_3$ |

**Figure 9**  C-16-substituted acid esters

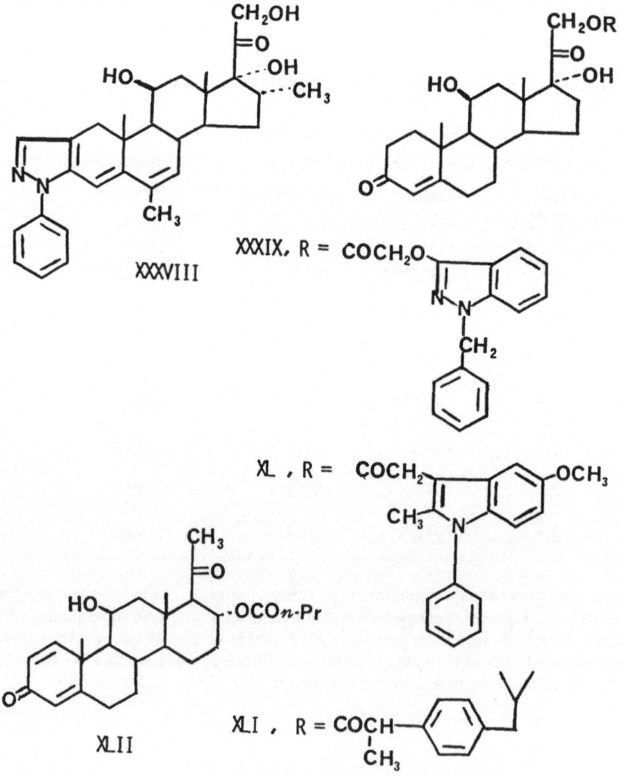

XXXVIII

XXXIX, R = $COCH_2O$

XL, R = $COCH_2$

XLI, R = $COCH-$

XLII

**Figure 10**  Miscellaneous new corticosteroids

172

## (c)  Miscellaneous compounds

*Cortivazole* (XXXVIII) is a corticosteroid in which a phenyl pyrazole ring is fused to the C-2,C-3 positions of ring A. The structure also incorporates a 6-methyl substituent and 6,7 unsaturation and a 16α-methyl substituent[63]. The combination of these structural features makes cortivazole a highly potent corticosteroid.

Esterification of the 21-hydroxyl group of a steroid with the carboxylic acid group of non-steroidal anti-inflammatory drugs such as benzadac, indomethacin and ibuprofen yielded the conjugated hydrocortisone esters (XXXIX, XL, XLI) that had low to moderate activities in the adjuvant arthritis and vasoconstriction assays[64].

*Domoprednate* (XLII), a new local steroid of moderate potency for dermatological use, has the unusual structural feature of being a D-ring homosteroid, in which the pregnane nucleus is replaced by a D-homopregnane nucleus, the first clinical steroid with this feature. In addition, it has a 17-oxobutoxy ester function. In a double-blind study in 20 volunteers with healthy skin, treatment with 5g of a 0.1% domoprednate ointment over a period of 2 weeks did not effect serum concentrations of cortisol, indicating a lack of suppressive effect of the drug on adrenal function[65].

## IV.  RECENT PROGRESS IN STEROID PHARMACOLOGY

Biological responses to the corticosteroids are biphasic: at the physiological level of hydrocortisone, < 30 mg/day in man, glucocorticoids are clearly homeostatic and essential for survival. However, at therapeutically effective doses, > 30 mg/day in man, glucocorticoids are predominantly catabolic and compromise the structural integrity of many tissues.

Though the pharmacological manner in which steroids express their activities after binding to the receptors remains largely unknown, significant progress has been made in: (1) the process of steroid-receptor binding and complexing with DNA, (2) receptor down regulation, and (3) induction of specific proteins such as phospholipase inhibitory proteins, vascular permeability regulatory proteins and angiotensin converting enzyme[66,67].

## (1)  Corticosteroid receptors

Glucocorticoids exert their anti-inflammatory activity by controlling the biosynthesis of certain proteins, probably as a result of alterations in gene expression in target tissues. The net result following steroid-receptor-chromosome interaction is accumulation of precursor mRNA which is spliced to mature mRNA which relocates to the cytoplasm, binds to ribosomes and directs synthesis of steroid-mediated effector proteins. Nuclear retention of the steroid-receptor complexes is believed to be required for maintenance of the steroid effect[68-70].

The traditional two-step model of steroid action, unoccupied cytosolic receptors which become occupied then translocate to the nucleus, has been recently challenged. Progesterone and oestrogen receptors may reside in the nuclear compartment, thus requiring no true nuclear translocation process. Unlike these, glucocorticoid receptors have been repeatedly observed in the cytoplasm, with an increase in nuclear receptor number after addition of glucocorticoids[71,72].

The magnitude of the biological responses of target cells to glucocorticoids correlates with the number of glucocorticoid receptors present. In several types of cell cultures, glucocorticoids have been shown to regulate their own receptor numbers. For example, in mouse AtT-20/D-1 pituitary tumour cells, prolonged incubation with glucocorticoid agonists resulted in a 75% reduction in total receptor number[73]. This down-regulation was not associated with a change in binding affinity but establishment of a new receptor equilibrium which remained stable until agonists were removed[74]. Similar down-regulation was observed in HeLA S3 human cells. Only those receptors which translocated to the nucleus were affected by the glucocorticoid treatment[75]. In glucocorticoid-responsive GH1 rat pituitary tumour cells, results of dense amine acid labelling studies suggested that as exposure to concentrations of glucocorticoids was increased, the amount of the monomeric (4S) cytosolic and nuclear receptors increased, while the amount of oligomeric (10S) cytosolic receptors decreased. The converse occurred following the removal of steroid[76,77]. Reversible binding of the monomeric form to DNA suggested that the monomer is the activated receptor form. The monomeric receptor may be regulated by reassociation to an oligomeric, non-steroid binding form, or degraded to an inactive receptor. Inactive steroid-binding sites have been described in nuclear extracts from female rat livers. Binding properties were clearly distinct from the nuclear high-affinity receptors since they exhibited moderate or low affinity with significant cross-reactivity between classes of steroids. Progesterone, oestradiol, testosterone and dexamethasone bound to the low-affinity binding sites. It has been postulated that these secondary binding sites may serve a protective physiological role[78].

*In vivo* studies which have shown neural glucocorticoid receptor down-regulation in rats subjected to sustained corticosterone secretion indicated that receptor number down-regulation constitutes a physiological phenomenon[79].

Under physiological conditions in glucocorticoid-responsive thymic cells, non-activated steroid-receptor complexes where necessary intermediates in initial formation of activated complexes. Greater efficacy of synthetic corticosteroids such as dexamethasone may be related to their ability to form increased ratios of active to non-active DNA-binding steroid-receptor complexes[80]. This suggests that cellular responses to glucocorticoids depend not only on the total number but the kind of steroid-receptor complexes formed.

Although most steroid hormone actions including anti-inflammatory actions of glucocorticoids involve genomic transcription, there are a few effects which appear to be unexplained non-nuclear actions. For example, glucocorticoids rapidly decrease ACTH release from AtT-20 cells. Little is known about how glucocorticoids mediate this response. A second, extensively studied effect is the glucocorticoid stabilization of lysosomes, an effect which requires high steroid concentrations.

## (2)  Steroid binding studies

Since interaction of a steroid with intracellular receptors is an obligatory step in the mechanism of action of glucocorticoids, the effectiveness of a steroid in eliciting or inhibiting a particular response has been explained by its intrinsic affinity for its receptor. Satisfactory parallelism between the affinities of a given new series of anti-inflammatory steroids has been reported except for a few exceptional cases where receptor accessibility is hindered by rapid metabolism and low lipid solubility.

Table 5. The relative binding affinity of steroid esters and amides to the cytosolic receptors of rat liver and thymus

| Compound | Liver | | Thymus | |
|---|---|---|---|---|
| | Relative affinity | $C_{50}$ | Relative affinity | $C_{50}$ |
| Dexamethasone | 100 | 32 nM | 100 | 138 nM |
| Prednisolone | 27 | 117 nM | 39 | 355 nM |
| XXV | 9 | 347 nM | 20 | 708 nM |
| XXVI | 2 | 1.6 $\mu$M | 5 | 2.8 $\mu$M |
| XXIII | 0.3 | 11.5 $\mu$M | 0.2 | 63.1 $\mu$M |
| XXIV | 0.1 | 31.6 $\mu$M | 0.1 | 89.1 $\mu$M |
| XXXc | 0.5 | 6.3 $\mu$M | 0.6 | 22.4 $\mu$M |
| XXXIc | 0.02 | 166 $\mu$M | 0.02 | 891.3 $\mu$M |

$C_{50}$ indicates the concentration required for 50% inhibition of the specific binding of 28 nM [$^3$H]dexamethasone to hepatic and thymus cytosol. For steroid nomenclature refer to Figure 7 and 8.

In mouse thymocytes, tixocortol pivalate, a moderately potent new steroid, was slightly less potent than cortisol. In intact rat renomedullary interstitial cells in culture, tixocortol pivalate was equipotent with cortisol acetate in displacing dexamethasone from the glucocorticoid receptor and in suppressing PGE$_2$ secretion[82].

Hydrocortisone 17-butyrate 21-propionate (HBP) has exhibited increased affinity for the glucocorticoid receptor of rat liver cytoplasmic fractions when compared with hydrocortisone. The increased affinity was attributed to the decreased dissociation rate at the receptor site. Likewise, esterification of the C-17 and/or C-21 hydroxyl groups of betamethasone or clobetasol significantly increased their affinities. The binding site of HBP appeared the same as the dexamethasone binding site and corresponded to the low-affinity hydrocortisone binding site[83]. These results suggest that esterification of the ketol group of corticoids may increase their affinities and potentiate their pharmacological activities.

The new ester and amide epimers of 20ξ-dihydroprednisolonic acid specifically bound to steroid receptors in both thymic and liver cytosolic preparations, as shown in Table 5. In the cotton pellet granuloma bioassay, calculated $ED_{50}$ for inhibition of granuloma formation is prednisolone 0.5 mg, XXV 1.0 mg, XXIV 1.3 mg, XXIII 5.8 mg and XXVI 6 mg. At the equipotent doses, in contrast to binding studies, the alpha epimers are not always more potent. Reasons for such a discrepancy may be due to metabolism, different receptor dissociation rates or binding to inactive versus active glucocorticoid receptors. Continuing investigations on metabolism of the esters, as well as cell binding studies, may account for this discrepancy.

Anti-glucocorticoids are steroidal or non-steroidal compounds which bind to the steroid receptor without eliciting normal steroidal responses of the cell. Recent results with L-929 mouse fibroblasts indicated that compounds RU486 bound to the glucocorticoid receptor with greater affinity than dexamethasone, but abolished the growth-arresting and decreasing adhesive responses normally seen when fibroblasts are treated with glucocorticoids[84]. Similarly, the anti-oestrogen tamoxifen inhibited cell growth and adhesiveness normally observed when L-929 cells were exposed to oestrogen[85]. Recently, 17β-carboxamide derivatives of dexamethasone behaved as antagonists in rat hepatoma cells, but acted as agonists by inhibiting the phytohaemagglutinin-mediated blastogenesis of normal human peripheral lymphocytes[86]. Expression of agonist versus antagonist activity for a given steroid-receptor complex is presumably determined by a balance of interactions between the receptor and several steroidal functional groups.

## (3)  Actions of glucocorticoids on leucocytes

Recent findings of the effects of glucocorticoids on leucocytes can be divided as follows: (1) effects on circulating cells, (2) effects on the vascular bed and (3) specific actions on leucocyte functions[87].

Following a moderate oral or parenteral dose of glucocorticoids, (50 mg prednisone or 350 mg hydrocortisone in man), effects on circulating white blood cells are neutrophilia, lymphopenia, monocytopenia, eosinopenia and basopenia. Lymphopenia, the result of a temporary redistribution of long-lived lymphocytes in tissues, is maximal at approximately 4 hours and returns to normal by 24 hours[88]. Since neutrophils are the predominant circulating white cell, total white counts may not change.

Results of *in vitro* studies with animals have shown that anti-inflammatory steroids reduce the margination and adherence of leucocytes to vascular endothelium following administration of an inflammatory stimulus[89]. Mechanisms by which steroids reduce margination and adherence or affect vasoconstriction are not well characterized; however, the overall observation in animal models of inflammation is decreases in exudate volume and in the number of leucocytes attracted to the site of inflammation.

**Table 6** Effects of steroids on leucocyte migration, exudate volume and circulating lymphocytes during carrageenan-induced pleurisy

| Treatment (mg/animal) | Leucocyte migration total cells (x 10 ) (% inhibition) | Exudate volume (ml) (% inhibition) | Percentage circulating lymphocytes |
|---|---|---|---|
| Control | $176.0 \pm 12.1$ | $2.7 \pm 0.3$ | $48.1 \pm 1.7$ |
| Prednisolone (0.5) | $70.6 \pm 8.1$*** (59.9) | $1.8 \pm 0.2$** (33.7) | $33.9 \pm 1.2$*** |
| XXV (1) | $97.9 \pm 9.5$*** (44.4) | $2.2 \pm 0.2$ (17.4) | $51.1 \pm 2.5$ |
| XIV (1.3) | $94.7 \pm 9.9$*** (46.2) | $1.7 \pm 0.1$*** (37) | $56.3 \pm 3.7$ |
| XXIII (5.8) | $107.3 \pm 11.9$*** (39.1) | $2.5 \pm 0.2$ (7.6) | $49.5 \pm 2.2$ |
| XXVI (6) | $120.2 \pm 11.7$*** (31.7) | $4.6 \pm -0.3$*** (-67.9) | $49.1 \pm 2.7$ |

Treatments (mg/animal) are equipotent doses which inhibit cotton pellet granuloma formation by 50% in a 7-day experiment with rats. Drugs were suspended in carboxymethylcellulose and injected into the pleural cavities just prior to injection of 0.2 ml of 0.5% carrageenan is saline. For steroid nomenclature, refer to Figure 7. Values are the means ± SEM for eight animals where ** ($p < 0.01$) and *** ($p < .005$) indicate differences significant from contols by the Student's $t$-test.

One well-characterized acute animal model for assessing potential anti-inflammatory drugs is caragenan (CGN)-induced pleurisy in the rat[90,91]. Although the model has been used less in the assesment of steroidal than non-steroidal anti-inflammatory agents, steroid data have been reported. When hydrocortisone or betamethasone was introduced into the pleural cavity at the time of carrageenan injection, dose-dependent reductions in the number of accumulated neutrophils and exudate volume were measured. The $ED_{50}$ values for these processes, 3 hours following injections were 100 μg/rat for hydrocortisone and 3 μg/rat for betamethasone. Since the ester derivatives of prednisolone were designed to be administered locally, we have adapted a similar model and injected steroidal suspensions followed by CGN directly into the pleural cavities. The numbers of cells (averaging 90% neutrophils) emigrating into the inflammatory site, exudate volumes and the percentage total circulating leucocytes which were lymphocytes were then measured 5 hours following local injections of steroids then CGN (Table

6). At doses which inhibit cotton pellet granuloma formation by 50%, all the ester derivatives of prednisolone significantly inhibited accumulation of neutrophils in the pleural cavities. Effects on exudate volume were more variable, however, as noted with budesonide in a pulmonary model of inflammation, oedema-blocking effects depend mainly upon systemic activity[93]. These derivatives of prednisolone, synthesized to maximise local activity, may be expected to have less effect on exudate volume. Similarly, the ester derivatives of $20\xi$-dihydroprednisolonic acid, in contrast to prednisolone and most classical steroids, did not induce lymphopenia; this may also be attributed to their enhanced local versus systemic activity.

Mechanisms which contribute to steroidal anti-inflammatory effects include induction of the synthesis of peptides such as lipomodulin or macrocortin (lipocortin) which block the phospholipase $A_2$-mediated release of arachidonic acid (AA) from membrane phospholipids. Recent evidence for phospholipase inhibition as a major mechanism of action of steroidal anti-inflammatory drugs has been concisely reviewed[89], as have the AA metabolites characteristic of distinct classes of leucocytes[94].

Inhibition of AA metabolites specifically by anti-inflammatory steroids has been reported for mast cells, endothelial cells, macrophages and synovial cells, among others. In mast cells, pretreatment with anti-inflammatory steroids such as fluocinolone, dexamethasone or hydrocortisone selectively inhibited IgE-mediated release of histamine and generation of AA and its metabolites (predominantly $PGD_2$). This inhibitory effect was consistent with induction of a phospholipase inhibitory protein[95,96]. In human endothelial cells, dexamethasone, hydrocortisone and triamcinolone were effective in suppressing release of $PGI_2$ and $PGE_2$. Presence of the glucocorticoid antagonist cortisol mesylate, which does not affect PG release alone, prevented the inhibitory action of the anti-inflammatory steroids[97].

Macrophages, which produce a number of inflammatory mediators that can be involved in tissue injury associated with inflammation as well as tissue repair mechanisms, are sensitive to anti-inflammatory steroids. In lipopolysaccharide-stimulated guinea-pig macrophages, therapeutically effective doses of dexamethasone inhibited the release of the proinflammatory mediators $PGE_2$ and collagenase. In contrast, macrophage-derived fibroblast-activating factor, which enhances connective tissue formation, was unaffected by dexamethasone at pharmacological concentrations[98]. While collagenase release by macrophages is dependent upon sequential events in the AA cascade, release of fibroblast-activating factor is independent of these events. Dissociation of regulatory mechanisms for release of macrophage pro-inflammatory mediators from tissue repair mediators might serve as a new rationale for the synthesis of anti-inflammatory steroids which do not jeopardise tissue repair.

Cells derived from cultured human synovium also release collagenase and prostaglandins, particularly $PGE_2$ and $PGF_{2\alpha}$. Synovial cells can be stimulated to synthesize and release these mediators by macrophage-derived interleukin 1 (IL-1)[99].

We have recently employed this system to study the effects of ester derivatives of prednisolone on $PGE_2$ synthesis by IL-1 stimulated human synovial cells in culture. When cells were pretreated with ester derivatives at $10^{-7}$ mol/l, XXV and the 16-carboxylate derivatives, XXXIII and XXXIV, were equipotent with prednisolone in inhibiting $PGE_2$ release, but XXIII and XXIV did not significantly alter its release (HJ Lee and JM Dayer, unpublished observations). These results suggest that there may be slightly differing mechanisms of action at the molecular level.

Both IL-1 and IL-2 have emerged as important mediators of immune responses. IL-1, found in many cell types, has emerged as a factor in the pathogenesis of rheumatoid arthritis since it induces release of collagenase and $PGE_2$ from cultured rheumatoid synovium fibroblast-type cells[100,101]. Chondrocytes derived from several species respond to human IL-1 by release of proteoglycan and collagenase-degrading enzymes. Chondrocytes derived from human osteoarthritic cartilage appear to be in an activated state and produce measurable amounts of proteoglycan- and collagen-degrading enzymes which can be further increased by exposure to human IL-1[102]. IL-1 has also been shown to mediate bone resorption[103]. The picture of IL-1 activities is complicated by recent evidence of *in vivo* generation of suppressive factors in human histiocyte cell line U937, cell line THP-1, glioblastoma cell line 308, EBV-transformed B cells and others. These suppressive factors may mask IL-1 activity in culture supernatants, inhibit T-cell IL-2 production and inhibit thymocyte proliferation. Their physiological functions are not well described[104]. A comparison between normal, recently active rheumatoid arthritic (RA) and stabilized RA people has shown that only monocytes from those having a recent RA exacerbation or onset exhibited elevated IL-1 release (twice the normal values). IL-2 release from peripheral blood mononuclear cells of all RA people were within normal range. This indicates that in RA, which may involve a disorder of macrophage-T cell interaction, elevated IL-1 is linked to an early event in onset of the disease[105]. The anti-inflammatory steroids hydrocortisone, dexamethasone and methyl-prednisolone have been shown to inhibit IL-2 production by mitogen-stimulated T-cell proliferation; this inhibition may involve corticosteroid-induced lipocortin which reduces $LTB_4$ generation[106,107].

The role(s) of anti-inflammatory steroids in suppressing inflammatory and immune responses are far from clear. However, there is much evidence that their effects are indirect actions via specific glucocorticoid receptors which interact with nuclear material in generating a network of mediators active in inflammation and immune responses. Two recently studied mediators include AA and its metabolites and IL-1. As better models for investigation become available, the network of glucocorticoid-controlled mediators central to specific inflammatory conditions will become characterized.

## V. CONCLUDING REMARKS

One of the remarkable aspects of the first decade that followed the historic discovery of cortisone as an anti-arthritis drug in 1948 was the rapidity with which major anti-inflammatory drugs were synthesized and put to therapeutic use. Initial success in the development of potent semisynthetic corticosteroids without salt-retaining activity was, however, quickly overshadowed by the fact that increases in anti-inflammatory activities were accompanied by proportional increases in various adverse effects. Despite the dramatic ability of the semisynthetic corticosteroids, the adverse effects preclude their routine therapeutic use. Apparently the nature of the corticosteroid molecule is such that the multiple glucocorticoid activities arise from common functional groups. Inseparability of anti-inflammatory from other glucocorticoid activities has led to efforts towards the synthesis of non-systemic corticosteroids.

The assertion that the multiplicity of steroid activities is only a different biological expression of a common mechanism of action, and that, therefore, separation of anti-inflammatory from other glucocorticoid activities is not possible, may not be tenable. With the corticosteroids of the 1980s exemplified in this review we have seen that from the chemist's viewpoint some degree of freedom is allowable in modifying the so-called untouchable functional groups of the molecule. From the pharmacologist's viewpoint there is evidence that not all the molecular mechanisms of action of anti-inflammatory steroids are identical.

Future breakthroughs in anti-inflammatory steroid drug development could arise with organized efforts of various research disciplines. Future research directions include the following:

1.   Steroids with bold structural changes should be synthesized and screened for structure-activity relationships. The retention of anti-inflammatory activity by steroids having modified so-called essential groups and/or functional groups at non-traditional positions provides a foundation upon which new avenues of steroid chemistry can be built.

2.   There is a need for development of new delivery systems for locally active anti-inflammatory steroids. Options in this area are liposomal delivery systems or conjugation of steroids to antibody Fab fragments somewhat akin to immunotoxin-targeting cancer therapy research.

3.   Since multiplicity of drug receptors is the rule for explaining the diversity of actions amongst most classes of drugs, exploration of possible diversity of tissue steroid receptor identity may lead to a basis for development of corticosteroids with selectivity.

4.     Continued discovery and characterization of the effector proteins induced by glucocorticoids which lead to amelioration of inflammation could have an important impact upon future drug design.

5.     Expanded investigations of the molecular mechanisms of action of new steroids, especially those with modified essential functional groups, are needed. Delineating such differences could evolve into the synthesis of rationally designed agents which uniquely modulate pathways of inflammation. Unfortunately, very few of the new corticosteroids have been tested for mechanisms of action other than the inhibition of AA release.

6.     There is a need for application of cell culture systems for screening, as well as testing specific biological activities of new anti-inflammatory steroids.

The recent achievements in the chemistry and pharmacotherapy of corticosteroids have been dominated by local anti-inflammatory steroidal compounds. Anti-inflammatory activities with concomitant reduction in side-effects, particularly for those steroids with non-traditional modifications, are significant advances, and should enliven interest and future research activities.

## REFERENCES

1.     Hench, PS, Kendall, EC, Slocumb, CH and Polley, HF (1950). Effects of cortisone acetate and pituitary ACTH on rheumatoid arthritis, rheumatic fever and certain other conditions. *Arch Intern Med,* **85,** 545-666

2.     Bernstein, S (1982). Glucocorticoids: past, present and future. In Lee, HJ and Fitzgerald, TJ (eds) *Progress in research and Clinical Applications of Corticosteroids*, pp. 230-42. (Philadelphia: Heyden and Sons)

3.     Lee, HJ, Khalil, MA and Lee, JW (1984). Antedrug: a conceptual basis for safer anti-inflammatory steroids. *Drugs Exp Clin Res,* **X,** 835-44

4.     Lee, HJ (1986). Anti-inflammatory carboxy pregnane derivatives. *US Patent* application No. 828, 460

5.     Thalen, A and Brattsand, E (1979). Synthesis and anti-inflammatory properties of Budesonide, a new non-halogenated glucocorticoid with high local activity. *Arzneim-Forsch Drug Res,* **29(II),** 687-90

6.     Brattsand, P, Thalen, A, Roempke, K *et al.* (1982). Influence of $16\alpha,17\alpha$-acetal substitution and steroid nucleus fluorination in the topical to systemic activity ratio of glucocorticoids. *J Steroid Biochem,* **16,** 779-86

7.     Anderson, P, Edsbacker, S, Ryrfeldt, L and von Bahr, C. (1982). In vitro biotransformation of glucorcorticoids in liver and skin homogenate fraction from man, rat and hairless mouse. *J.Steroid Biochem,* **16,** 778-95

8.     Bush, IE (1962). Chemical and biological factors in the activity of adrenocortical steroids. *Pharmacol Rev,* **14,** 374-92

9.     Ryrfeldt, L, Andersson, P, Edsbacker, S *et al.* (1982). Pharmacokinetics and metabolism of Budesonide, a selective glucocorticoid. *Eur J Resp Dis,* **63** (Suppl.122), 86-95

10.    Adelroth, E, Rosenhall, L and Glennon, C. (1985). High dose inhaled Budesonide in the treatment of severe steroid dependent ashmatics; a two year study. *Allergy,* **40,** 58-64

11.    Webb, DR, Mullarkey, MF and Freeman MJ (1979). Flunisolide in chronic bronchial asthma. *Ann Allergy,* **42,** 80-2

12.    Sarsfield, JK and Thompson, GE (1979). Flunisolide nasal spray in perennial rhinitis in children. *Br Med J,* **2,** 95-7

13.    Criscuolo, D, Fraioli, F, Bonifacio V, *et al*. (1980). Effects of a new glucocorticoid, deflazacort on pituitary-adrenal function in man: a comparison with prednisolone. *Int J Clin Pharmacol Ther Toxicol,* **18,** 37-41

14.    Barbieri, C, Baruto, C, Sala M, *et. al*. (1985). Lack of effect of deflazacort, a novel glucocorticoid on basal and TRH-stimulated prolactin and thyrotropin levels in healthy human adults. *Eur J Clin Pharmacol,* **29,** 123-5

15.    Wojnar, RJ, Alpaugh, WC and Dzelzkalns, E. (1985). Characterization of the anti-inflammatory activity and reduced potential for dermal atrophy of (11β, 16β)-9-fluoro-1',2',3'4'-tetrahydro-11,21-dihydroxypregna-1,4-dieno[16,17]naphthalene-3,20-dione hydrate (1:1), a topically active corticoid. *Arzneim-Forsch /Drug Res,* **35(II),** 1264-8.

16.    Ponec, M, Kempenaar, JA and Shroot, B (1986). Glucocorticoids; binding affinity and lipophilicity. *J Pharm Sci,* **75,** 973-5

17.    Shroot, B, Caron, JC and Ponec, M (1982). Glucocorticoid-specific binding. Structure-activity relationships. *Br J Dermatol,* **107,** (Suppl 23), 30-4

18.    Ponec, M, Kempenaar, JA and Kloet, ER (1981). Corticoids and cultured human epidermal keratinocytes: Specific intracellular binding and clinical efficacy. *J Invest Dermatol,* **76,** 211-14

19.    Ponec, M (1982). Glucocorticoids and cultured human skin cells. Specific intracellular binding and structure-activity relationships. *Br J Dermatol,* **107,** (Suppl 23), 24-9

20.    Alperman, HG, Sandow, J and Vogel, HG (1982). Tierexperimentelle Untersuchungen zur topischen und systemischer Wirksamkeit von Prednisolon-17-ethylcarbonat-21-propionat. *Arzneim-Forsch /Drug Res,* **32,** 633-8

21.    Stache, U, Fritsch, W, Rupp, H *et al*. (1985). Synthese von Prednicarbat, einem halogenfrein topisch anti-inflammatorisch wirksamen Derivat des Prednisolon-17-ethylkohlrensaureesters. *Arzneim-Forsch/Drug Res,* **35 (II),** 1753-7

22.    Sugai, S, Okazaki, T, Kajiwara, Y, *et al*. (1985). Studies on topical anti-inflammatory corticosteroids. I Syntheses and vasoconstrictive activities of 11β, 17β, 21-trihydroxy-6α methyl-1,4-pregnadiene-3,20-dione 17-ester and 17,21-diester derivatives. *Chem Pharm Bull,* **33,** 1889-98

23.    Sugai, S, Okazaki, T, Kajiwara, Y, *et al*. (1986). Studies on topical anti-inflammatory corticosteroids. II-Synthesis and vascoconstrictive activity of 11β,17β,21-trihydroxy-6α-methyl-1,4-pregnadiene-3,20-dione 17-methoxy and (methylthio) acetates. *Chem Pharm Bull,* **34,** 1607-12

24.    Sota, K, Mitsukuchi, M, Nakagami, T, *et al*. (1982). Synthesis and anti-inflammatory activity of hydrcortisone-17,21-diester, *Yakugaku Zasshi 102,* 365-70

25.    Kimura, M, Tarumoto, Y, Nakane, S and Otomo, S (1986). Comparative toxicity study of hydrocortisone-17-butyrate-21-proprionate (HBP) ointment and other topical corticosteroids in rats. *Drugs Exp Clin Res,* **12,** 643-52

26.    Kitano, Y (1986). Hydrolysis of hydrocortisone-17-butyrate-21-proptionate by cultured human keratinocytes. *Acta Dermatol Venereol, (Stockh),* **66,** 98-102

27.    Lutsky, BN, Berkenkopf, J, Fernandez, X, *et al*. (1979). Selective effects of 7α-halogeno substitution on corticosteroid activity. Sch. 22209 and Sch. 23409. *Arzneim-Forsch/Drug Res,* **29(I),** 992-8

28. Green, MJ, Berkenkopf, J, Fernandez, X, *et al.* (1970). Synthesis and structure-activity relationships in a novel series of topically active corticosteroids. *J Steroid Biochem*, **11**, 61-6

29  Shue, H-J, Green, MJ, Berkenkopf, J, *et al.* (1980). Synthesis and structure-activity studies of 7α-halogeno corticosteroids. *J Med Chem*, **23**, 430-7

30. Lutsky, BN, Berkenkopf, J, Fernandez, X, *et al.* (1979). A novel class of potent topical anti-inflammatory agents. *Arzneim-Forsch /Drug Res*, **29**(I), 1662-7

31. Green, MJ, Shue, H-J,. Tiberi, R, *et al.* (1980). The influence of esterification on the topical anti-inflammatory activity of 7α-chloro and 7α-bromo-16α-methyl-prednisolones. *Arzneim-Forsch/Drug Res*, **30**(II), 1618-20

32. Mizushima, Y, Hoski, K and Kaneko, K (1981). Intra-articular injection of a highly topical corticosteroid in rheumatoid arthritis. *Drugs Exp Clin Res*, **7**, 633-5

33. Kiniwa, M and Miyake, M (1986). Selective local anti-inflammatory activity of THS-201, new intra-articular steroid in cotton pellet granuloma and monoarticular arthritis. *Arch Int Pharmacodyn Ther*, **200**, 153-64

34. Ortega, E, Rodriquez, C, Strand, L and Segre, E (1986). Effects of cloprednol and other corticosteroids on hypothalmic-pituitary-adrenal axis function. *J Int Med Res*, **4**, 326-30

35. Schwarz, K, Konzelman, M, Yawalkar, SJ and Schonenberger, PM (1982). A double blind comparison between a new trihalogenated dermatocorticosteroid (Halometasone) cream and clobetasol-17-propionate (Dermovate) cream. *Br J Clin Pract*, **36**, 192-6

36. Blum, G and Yawalkar, SJ (1983). Evaluation of Halometasone cream in the treatment of paediatric patients with acute excematous dermatoses. *J Int Med Res*, **11**, (Suppl. 1), 8-12

37. Tomasini, C and Castiglioni, G (1983). Plasma cortisol studies with 0.05% Halometasone cream and ointment in patients with psoriasis. *J Int Med Res*, **11**, (Suppl. 1), 38-42

38. Davies, JE, Kellet, DN, Staniforth, MW, *et al.* (1981). Pharmacological study on a new anti-inflammatory steroid. Tixocortol Pivalate (JO 1016). *Arzneim-Forsch/Drug Res*, **31**(I),453-59

39. Larochelle, P, DuSouith, B, Bolte, E, *et al.* (1983). Tixocortol pivalate: a corticosteroid with no systemic glucocorticoid effect after oral, intrarectal and intranasal application *Clin Pharmacol Ther*, **33**, 343-56

40. Uphill, PF (1981). A comparison of the effects of tixocortol pivalate and beclomethasone dipropionate and hydrocortisone acetate on the activation of lymphocytes. *Arzneim-Forsch/Drug Res*, **31**(I), 459-62

41. Uphill, PF and Daniel, MR (1981). A comparison of the effects of tixocortol pivalate, hydrocortisone acetate and declomethasone diproprionate on collagen synthesis and degradation. *Arzneim-Forsch/Drug Res*, **31**(I), 467-9

42. Teitelbaum, PJ and Ho, WK (1985). Metabolism of RS-35909. A novel thioester containing corticosteroid,. *Fed Proc*, Suppl. 4(C), Abstr. 8552, 1732

43. Devlin, RG, Dean, A, Kriplani, K, *et al.* (1986). Percutaneous absorption and adrenal suppressive potency of Tipredane, a new topical corticosteroid, *J Toxicol-Cut Ocular Toxicol*, **5**, 35-43

44. Fox, PK, Lewis, AJ, Rae, RM, *et al.* (1980). The biological properties of Org 6216, a new type of steroid with a selective local anti-inflammatory action. *Arzneim-Forsch/Drug Res*, **30**(I), 55-9

45. Lewis, AJ (1980). The local anti-inflammatory activity of Rimexolone (Org 6216) in fibrin-induced monoarticular arthritis and adjuvant induced arthritis. *Agents Actions*, **10**, 258-65

46. Rapi, G, Chelli, M, Ginanneschi, M *et al.* (1985). Synthesis of new aminooxazolyl 17-steroids and pharmacological studies on the whole series. *J Med Chem-Chim Ther*, **20**, 277-82

47.  Rapi, G, Ginanneschi, M, Chelli, M and Chimichi, S (1985). Reaction of some anti-inflammatory 17β-(2-aminooxazol-4-yl) steroids with hydrogen peroxide. Synthesis of steroid 17-spiro-5'-oxazolidino-2'4-diones. *Steroids,* **46,** 665-76

48.  Stonner, FW (1972). 17-hydroxy-17-ethynyl-4-androsteno-[3,2-c]-2'9(p-fluorophenyl) pyrazole and compositions containing same. *U.S. Patent* 3, 657,435

49.  Schane, HP, Harding, HR, Creange, JE *et al.* (1984). Nivazol: a glucocorticoid in rats with only hypothalmic-pituitary-adrenal inhibitory activity in primates. *Endocrinology,* **114,** 1983-9

50.  Winneker, RC, Russel, MM, Might, CK and Schane, HP (1984). The interaction of nivazol with the glucocorticoid receptor from rat and rhesus monkey target tissues. *Steroids,* **44,** 447-52

51.  Popper, TL and Watnick, AS (1984). Anti-inflammatory steroid. In Scherrer RA and Whitehouse, MW (eds). *Anti-inflammatory Agents - Chemistry and Pharmacology.* Vol I, pp 245-94. (New York: Academic Press)

52.  Soliman, MRI and Lee, HJ (1981). Local anti-inflammatory activity of acid ester derivatives of prednisolone. *Res Commun Chem Pathol Pharmacol,* **33,** 357-60

53.  Lee, HJ and Soliman MRI (1982). Anti-inflammatory steroids without pituitary-adrenal suppression. *Science,* **215,** 989-991

54.  DiPetrillo, L, Lee, HJ and Cutroneo, KR (1984). Anti-inflammatory steroids that neither inhibit collagen synthesis nor cause dermal atrophy. *J Invest Dermatol,* **19,** 878-83

55.  Lee, JW and Lee, HJ (1985). Binding of ester and amide epimers of 20ξ -dihydro-prednisolonic acid to cytosol receptors and their acute pharmacological activities in rats. *J Steroid Biochem,* **23,** 943-48

56.  Bird, J, Kim, HP and Lee, HJ (1986). Topical anti-inflammatory activity of esters of steroid-21-oic acids. *Steroids,* **47,** 35-45

57.  Kumari, D and Lee, HJ (1985). Hydrolysis of methyl steroid 21-oates and acetyl steroid 21-ols by rat liver microsomes. *Drug Metab Disp,* **13,** 627-9

58.  Bird, J, Lay, JC and Lee, HJ (1986). The effects of new local anti-inflammatory steroids on leucocyte migration and prostanoid liberation in rats. *J Pharm Pharmacol,* **38,** 589-94

59.  Olejniczak, E and Lee, HJ (1984). Systemic effects of chronically administered methyl prednisolonate and methyl 17-deoxyprednisolonate. *Steroid,* **43,** 657-62

60.  Gorsline, J, Bradlow, HL and Sherman, MR (1985). Triamcinolone acetonide methyl ester, a potent local anti-inflammatory steroid without detectable side-effects. *Endocrinology,* **116,** 263-73

61.  Kim, HP, Bird, J, Heiman, AS, *et al.* (1987). Manuscript submitted to *J Med Chem*

62.  Rousseau, GG and Schmidt, JP (1977). 17β-carboxamide steroids are a new class of glucocorticoid antagonists. *Nature,* **279,** 158-60

63.  Steelman, SDI, Morgan, ER and Glitzer, MS (1971). Heterocyclic corticosteroids. I Biological properties of the 6,16-dimethyl-4,6-pregnadiene-11β-17,21-triol-20-one-[3,2-c]-2'-phenylpyrazole. *Steroids,* **18,** 129-33

64.  Laurent H, Albring, M and Wendt H (1984). Syntheses und antiinflammatorische Wirking vor Estern entzundungshemmender Carbonsauren mit Hydrocortison. *Arch Pharm (Weinheim),* **317,** 421-4

65.  Schmidt, H and Holm, P (1985). Domoprednate, R012-7024 (Stermonid), a topical D-homocorticosteroid and andrenocortical function: a double blind randomized comparison with betamethasone valerate in volunteers. *Curr Ther Res,* **37,** 207-12

66.  DiRosa, M, Calignana, A, Carnuccio, R, *et al.* (1985). Multiple control of inflammation by glucocorticoids, *Agents Actions,* **17,** 284-9

67.  Dupont, E and Wybron, J (1985), Mechanisms of action of corticosteroids. *Int J Immunother,* **1,** 135-8

68.  Schmidt, TJ and Litwack, GL (1982). Activation of the glucocorticoid receptor complex. *Physiol Rev,* **62,** 1131-92

184

69. Johnson, LK, Longnecker, JP, Baxter, JD et al. (1982). Glucocorticoid action: a mechanism involving nuclear and non-nuclear pathways. Br J Dermatol, 107, Suppl. 23, 6-23

70. Yamamoto, KR (1985). Steroid receptor regulated transcription of specific genes and gene networks. Ann Rev Genet, 19, 209-52

71. Gasc, J-M and Baulieu, E-E (1986). Steroid hormone receptors: intracellular dsitribution. Biol Cell, 56, 1-6

72. Antakly, T and Eisen, HJ (1984). Immunocytochemical localization of glucocorticoid receptor in target cells. Endocrinology, 115, 1984-9

73. Svec, F and Rudis, M (1981). Glucocorticoids regulate the glucocorticoid receptor in the AtT-20 cell. J Biol Chem, 256, 5984-7

74. Svec, F (1985). Biopotency of corticosterone and dexamethasone in causing glucocorticoid receptor down regulation. J Steroid Biochem, 23, 669-71

75. Cidlowski, JA and Cidlowski, NB (1981). Regulation of glucocorticoid receptors by glucocorticoids in cultured HeLA S₃ cells. Endocrinology, 109, 1975-82

76. Raaka, BM and Samuels, HH (1983). The glucocorticoid receptor in GH1 cells. J Biol Chem, 208, 417-25

77. McIntre, WR and Samuels, HH (1985). Triamcinolone acetonide regulates glucocorticoid receptor levels by decreasing the half-life of the activiated nuclear-receptor form. J Biol Chem, 260, 418-27

78. Bechet, DM and Perry, BN (1986). A novel class of inactive steroid-binding sites in female rat liver nuclei. J Endocrinol, 110, 27-36

79. Sapolsky, RM, Krey, LC and McEwen, BS (1984). Stress downregulates corticosterone receptors in a site-specific manner in the brain. Endocrinology, 114, 287-92

80. Guyre, P, Bodwell, J, Holbrook, NJ, et al. (1982). Glucocorticoids and the immune system: activation of glucocorticoid-receptor complexes in thymus cells; modulation of Fc-receptors of phagocytic cells. In Lee, HJ and Fitzgerald, TJ (eds) Progress in Research and Clinial Applications of Corticosteroids, pp. 14-27. (London: Heyden)

81. Lee, HJ, Bradlow, HL, Moran, MC and Sherman, MR (1981). Binding of glucocorticoid 21-oic acids and esters to molybdate-stabilized hepatic receptors. J Steroid Biochem, 14, 1325-35

82. Lelievre, V, Junien, JL, Goyer, R and Russo-Marrie, F (1984). Affinity of tixocortol pivalate (Jo 1016), tixocortol, cortisone acetate and cortisol for dexamethasone receptors of mouse thymus cells and rat renomedullary interstitial cells in culture. Correlation with their biological activities. J Steroid Biochem, 20, 363-6

83. Muramatsu, M, Fujita, A, Tanaka, M, et al. (1986). Enhancement of affinity to receptors in the esterified glucocorticoid, hydrocortisone 17-butyrate 21-proprionate (HBP) in the rat liver. Biochem Pharmacol, 35, 1933-7

84. Bertagna, X, Bertagna, C, Luton, JP, et al. (1984). The new steroid analog RU486 inhibits glucocorticoid action in man. J Clin Endocrinol Metab, 59, 25

85. Jung-Testas, I and Baulieu, E-E (1984). Anti-steroid action in cultured L-929 mouse fibroblasts. J Steroid Biochem, 20, 301-6

86. Manz, B, Rehder, M, Heubner, A, et al. (1984). 17-carboxamide steroids: highly effective inhibitors of the phytohaemagglutinin mediated blastogenesis of normal human peripheral lymphocytes. J Clin Chem Clin Biochem, 22, 209-14

87. Meulesman, J and Katz, P (1985). The immunologic effects, kinetics and use of glucocorticosteroids. Med Clin, 69, 805-16

88. Claman, HN (1984). Anti-inflammatory effects of corticosteroids. Clin Immunol Allergy, 4, 317-29

89. Schleimer, RP (1985). The mechanisms of anti-inflammatory steroid action in allergic diseases. Ann Rev Pharmacol Toxicol, 25, 381-412

90. Taylor, BM and Sun, FF (1985). Disappearance and metabolism of leukotriene B 4 during carrageenan-induced pleurisy. Biochem Pharmacol, 34, 3495-8

91.  Almeida, AP, Bayer, BM, Horakova, Z and Beaven MA (1980). Influence of indomethacin and other anti-inflammatory drugs on mobilization and production of neutrophils: studies with carrageenan-induced inflammation in rats. *J Pharmacol Exp Ther*, **214**, 74-9

92.  Vinegar, R, Truax, JF and Selph, JL (1976). Quantitative studies of the pathway to acute carrageenan inflammation. *Fed Proc*, **35**, 2447-54

93.  Brattsand, R, Kallstrom, L, Johansson, U and Dahlback, M (1985). Route of administration and rapid inactivation as determinants of the lung-specific actions of glucocortocosteroids. *In Glucocorticosteroids, Inflammation and Bronchial Hyperactivity*, pp. 145-155. (Symposium at the 3rd Congress of the European Society of Pneumonology, Basel). (Amsterdam:Excerpta Medica)

94.  Goetzl, E (1981), Oxygenation products of arachidonic acid as mediators of hypersensitivity and inflammation. *Med Clin N Am*, **65**, 809-28

95.  Heiman, AS and Crews, FT (1984). Inhibition of immunoglobulin but not peptidebase stimulated release of histamine and arachidonic acid by anti-inflammatory steroids. *J Pharmacol Exp Ther*, **230**, 175-82

96.  Daeron, M, Sterk, A, Hirata, F and Ishizaka, T (1982). Biochemical analysis of glucocorticoid-induced inhibition of IgE-mediated histamine release from mouse mast cells. *J Immunol*, **129**, 1212-18

97.  Lewis, GA, Campbell, WB and Johnson, AR (1986). Inhibition of prostaglandin synthesis by glucocorticoids in human endothelial cells. *Endocrinology*, **119**, 62-9

98.  Wahl, SM and Wahl, LM (1985). Regulation of macrophage collagenase, prostaglandin and fibroblast-activating-factor production by anti-inflammatory agents: different regulatory mechanisms for tissue injury and repair. *Cell Immunol*, **92**, 302-12

99.  Nardella, FA, Dayer, J-M, Roelke, M, *et al*. (1983). Self-associating IgG rheumatoid factors stimulate monocytes to release prostaglandins and mononuclear cell factor that stimulates collagenase and prostaglandin production by synovial cells. *Rheumatol Int*, **3**, 183-6

100. Oppenheim, JJ, Kovacs, EJ, Matsushima, K and Durum, SK (1986). There is more than one interleukin 1. *Immunol Today*, **7**, 45-56

101. Balavoine, J-F, deRochemonteix, B, Williamson, K. *et al*. (1986). Prostaglandin E2 and collagenase production by fibroblasts and synovial cells is regulated by urinederived human interleukin 1 and inhibitors. *J Clin Invest*, **78**, 1120-4

102. DiPasquale, G, Caccese, R, Pasternak, R, *et al*. (1986). Proteoglycan- and collagendegrading enzymes from human inteleukin-1 stimulated chondrocytes from several species: proteoglycanase and collagenase inhibitors as potentially new disease-modifying antiarthritic agents. *Proc Soc Exp Biol Med*, **183**, 262-7

103. Gowen, M, Wood, DD, Ihrie, EJ, *et al*. (1983). An interleukin 1-like factor stimulated bone resorption in vitro. *Nature*, **306**, 378-80

104. Krakauer, T (1986). Human interleukin 1, *CRC Crit Rev Immunol*, **6**, 213-44

105. Shore, A, Jaglal, S and Keystone, EC (1986). Enhanced interleukin 1 generation by monocytes *in vitro* is temporaily linked to an early event in the onset or exacerbation of rheumatoid arthritis. *Clin Exp Immunol*, **65**, 293-302

106. Randazzo, B, Hirschberg, T and Hirschberg, H (1984). Inhibition of the antigen-activated T cell response by methylpredinsolone is caused by inhibition of interleukin-2 production. *Int J Immunopharmacol*, **6**, 419-29

107. Goodwin, JS, Atlura, D, Sierakowski, S and Lianos, EA (1986). Mechanism of action of glucocorticosteroids. Inhibition of T cell proliferation and interluekin 2 production by hydrocortisone is reversed by leukotriene B4. *J Clin Invest*, **77**, 1244-50

# 7
# Oxyradicals, inflammation and drugs acting on oxyradical production

**Dennis V. Parke, Andrew M. Symons and Ann L. Parke**
Department of Biochemistry, University of Surrey, Guildford, Surrey, UK
and Division of Rheumatic Diseases, University of Connecticut Health
Center, Farmington, Connecticut, USA

Rheumatoid arthritis is a chronic systemic disease, with an autoimmune component, involving both humoral and cellular mechanisms. The biochemical mechanisms concerned are esoteric and involve the formation of immune complexes resulting in the production of oxygen radicals, with consequent damage of membranes, and activation of phospholipase $A_2$. The subsequent release of arachidonate from membrane phospholipids leads to increased production of prostanoids. The production of oxygen radicals also results in the destruction of microsomal cytochromes, with impairment of corticosteroid biosynthesis, anaemia and accumulation of inorganic iron. All these molecular events, comprising a partly self-promoting cascade of chronic immunological injury, are considered to be initiated, at least originally, by an immune response to some infectious agent or ingested antigen and to be mediated by oxygen radicals (see Figure 1). However, although recent trends have been for physicians and pharmaceutical companies to exploit possible therapeutic benefits of oxygen radical scavengers and antioxidants in the treatment of rheumatoid disease, unequivocal evidence *in vivo* of oxygen radical involvement in arthritic tissue damage, and of therapeutic benefit of radical scavengers, is somewhat lacking[1]. This chapter is therefore directed to reviewing existing evidence for the participation of oxygen radicals in rheumatoid disease, and to consider the possible forms of treatment which involve inhibition of oxyradical production and prevention of oxyradical tissue damage.

*New Developments in Antirheumatic Therapy.* Rainsford, KD and Velo, GP (eds),
Inflammation and Drug Therapy Series, Volume III.

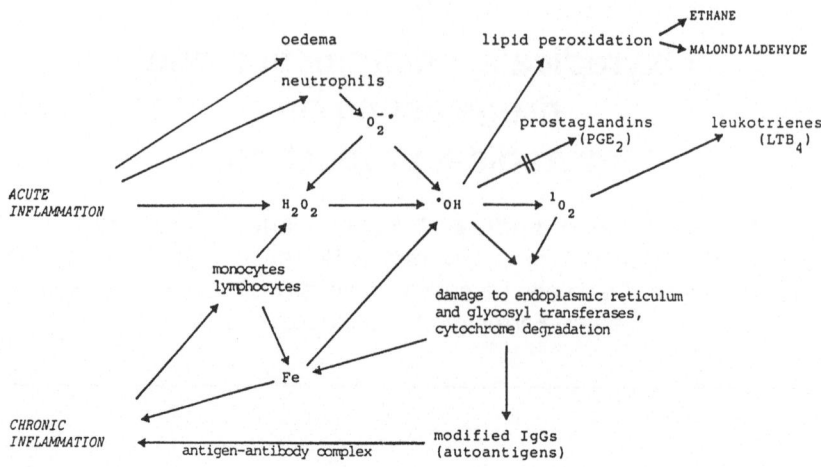

**Figure 1**  Oxyradical mediation of acute and chronic immunological injury. Key to abbreviations: $O_2^{-\cdot}$, superoxide radical; $H_2O_2$, hydrogen peroxide; $^1O_2$, singlet oxygen; $^\cdot OH$, hydroxyl radical

## I.  PATHOGENESIS OF RHEUMATOID DISEASE

In rheumatoid arthritis, a systemic autoimmune disease, immune complexes consisting exclusively of immunoglobulin are present, indicating that both antigen (mostly IgG) and antibody (rheumatoid factor) are derived from endogenous immunoglobulins. Although no polypeptide determinant for auto-antigenicity in the IgGs has been detected, carbohydrate changes have been reported, and extensive studies of IgG samples from 46 rheumatoid arthritis patients, normal individuals, and patients with osteoarthritis, from Oxford and Tokyo, have confirmed changes in the extents of glycosylation of these immunoglobulins, though no novel oligosaccharides were found[2]. IgGs containing oligosaccharide chains lacking galactose and, consequently, lacking one or both terminal sialic acid moieties, are increased in both rheumatoid arthritis ($51\pm8\%$ total IgGs) and osteoarthritis ($35\pm5\%$) over control ($25\pm5\%$). This could explain the persistence of IgG complexes in rheumatoid disease, which may or may not involve true autoimmune response. Although osteoarthritis is clinically distinct from rheumatoid arthritis, and is not associated with autoimmunity or with pathological levels of immune complexes in the serum, it is associated with an altered glycosylation pattern of serum IgG. This might also extend to the proteoglycans of the joints and hence result in increased susceptibility to degradation, characteristic of osteoarthritis. Similarly, it is probable that the glycosylation of other glycoproteins in rheumatoid patients, such as cell-surface major histocompatibility antigens, are likewise affected, thus explaining the known relationships between rheumatoid arthritis and certain HLA antigens[2].

The glycosyl side-chains of the glycoproteins of the cell-surface gly-cocalyx, and of the lysosomal enzymes, also undergo changes in malignancy and in cell transformation[3]. A common feature of rheumatoid arthritis and malignancy is the increased production of oxygen radicals, which is known to damage the endoplasmic reticulum, the site of glycosylation and glycopro-tein synthesis. Hence, whatever the initiating antigen, the prolonged produc-tion of oxygen radicals in rheumatoid disease could damage the endoplasmic reticulum and certain glycosyl transferases, resulting in the synthesis of ab-normally high amounts of IgG with deficient oligosaccharides that could con-sequently act immunogenically to produce the chronic immunological condition of rheumatoid arthritis (see Figure 1).

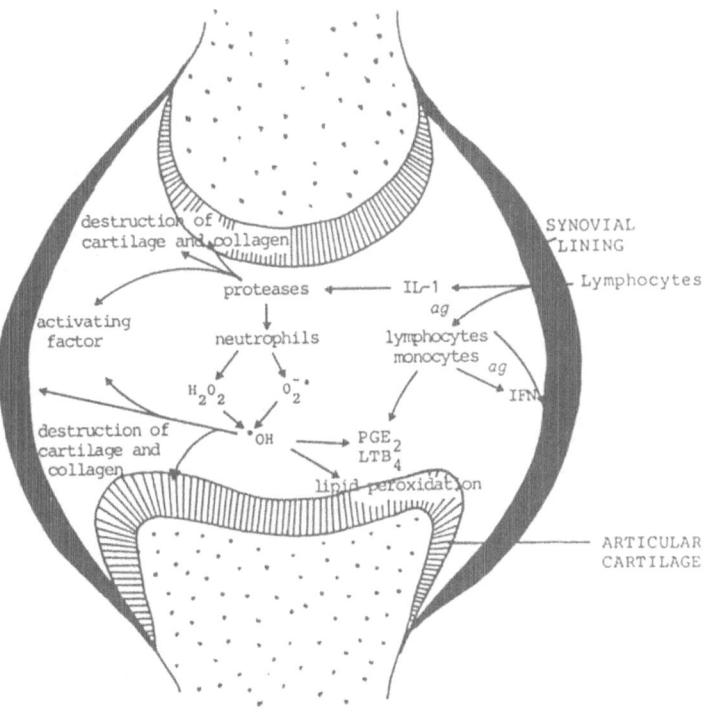

**Figure 2** Oxyradicals and interleukin 1 in the rheumatoid synovium. Key to abbreviations: $ag$, antigen; IL-1, interleukin 1; IFN, $\gamma$-interferon; PGE$_2$, prostaglandin E$_2$; LTB$_4$, leukotriene B$_4$; H$_2$O$_2$, hydrogen peroxide; O$_2^{-\cdot}$, superoxide radical

The absence of any 'active' cell-mediated immune response in pa-tients with rheumatoid arthritis is in contrast to the involvement of the cell-mediated response seen in reactive arthritis, in which antibodies to the initiating infectious agent (*Yersinia, Salmonella*, etc) can be demonstrated. By the use of monoclonal antisera to several lymphocyte activation markers (Tac, T9, 4F2), synovial fluid lymphocytes from patients with reactive arth-ritis have been shown to be 'activated', whereas those from rheumatoid arth-

189

ritis were 'non-activated', being 'innocent bystanders' instead of 'active participants' in the local immune inflammation[4]. Similarly, the small number of lymphocytes (blasts) in the S phase of the cell cycle, found in the synovial fluid of rheumatoid arthritis patients, indicates the absence of a cell-mediated immune response[5].

In the chronic inflammatory condition of rheumatoid synovitis the mechanism of lymphocyte migration into the synovium involves firstly the binding of the lymphocytes to the endothelial cells and then their traversing the endothelial barrier. Both the monokine, interleukin-1 (IL-1), and the lymphokine, γ-interferon (IFNγ), formed by histocytes, macrophages and lymphocytes in the presence of antigen (ag), are involved in these processes of initiating and maintaining chronic inflammation[6,7]. The cytokine, IL-1, which induces the signs of chronic arthritis, is present in the synovial fluid of rheumatoid patients, is produced also by endothelial cells, and is chemotactic for both T and B lymphocytes (see Figure 2). The lymphokine, IFNγ, acts by enhancing the binding of lymphocytes to the endothelial cells. The IL-1 of rheumatoid synovial fluid stimulates synovial cell production of the serum protease, plasminogen activator, which together with other synovial proteases such as collagenase and neutral proteoglycanase, result in cartilage destruction[8].

## II. OXYGEN RADICAL PRODUCTION

Tissue oxygen is readily reduced in biological systems to superoxide radical ($O_2^{\cdot-}$) and peroxide anion ($O_2^{--}$) which, under the catalytic influence of inorganic iron and other transition metal ions, can yield the more toxic hydroxyl radical ($^{\cdot}OH$) and singlet oxygen ($^1O_2$). These oxygen radicals are formed continuously in biological systems, from (1) one-electron reductions of oxygen by flavoprotein oxidoreductases such as NADPH-cytochrome P-450 reductase, or xanthine oxidase; (2) one- or two-electron reductions of oxygen by the cytochromes P-450 in preference to the insertion of the activated oxygen into a substrate; (3) redox cycling of quinones or quinonimines, and (4) prostanoid biosynthesis in the conversion of $PGG_2$ to $PGH_2$. In the inflammatory process, superoxide radicals are produced by neutrophils and macrophages, via an NADPH-dependent oxidase, and by conversion to hydrogen peroxide and hypochlorous acid (by myeloperoxidase) constitute a natural defence system against bacterial infection[9]. Hydroxyl radicals result in destruction of endothelial cells, increased vascular permeability, release of chemotactic factors and other mediators of tissue inflammation and, subsequent to autoxidative injury including lipid peroxidation, result in membrane damage, oxidative destruction of pyridine nucleotides, denaturation of enzymes, and degradation of DNA and hyaluronic acid[10].

Oxygen radicals are also closely associated with the production of the prostanoids, which are now regarded as classical mediators of inflammation. Singlet oxygen can initiate the lipoperoxidation of arachidonic acid, but the hydroxyl radical results in the inactivation of prostaglandin synthetase, and hydroxyl radical scavengers stimulate the synthesis of prostaglandins[10]. Excessive production of oxygen free radicals is prevented by an elaborate defence system comprising the enzymes superoxide dismutase (SOD), catalase, glutathione peroxidase, and glutathione reductase, the natural antioxidants and radical scavengers including the tocopherols, ascorbic acid and the retinoids, and the ubiquitous intracellular redox buffer, glutathione (GSH) (see Figure 3).

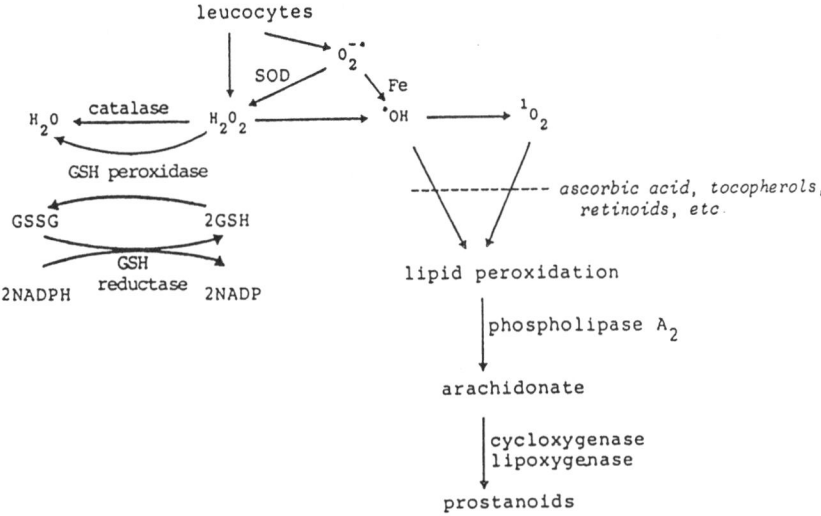

**Figure 3** Oxyradicals and biological defence against lipid peroxidation. Key to abbreviations: $O_2^{-\bullet}$, superoxide radical; $H_2O_2$, hydrogen peroxide; $^1O_2$, singlet oxygen; $^\bullet OH$, hydroxyl radical; SOD, superoxide dismutase; GSH, glutathione; GSSG, oxidized glutathione; NADP, nicotinamide adenine dinucleotide phosphate

Evidence for the fundamental involvement of reactive oxyradicals in inflammatory injury has been established both *in vitro* and *in vivo* using the rat footpad oedema (Koch) model[11-13]. The sequence of the molecular mechanisms of the acute inflammatory reaction in this model was studied using luminol-amplified chemiluminescence to detect specific reactive oxygen species, to determine malondialdehyde by the thiobarbituric acid method and exhalation of ethane as an index of lipid peroxidation, and quantification of the prostanoids $PGE_2$, $TXB_2$ and 6-oxo-$PGF_{1\alpha}$ by specific radioimmunoassay. Rats inoculated in the scruff with Freund's complete adjuvant and challenged 6 days later with Freund's adjuvant in one hind paw, developed footpad oedema in a biphasic manner over the initial 24 hours, after which oedema persisted for a further 72 hours, when the experiment was terminated. Alkane exhalation by the live animal was significantly increased 2 hours after challenge, and then progressively declined (AM Symons and EJ Dowling, unpublished). The tissue malondialdehyde content of the footpad, post-mortem, increased biphasically simultaneously with the occurrence of oedema. Luminol-amplified chemiluminescence was also increased, achieving peak levels just before each of the two phases of oedema and increased tissue malondialdehyde content. $PGE_2$ attained a maximum coincident with the first phase of oedema, whereas $TBX_2$ and 6-oxo-PG-$F_{1\alpha}$ rose to maxima before the second phase of oedema, indicating that prostanoids appear to contribute to initiation of the second phase only[11]. Using luminol-amplified chemiluminescence in the presence of catalase and mannitol respectively to quantify hydrogen peroxide ($H_2O_2$) and hydroxyl radicals ($^\bullet OH$), and DABCO-enhanced chemiluminescence to quantify singlet oxygen ($^1O_2$), it was shown that catalase maximally inhibited the $H_2O_2$ contribution to the chemiluminescence at 4 hours and mannitol showed maximal inhibition of $^\bullet OH$ at 6 hours, post-challenge. The DABCO-enhanced measurement of $^1O_2$-associated chemiluminescence showed a peak at 8 hours post-challenge. It may be concluded from this study that the contribution of $H_2O_2$ and $^\bullet OH$ to tissue damage[12,13] occurred before significant production of $^1O_2$. Similar groups of rats treated with the anti-inflammatory agents, diclofenac, indomethacin, piroxicam, prednisolone, or the iron chelator, desferrioxamine, 1 hour before challenge, all exhibited inhibition of the chemiluminescence at 4 hours post-challenge, although significant inhibition of the oedema was not observed until 24 hours post-challenge. Thus despite the different modes of action of the various drugs administered (prostaglandin synthesis inhibitors, lipocortin synthesis inducer, and an iron chelator) all resulted in a decrease in the generation of reactive oxygen species and the associated lipid peroxidation and inflammatory injury[14].

Oxygen radicals are produced in enhanced amounts by neutrophils of subjects with rheumatoid arthritis, osteoarthritis, systemic lupus erythematosus, and scleroderma. The production of oxygen radicals from neutrophils of patients with bacterial infection was studied and the release of hydrogen peroxide by zymosan treatment was considered to be the most reliable indicator of the disease process[15]. Using this procedure it was found that hydrogen peroxide production by neutrophils from rheumatoid arthritis patients was not significantly different from that of normal control subjects[15]. In contrast, other workers found that PMA- or zymosan-stimulated neutrophils from rheumatoid arthritis and osteoarthritis patients exhibited significantly increased production of superoxide radicals (20 to 100%) over those of neutrophils from healthy control subjects[16]. Moreover, the large number of neutrophils, and the high titre of neutrophil-derived lysosomal enzymes, in the synovial fluid[17], together with the greater potential radical-generating function of the neutrophils of synovial fluid compared with circulating leucocytes[18] indicates that in rheumatoid arthritis a potentiation of neutrophil oxygen production occurs. More recently, synovial fluid has been shown to contain a factor which activates neutrophils to enhance the release of oxygen radicals and also to enhance myeloperoxidase activity[19]. Similarly, neutrophils from patients with systemic lupus erythematosus (SLE) showed high levels of oxygen radical production, as did normal neutrophils treated with serum from SLE patients, indicating that tissue damage in SLE may be due to excessive production of oxygen radicals which results from the neutrophils themselves and from a serum factor which further activates the leucocytes[20]. Likewise neutrophils and serum from patients with systemic sclerosis (scleroderma), a disease of vascular damage with connective tissue disease symptoms, exhibited enhanced chemiluminescence associated with increased production of reactive oxygen, especially hydrogen peroxide[21].

The destruction of joint tissues in rheumatoid arthritis is effected largely by oxygen free radicals and leucocyte proteases and collagenase (see Figure 2), and the destructive effects of superoxide radicals on the proteoglycans and collagen of connective tissue, and on the hyaluronic acid of synovial tissue, are well established[22]. Oxygen radicals have also been shown to result in the degradation of intact cartilaginous matrix, both by a direct action and indirectly by activation of the latent collagenase activity present in neutrophils. Both of these activities were inhibited by either superoxide dismutase or catalase, which indicates that a product from both superoxide anion and peroxide, namely hydroxyl radical, is the active agent, and that iron, the necessary catalyst, must also be involved[23]. Synovial fluid from rheumatoid patients was found to be deficient in superoxide dismutase, catalase and caeruloplasmin activities and consequently had limited ability to scavenge superoxide and hydrogen peroxide[24].

## III. PROSTANOID PRODUCTION

Prostaglandins and other prostanoids, oxygenated products of arachidonic acid and other polyunsaturated fatty acids (PUFAs), are important regulators of immune and inflammatory responses. They are formed by the actions of the enzymes cyclo-oxygenase and lipoxygenase on arachidonate and other PUFAs released from the phospholipids of the endoplasmic reticulum of cells by the action of phospholipase $A_2$ (see Figure 4). The preferential release of peroxidized fatty acids from phospholipid membranes by phospholipase $A_2$ is an absolute requirement for the detoxication of membrane fatty acid hydroperoxides by glutathione peroxidase. Phospholipase $A_2$ is thus considered to play a major role in the protection of membranes from lipid peroxidation damage[25]. High concentrations of prostanoids are present in the synovial fluid of patients with rheumatoid arthritis[26], and increased amounts of prostanoids are produced by rheumatoid arthritis[26], and increased amounts of prostanoids are produced by rheumatoid synovium in organ culture[27,28] (see Figure 2). Prostaglandin $E_2$ ($PGE_2$) is the most potent mediator of inflammation formed from arachidonic acid by the cyclo-oxygenase pathway, and peripheral monocytes from rheumatoid patients have been shown to produce greater amounts of $PGE_2$ than do normal leucocytes[29]. Peripheral monocytes from rheumatoid patients exhibit greater phospholipase $A_2$ and phospholipase C activities[30], which would lead to increased release of arachidonic acid and increased formation of prostanoids. Furthermore, antibodies to lipocortin, the natural inhibitor of phospholipase activity and the second messenger of the immunosuppressive, phospholipase-inhibiting corticosteroids[31], have been found in the serum of rheumatoid arthritis patients, which could account for the increased phospholipase activity and prostanoid formation associated with this disease state[32] (see Figure 4). The biosynthesis of the phospholipids themselves may undergo changes in systemic inflammatory conditions, and induction of adjuvant arthritis in rats decreased the liver microsomal phosphatidylcholine and phosphatidylethanolamine contents, which might also be associated with the loss of microsomal cytochrome P-450 activity[33].

Leukotrienes, the products derived from arachidonic acid by the ac-

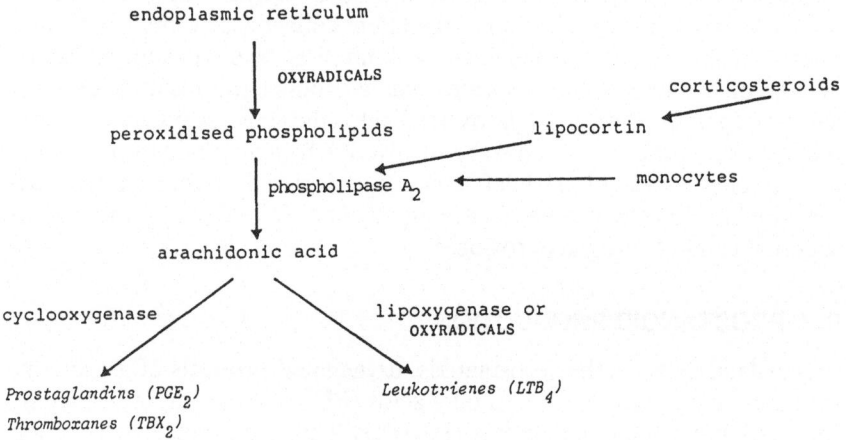

**Figure 4** Oxyradicals and prostanoid formation

tion of lipoxygenase, are also potent mediators of inflammation, the most active being $LTB_4$, one of the most potent leucotactic substances known. $LTB_4$ and $LTC_4$ (a glutathione analogue) have been shown to be present in the synovial fluid of rheumatoid arthritis patients[34] (see Figure 2).
Patients with systemic sclerosis complicated by Raynaud's phenomenon exhibit increased biosynthesis of thromboxane $A_2$, the predominant cyclooxygenase metabolite of arachidonic acid in blood platelets, and potent vasoconstrictor and platelet aggregatory factor[35].

194

## IV.  EFFECTS OF IRON

Ferrous ion is the most active catalyst known for the dismutation of superoxide radical and peroxide anion to the highly toxic hydroxyl radical, and therefore greatly potentiates the toxic effects of oxygen radicals. Furthermore, the destructive effects of oxygen radicals on the microsomal and mitochondrial cytochromes and on haemoglobin results in a diminution of the haem pool and an accumulation of inorganic iron. Iron is therefore concerned in the initiation of autoxidative injury and is also a product, thus providing a mechanism of autocatalysis. Iron has long been known to have a role in the pathogenesis of rheumatoid disease[36].

Significant quantities of iron accumulate in the synovial membranes, synovial fluid and lymph nodes of rheumatoid patients, some as free iron, but mainly in the form of iron complexes, such as ferritin. Sufficient ferritin loaded with iron is available in the joints of rheumatoid arthritic patients to stimulate oxygen free radical production[37] (see Figure 2). The accumulated iron in the synovium has two implications for this disease state. Firstly, it catalyses the reduction of tissue oxygen to the superoxide radical, and the dismutation of the superoxide radical and hydrogen peroxide to the more destructive hydroxyl radical, thus mediating the acute stages of inflammation. Secondly, it is chemotactic to the inflammatory lymphocytes and macrophages, for the lymphoid cells have iron-binding receptors and migrate not towards an antigen but towards reticuloendothelial iron deposits[38], so that it also mediates the subsequent chronic phase of inflammation. As the protective enzymes, superoxide dismutase and catalase, which scavenge superoxide radical and peroxide respectively, are absent from the synovial fluid of rheumatoid patients, the presence of even traces of iron results in the production of hydroxyl radicals, lipid peroxidation of the membranes of the reticuloendothelial synovial cells, release of lysosomes and lysosomal enzymes, and the enzymic and radical degradation of collagen and cartilage. The knee-joint synovial fluid of rheumatoid patients contains lipid peroxidation products (TBA-reactive material), which have been shown to correlate with the content of bleomycin-iron and with the clinical and laboratory assessment of the arthritic disease[39] (see Figure 2). It is perhaps significant that in populations where malnutrition and parasitic infestations result in low levels of iron, severe rheumatoid disease is rarely reported[38].

In support of these views on the importance of iron in mediating the inflammatory injury of rheumatoid arthritis, an exacerbation of rheumatoid synovitis has been described in a long-standing rheumatoid patient treated with iron–dextran intravenous infusion for treatment of an accompanying anaemia[40]. On the first day after infusion the iron–binding capacity of the serum and synovial fluid became saturated and low molecular complexes of iron ('bleomycin–iron') appeared, lipid peroxidation and dehydroascorbic acid (oxidized vitamin C) in the serum and synovial fluid increased, erythrocyte glutathione (GSH) decreased, and the plasma acute-phase proteins, ferritin and caeruloplasmin, showed marked but slower increases. These related indications of iron loading and autoxidative damage paralleled a swelling of the peripheral joints and a pronounced effusion of the right knee which remained until the 8th day after infusion, when total iron, erythrocyte GSH and 'thiobarbiturate-reactive substances', an index of lipid peroxidation, returned to normal.

High iron content in leucocytes and platelets are also associated with chronic inflammatory conditions. Patients with ankylosing spondylitis have granulocyte and platelet concentration of iron of $32 \pm 3$ and $11 \pm 2.6$ $\mu$g/g dry weight respectively, compared with $5.2 \pm 1.9$ and $4.6 \pm 0.8$ $\mu$g/g for sex- and age-matched healthy controls. Correlations were found between the granulocyte iron concentration and circulating levels of total iron, transferrin and lactoferrin, and the degree of inflammatory activity as measured by the erythrocyte sedimentation rate, and immunoglobulins A and G.

## V.   TREATMENTS OF FREE RADICAL DAMAGE

Clinical treatments available to prevent oxyradical tissue damage in rheumatoid arthritis include drugs which act to inhibit oxyradical production by leukocytes, drugs which act as antioxidants and radical scavengers thereby diminishing the tissue destructive effects of oxyradicals, complexing agents to remove iron and its catalytic effects in forming the more toxic hydroxyl radical ($^{\bullet}$OH) and singlet oxygen ($^{1}O_2$), drugs which protect against the adverse effects of prostanoids, and nutritional factors such as eicosapentaenoic acid and antioxidants which moderate the adverse effects of the prostanoids or enhance the body's natural defence against oxyradical toxicity.

### (1)   Protection against oxygen radicals

Radical scavenging and antioxidant drugs may act in several ways, by (a) inhibiting the production of oxygen radicals ($O_2^{-}$, $O_2^{-\bullet}$, and $^{\bullet}$OH) by neutrophils and macrophages; (b) inhibiting leucocyte myeloperoxidase, an enzyme which generates hypochlorite; or by (c) scavenging the oxygen radicals or hypochlorite after their release from the leucocytes (see Figure 5).

### (a) Inhibition of oxygen radical production

Although the inhibition of prostaglandin biosynthesis by the non-steroidal anti-inflammatory drugs (NSAIDs), due to their inhibition of the enzyme cyclo-oxygenase[41], is undoubtedly the major mode of action of these anti-inflammatory drugs, it is most likely that other mechanisms are also involved. The NSAIDs, indomethacin, ibuprofen, phenylbutazone and piroxicam, also act by inhibiting oxygen radical production from activated neutrophils[42]. Piroxicam achieves this by interfering with the mechanism by which the NADPH-oxidase of the leucocyte plasma membrane and phagosome is acti-

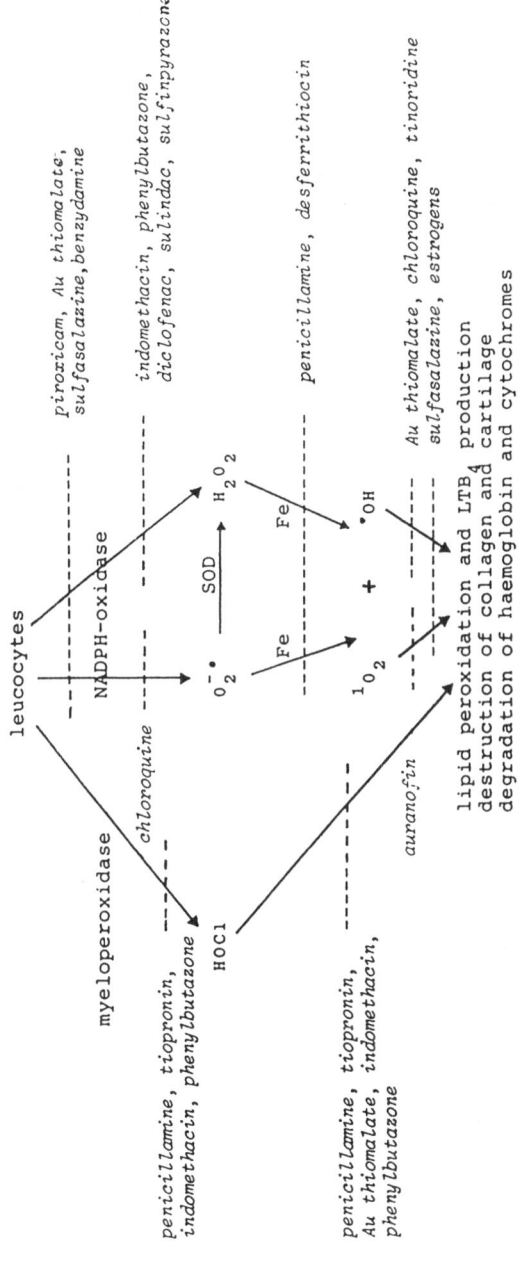

**Figure 5**  Modes of action of drugs acting on oxyradical production. Key to abbreviations: HOCl, hypochlorite; $O_2^{-\bullet}$, superoxide radical; $H_2O_2$, hydrogen peroxide; $^1O_2$, singlet oxygen; $^{\bullet}OH$, hydroxyl radical, SOD, superoxide dismutase

197

vated to generate superoxy radicals[16]. Gold sodium thiomalate also exerts its beneficial effect in rheumatoid arthritis[43], at least in part, by inhibition of monocyte- and macrophage-dependent generation of oxygen radicals, and inhibited the chemiluminescence of stimulated peripheral blood monocytes from rheumatoid arthritic patients *in vitro* (see Figure 5).

Sulfasalazine, a drug initially intended for the treatment of rheumatoid arthritis, but which has been used mainly in the treatment of ulcerative colitis, has been reinstated recently as an anti-rheumatoid agent[44]. It is an azo compound, which is reduced to its constituent 5-aminosalicyclic acid (5-ASA) and sulphapyridine (SP) in the colon, with all three moieties being absorbed, at least to certain extents. Sulfasalazine, 5-ASA and SP all show antioxidant effects with zymosan-stimulated neutrophils and with a cell-free xanthine–xanthine oxidase system. The most significant of these is the inhibition of hydroxyl radical generation and chemiluminescence by 5-ASA in the leucocyte system, the inhibition by sulfasalazine and 5-ASA of $H_2O_2$ generation in both the leucocyte and cell-free systems, and the inhibition of superoxide radical production in leucocytes by SP and in the cell-free system by sulfasalazine[45] (see Figure 5). A double-blind, placebo-controlled, clinical trial of sulfasalazine, 3 g daily, in 50 rheumatoid arthritis cases of >6 years duration, and 36 controls, showed significant clinical benefit after 15 weeks of treatment, but adverse reactions led to drug withdrawal by 28% of the patients[44]. Sulfasalazine has been associated with folate deficiency and macrocytic anaemia, both of which are dose-dependent[46].

Inhibition of oxygen radical production by activated neutrophils/macrophages *in vitro* has been studied by chemiluminescence amplified by lucigenin to detect $O_2{}^{\bullet-}$ and by luminol to detect $H_2O_2$. The most active inhibitors for both $O_2{}^{\bullet-}$ and $H_2O_2$ were the antioxidants nordihydroguaiaretic acid (NDGA) and N-propyl gallate, the NSAID benzydamine, the lipoxygenase inhibitor sulfasalazine, and the enzymes SOD and catalase. The lipoxygenase inhibitors CBS 1108 and CBS 1114 (Chauvin Blache) and BW 755C (Wellcome), the NSAIDs metamizole, indomethacin, phenylbutazone, diclofenac and sulindac, and the anti-gout drugs allopurinol and sulfinpyrazone were more effective with luminol ($H_2O_2$) than with lucigenin ($O_2{}^{\bullet-}$). Chloroquine was effective with lucigenin ($O_2{}^{\bullet-}$) but not with luminol. Inactive in this system were most NSAIDs (ibuprofen, benoxaprofen, aspirin, ketoprofen), corticosteroids, and the disease-modifying drugs, D-penicillamine, levamisole, and gold thiomalate[47] (Figure 5).

## (b) Inhibition of myeloperoxidase

D-Penicillamine and other thiol-containing anti-arthritic drugs, such as tiopronin (N-2-mercaptopropionyl glycine), inhibit the action of myeloperoxidase, and together with sodium aurothiomalate and aurothioglucose, have also been shown to scavenge hypochlorite[48] (see Figure 5). All four drugs develop their beneficial effects over a period of weeks, and these therapeutic effects do not necessarily correlate with the serum levels of the drugs. This may be because the gold complexes dissociate, losing the metal and thereby freeing the thiol groups, which are considered to be the active moieties of these drugs. Sodium aurothiomalate, other gold complexes, penicillamine and captopril, all have a sulphydryl group, and have the same profile of toxic reactions (dermatitis, bone-marrow depression and nephrotoxicity) which may develop in up to 45% of the patients. This drug toxicity has recently been shown to be associated with impaired ability to oxidize sulphides to sulphoxides and consequently with drug detoxication[49].

A number of NSAIDs of various classes have been shown to be effective in the inhibition of myeloperoxidase-catalysed hypochlorite production, either through inhibition of the enzyme or scavenging of the product; among the most potent, as determined by luminol-enhanced chemiluminescence, were BW 755C ($ID_{50} = 5 \times 10^{-8}$ M), indomethacin ($8 \times 10^{-7}$ M), phenylbutazone ($3 \times 10^{-6}$ M) and sulindac sulphide ($6 \times 10^{-6}$ M)[49a].

## (c) Scavenging of oxygen radicals

D-Penicillamine, a so-called disease-modifying antirheumatic drug, can scavenge or produce $H_2O_2$, according to the ratio of penicillamine to $Cu^{2+}$ ions present in the tissue. At $Cu^{2+}$ concentrations which occur in rheumatoid arthritis serum and synovial fluid, penicillamine plus $Cu^{2+}$ produce $H_2O_2$, which suppresses lymphocyte proliferation resulting in immunosuppression. However, penicillamine present in excess of $Cu^{2+}$, rapidly scavenges $H_2O_2$, and may also lead to an increase in intracellular glutathione in patients responding to treatment[50] (see Figure 5).

Other disease-modifying antirheumatoid drugs, such as various gold (Au-I) compounds also act by scavenging oxygen radicals, and Auranofin (tetra-O-acetylglucose-1-thiol gold triethylphosphine complex) has been shown to be a highly effective deactivator *in vitro* of singlet oxygen, a potent initiator of lipid peroxidation[51]. Gold sodium thiomalate and chloroquine[52] have also been shown to be effective scavengers of hydroxyl radicals *in vitro* (see Figure 5).

Tinoridine, a NSAID, has potent antiperoxidative activity, about 50 times greater than that of α-tocopherol, and has also been shown[52] to be a potent scavenger of hydroxyl radicals *in vitro* (see Figure 5).

The oestrogens, oestradiol, oestrone and oestriol, are weak antioxidants which inhibit the peroxidation of phospholipid membranes, and may be metabolized to catechol derivatives which are far more effective antioxidants[54]. This may give some rationale to the long-observed female association of rheumatoid arthritis, its remission during pregnancy, and to the evidence that oral contraceptives and hormonal replacement therapy appear to exert a protective effect against rheumatoid disease[55] (see Figure 5).

## (2)  Removal of iron

A major determinant of the cytotoxicity of oxygen radicals is the presence of iron, including ferritin and loosely bound iron complexes termed 'bleomycin iron'. Lactoferrin released from neutrophils, unlike transferrin, retains its iron even at low pH values, so that it may act to protect against the catalytic action of iron on hydroxyl radical production[55,56]. Treatment of rheumatoid arthritis with the iron chelating agent, desferrioxamine, (1 g/day intramuscularly, for 14 days) available as the mesylate salt (Desferal, Ciba-Geigy) resulted in moderate clinical improvement (less pain, morning stiffness and lower Ritchie's index), and to release of iron from synovial tissue, increased urinary excretion of iron, increased serum iron and haemoglobin, and decreased serum ferritin[57]. In another study of desferrioxamine administered subcutaneously (2 g daily for 5 days/week for 4 weeks), serum ferritin was decreased but no clinical improvement was seen or improvement was only temporary[58]. However, adverse reactions may occur by removal of iron from the central nervous system with consequent ocular and auditory toxicity[59], or by an inhibitory effect on the gastrointestinal mucosa resulting in nausea and vomiting, indicating that the rate and route of dosage are critical and should be determined by the pretreatment concentration of serum iron[60].

More recent iron-chelating agents, such as desferrithiocin (DFT, Ciba-Geigy) have also produced promising results. While Desferal is active only when administered by i.p. or i.m. injection, and is inactive when given orally, desferrithiocin stimulates ferritin iron mobilization when administered by either route but is most effective when given orally[61]. Although toxic at high dosage (100 mg/kg to rats) DFT is more efficacious as an iron chelator at low doses (10–30 mg/kg) which are non-toxic to animals, and would thus appear to represent a considerable advance in the development of iron-chelating agents, which may find future use in the treatment of rheumatoid arthritis and other inflammatory conditions (see Figure 5). There is thus a need for more new iron-chelating drugs, that can be administered orally and are safer than desferrioxamine[36].

## (3)  Enhanced defence against oxygen radicals

Increase of disease activity in rheumatoid arthritis has been found to parallel a decrease in serum sulphydryl compounds, and a good response to treatment[62] with sulphydryl-stimulating drugs such as chloroquine or corticosteroids, is paralleled by an increase in extracellular thiol levels *in vivo*. Glutathione (GSH) protects against oxygen radical damage, inhibits lipid peroxidation, inhibits prostaglandin biosynthesis, and stabilizes lysosomal and other cellular membranes. Extracellular GSH is not as important as intracellular GSH as it cannot penetrate the plasma membrane, and a good index of intracellular GSH is erythrocyte GSH. Although erythrocyte GSH is not decreased in rheumatoid disease, treatment with penicillamine for 2 to 8 weeks increased erythrocyte GSH by 30% in those patients showing good clinical response, but produced a slight decrease in those who showed no response. However, when L-cysteine was given with the penicillamine, there was a marked clinical improvement and an increase in erythrocyte GSH in the previous non-responders, while the responders showed even greater clinical improvement and further increases in erythrocyte GSH[63]. The antioxidant effect of the immunopotentiating drug, levamisole, is due to its hydrolytic product formed on metabolism by ring opening to give the water-soluble sulphydryl compound, DL-2-oxo-3-(2-mercaptoethyl)-5-phenylimidazolidine (OMPI)[64].

Selenium, an essential component of the enzyme GSH peroxidase, which protects against peroxides, is reported to be low in rheumatoid arthritis. Dietary supplementation with Se(250 μg/day) increased the serum and erythrocyte levels of Se in rheumatoid patients some 3- to 4-fold, but had no significant effects on the clinical conditions of the patients[65]. Superoxide dismutase protects against the toxic oxygen radical, superoxide anion, and although superoxide dismutases with long half-lives have been shown to inhibit immune complex-induced inflammation in experimental animals[66] no therapeutic benefit has been seen in rheumatoid patients.

## (4) Protection against adverse effects of prostanoids

Oxygen radicals are closely interrelated with prostanoid biosynthesis. Singlet oxygen may initiate the peroxidation of arachidonic acid, hydroxyl radicals are formed in the degradation of the initial prostanoid hydroperoxides to the corresponding alcohols, and peroxide and hydroxyl radicals inhibit prostaglandin synthetase. Factors affecting prostanoid biosynthesis may therefore have an effect on oxygen radical production, and vice-versa. The antioxidant, NDGA[67], and the flavonoid, quercetin, are specific potent inhibitors of lipoxygenase activity[68]. With a rat colon preparation and $^{14}$C-arachidonic acid in vitro, D-pencillamine showed selective inhibition of lipoxygenase activity, decreasing the formation of the leukotriene $LTB_4$ and 5-HETE, while levamisole and tiopronin showed more pronounced inhibition of lipoxygenase but also inhibited cyclo-oxygenase activity[69].

The modulation of dietary fatty acids to modify prostanoid formation from arachidonic acid has been studied using the fish oil polyunsaturated fatty acids, eicosapentaenoic acid (EPA, a 20:5 ω-3 PUFA) and docosahexaenoic acid (DHA, a 22:6 ω-3 PUFA), which are metabolized to prostanoids that have less adverse biological activities than those derived from arachidonic acid. Dietary enrichment with EPA and DHA over several weeks led to incorporation into human neutrophils and monocytes with diminution in the production of arachidonic acid metabolites[70], and dietary fish oil decreased the frequency and severity of collagen-induced arthritis in a study in mice[71] but increased it in another study in rats[72]. Dietary supplementation with fish oil slightly decreased the joint symptoms of rheumatoid arthritis patients[73], and in a subsequent double-blind, controlled, cross-over study[74] with 40 rheumatoid arthritis patients, in 14-week treatment periods, daily supplementation with 2.7 g EPA plus 1.8 g DHA resulted in subjective alleviation of active rheumatoid arthritis and a 50% decrease in the production of neutrophil leukotriene, $LTB_4$.

## ACKNOWLEDGEMENT

The original experimental studies described in this paper were financially supported by the Sir Halley Stewart Trust, for which the authors DVP and AMS are most grateful.

## REFERENCES

1. Greenwald, RA (1985). Therapeutic benefits of oxygen radical scavenger treatments remain unproven. *J Rheumatol*, 7, 212–14
2. Parekh, RB, Dwek, RA, Sutton, BJ *et al.* (1985). Association of rheumatoid arthritis and primary osteoarthritis with changes in the glycosylation pattern of total serum IgG. *Nature (London)*, 316, 452–7
3. Parke, DV and Symons, AM (1977). The biochemical pharmacology of mucus. In Elstein, D and Parke, DV (eds) *Mucus in Health and Disease.* pp. 423–41 (New York: Plenum)
4. Konttinen, YT, Nordstrom, D, Bergroth, V *et al.* (1986). Cell-mediated immune response in the diseased joints in patients with reactive arthritis. *Scand J Immunol*, 23, 685–91
5. Bergroth, V, Konttinen, YT, Nykanen, P *et al.* (1985). Proliferating cells in the synovial fluid in rheumatic disease. Analysis with autoradiography–immunoperoxidase double staining. *Scand J Immunol*, 22, 383–391
6. Cavender, D, Haskard D, Yu, C-L *et al.* (1987). Pathways to chronic inflammation in rheumatoid synovitis. *Fed Proc*, 46, 113–17
7. Henderson, B, Pettipher, ER and Higgs, GA (1987). Mediators of rheumatoid arthritis. *Br Med Bull*, 43, 415–28
8. Mochan, E, Uhl, J and Newton, R (1986). Interleukin I stimulation of synovial cell plasminogen activator production. *J Rheumatol*, 13, 15–19
9. Prince, RC and Gunson, DE (1987). Superoxide production by neutrophils. *Trends Biochem Sci*, 12, 86–7
10. Vapaatalo, H (1986). Free radicals and anti-inflammatory drugs. *Med Biol*, 64, 1–7
11. Dowling, EJ, Jasani, MK, Parke, DV *et al.* (1985a). Free radicals lipid peroxidation and prostaglandins during the development and maintenance of foot-pad oedema in the Koch model. *Br J Pharmacol*, 84, 35P
12. Dowling, EJ, Jasani, MK, Parke, DV *et al.* (1985b). Characterisation of ex-vivo luminol-amplified chemiluminescence accompanying the initiation of foot-pad oedema in the Koch model. *Br J Pharmacol*, 84, 79P
13. Dowling, EJ, Symons, AM and Parke, DV (1986). Free radical production at the site of an acute inflammatory reaction as measured by chemiluminescence. *Agents and Actions*, 19, 203–7.
14. Dowling, EJ, Symons, AM, Andrews, FJ and Blake, DR (1987). Reactive oxygen species, inflammation and drug evaluation. *Br J Rheumatol*, 26, *Abstr Suppl*, No.1, p. 19

202

15. Ozaki, Y, Ohashi, T and Niwa, Y (1986). Oxygen radical production by neutrophils from patients with bacterial infection and rheumatoid arthritis. *Inflammation*, 10, 119–30

16. Biemond, P, Swaak, AJG, Penders, JMA *et al.* (1986). Superoxide production by polymorphonuclear leucocytes in rheumatoid arthritis and osteoarthritis: *in vivo* inhibition by the antirheumatic drug piroxicam due to interference with the activation of the NADPH-oxidase. *Ann Rheum Dis*, 45, 249–55

17. Janoff, A (1975). At least three human neutrophil lysosomal proteases are capable of degrading joint connective tissues. *Ann NY Acad Sci*, 256, 402–8

18. Niwa, Y, Sakane, T, Shingu, M and Yokoyama, M (1983). Effect of stimulated neutrophils from the synovial fluid of patients with rheumatoid arthritis on lymphocytes. A possible role of increased oxygen radicals generated by neutrophils. *J Clin Immunol*, 3, 228–40

19. Bender, JG, van Epps, DE, Searles, R and Williams, RC Jr (1986). Altered function of synovial fluid granulocytes in patients with acute inflammatory arthritis: Evidence for activation of neutrophils and its mediation by a factor present in synovial fluid. *Inflammation*, 10, 443–53

20. Niwa, Y, Sakane, T, Shingu, M and Miyachi, Y (1985). Role of stimulated neutrophils from patients with systemic lupus erythematosus in tissue injury, with special reference to serum factors and increased active oxygen species generated by neutrophils. *Inflammation*, 9, 163–72

21. Kovacs, IB, Meyrick Thomas, RH, Mackay, AR *et al.* (1986). Increased chemiluminescence of polymorphonuclear leucocytes from patients with progressive systemic sclerosis. *Clin Sci*, 70, 257–61

22. Monboisse, JC, Braquet, P, Randoux, A and Borel, JP (1983). Non-enzymatic degradation of acid soluble calf skin collagen by superoxide ion: protective effects of flavonoids. *Biochem Pharmacol*, 32, 53–8

23. Burkhardt, H, Schwingel, M, Menninger, H *et al.* (1986). Oxygen radicals as effectors of cartilage destruction: Direct degradative effect on matrix components and indirect action via activation of latent collagenase from polymorphonuclear leukocytes. *Arthritis Rheum*, 29, 379–87

24. Blake, DR, Hall, ND, Treby, DA *et al.* (1981). Protection against superoxide and hydrogen peroxide in synovial fluid from rheumatoid patients. *Clin Sci*, 61, 483–86

25. van Kuijk, FJGM, Sevanian, A, Handelman, GJ and Dratz, EA (1987). A new major role for phospholipase A$_2$: protection of membranes from lipid peroxidation damage. *Trends Biochem Sci*, 12, 31–4

26. Trang, LE, Granstrom, E and Lovgren, O (1977). Levels of prostaglandins F$_2$ and E$_2$ and thromboxane B$_2$ in joint fluid in rheumatoid arthritis. *Scand J Rheumatol*, 6, 151–4

27. Salmon, JA, Higgs, GA, Vane, JR *et al.* (1983). Synthesis of arachidonate cyclooxygenase products by rheumatoid and non-rheumatoid synovial lining in non-proliferative organ culture. *Ann Rheum Dis*, 42, 36–9

28. Moilanen, E, Seppala, E, Nissila, M and Vapaatalo, H (1987). Differences in prostanoid production between healthy and rheumatic synovia *in vitro*. *Agents Actions*, 20, 98–103

29. Seitz, M, Deimann, W, Gram, N *et al.* (1982). Characterisation of blood mononuclear cells of rheumatoid arthritis patients. I. Depressed lymphocyte proliferation and enhanced prostanoid release from monocytes. *Clin Immunol Immunopathol*, 25, 405–16

30. Bomalaski, JS, Clark, MA and Zurier, RB (1986). Enhanced phospholipase activity in peripheral blood monocytes from patients with rheumatoid arthritis. *Arthritis Rheum*, 29, 312–18

31. Flower, RJ (1985). Background and discovery of lipocortins. *Agents Actions*, 17, 255–62

32. Hirata, F, del Carmine, R, Nelson, CA *et al.* (1981). Presence of autoantibody for phospholipase inhibitory protein, lipomodulin, in patients with rheumatic diseases. *Proc Natl Acad Sci, USA*, **78**, 3190–4

33. Buchar, E and Janku, I (1985). The effect of adjuvant-induced arthritis on rat liver microsomal phospholipid metabolism. *Methods Findings Exp Clin Pharmacol*, **7**, 469–72

34. Salmon, JA and Higgs, GA (1987). Prostaglandins and leukotrienes as inflammatory mediators. *Br Med Bull*, **43**, 285–96

35. Reilly, IAG, Roy, L and Fitzgerald, GA (1986). Biosynthesis of thromboxane in patients with systemic sclerosis and Raynaud's phenomenon. *Br Med J*, **292**, 1037–9

36. Editorial (1985). Metal chelation therapy, oxygen radicals and human disease. *Lancet*, **i**, 143–5

37. Biemond, P, Swaak, AJG, van Eijk, HG and Koster, JF (1986). Intraarticular ferritin-bound iron in rheumatoid arthritis. *Arthritis Rheum*, **29**, 1187–93

38. Blake, DR, Hall, ND, Bacon, PA *et al.* (1981). The importance of iron in rheumatoid disease. *Lancet*, **ii**, 1142–4

39. Rowley, D, Gutteridge, JMC, Blake, D *et al.* (1984). Lipid peroxidation in rheumatoid arthritis: thiobarbituric-acid reactive material and catalytic iron salts in synovial fluid from rheumatoid patients. *Clin Sci*, **66**, 691–5

40. Winyard, PG, Blake, DR, Chirico, S *et al.* (1987). Mechanism of exacerbation of rheumatoid synovitis by total-dose iron-dextran infusion: *in vivo* demonstration of iron-promoted oxidant stress. *Lancet*, **i**, 69–72

41. Vane, JR (1971). Inhibition of prostaglandin synthesis as a mechanism of action for aspirin like drugs. *Nature New Biol*, **231**, 232–5

42. Gay, JC, Lukens, JN and English, DK (1984). Differential inhibition of neutrophil superoxide generation by non-steroidal anti-inflammatory drugs. *Inflammation*, **8**, 209–22

43. Harth, M, Keown, PA and Orange, JF (1983). Monocyte dependent excited oxygen radical generation in rheumatoid arthritis: inhibition by gold sodium thiomalate. *J Rheumatol*, **10**, 701–7

44. Pinals, RS, Kaplan, SB, Lawson, JG and Hepburn, B (1986). Sulfasalazine in rheumatoid arthritis. A double-blind, placebo-controlled trial. *Arthritis Rheum*, **29**, 1427–34

45. Miyachi, Y, Yoshioka, A, Imamura, S and Niwa, Y (1987). Effect of sulphasalazine and its metabolites on the generation of reactive oxygen species. *Gut*, **28**, 190–5

46. Prouse, P, Shawe, D and Gumpel, JM (1987). Macrocytic anaemia in patients treated with sulphasalazine for rheumatoid arthritis. *Br Med J*, **294**, 904–5

47. Muller-Peddinghaus, R and Wurl, M (1987). The amplified chemiluminescence test to characterize antirheumatic drugs as oxygen radical scavengers. *Biochem Pharmacol*, **36**, 1125–32

48. Cuperus, RA, Muijsers, AO and Wever, R (1985). Antiarthritic drugs containing thiol groups scavenge hypochlorite and inhibit its formation by myeloperoxidase from human leukocytes. *Arthritis Rheum*, **28**, 1128–33

49. Madhok, R, Capell, HA and Waring, R (1987). Does sulphoxidation state predict gold toxicity in rheumatoid arthritis. *Br Med J*, **294**, 483

49a Pekoe, G, Van Dyke, K, Peden, D *et al.* (1982). Antioxidant theory of non-steroidal anti-inflammatory drugs based on the inhibition of luminol-enhanced chemiluminescence from the myeloperoxidase reaction. *Agents Actions*, **12**, 371–6

50. Staite, ND, Messner, RP and Zoschke, DC (1985). In vitro production and scavenging of hydrogen peroxide by D-penicillamine. *Arthritis Rheum*, **28**, 914–21

51. Corey, EJ, Mehrotra, MM and Khan, AU (1987). Antiarthritic gold compounds effectively quench electronically excited singlet oxygen. *Science*, **236**, 68–9

52. Cleland, LG, Betts, WH, Vernon-Roberts, B and Bielicki, J (1982). Role of iron and influence of anti-inflammatory drugs on oxygen-derived free radical production and reactivity. *J Rheumatol*, **9**, 885–92

53. Shimada, O and Yasuda, H (1986). Hydroxyl radical scavenging action of tinoridine. *Agents Actions*, **19**, 208–14

54. Sugioka, K, Shimosegawa, Y and Nakano, M (1987). Estrogens as natural antioxidants of membrane phospholipid peroxidation. *FEBS Lett*, **210**, 37–9

55. Parke, AL (1985). Rheumatoid arthritis and oral contraceptives. *Intern Med*, **6**, 105–11

56. Halliwell, B, Gutteridge, JMC and Blake, D (1985). Metal ions and oxygen radical reactions in human inflammatory joint disease. *Phil Trans R Soc, Lond*, B, **311**, 659–71

57. Giordano, N, Sancasciani, S, Borghi, C *et al*. (1986). Antianaemic and potential anti-inflammatory activity of desferrioxamine: possible usefulness in rheumatoid arthritis. *Clin Exp Rheumatol*, **4**, 25–9

58. Polson, RJ, Jawad, ASM, Bomford, A *et al*. (1986). Treatment of rheumatoid arthritis and desferrioxamine. *Q J Med*, N.S., **61**, 1153–8

59. Orton, RB, de Veber, LL and Sulh, HMB (1985). Ocular and auditory toxicity of long-term, high-dose, subcutaneous desferrioxamine therapy. *Can J Ophthalmol*, **20**, 153–6

60. Polson, RJ, Jawad, A, Bomford, A *et al*. (1985). Treatment of rheumatoid arthritis with desferrioxamine: relation between stores of iron before treatment and side effects. *Br Med J*, **291**, (ii), 448

61. Longeville, A and Crichton, RR (1986). An animal model of iron overload and its application to study hepatic ferritin iron mobilisation by chelators. *Biochem Pharmacol*, **35**, 3669–78

62. Haataja, M, Nissila, M and Ruutsalo, H-M (1978). Serum sulphydryl levels in rheumatoid patients treated with gold thiomalate and penicillamine. *Scand J Rheumatol*, **7**, 212–14

63. Munthe, E, Kass, E and Jellum, E (1981). D-Penicillamine-induced increase in intracellular glutathione correlating to clinical response in rheumatoid arthritis. *J Rheumatol*, **8**, Suppl. 7, 14–19

64. Sree Kumar, K, Chirigos, MA and Weiss, JF (1979). Protection of rat liver microsomes from NADPH-, ascorbate-, and X-irradiation-induced lipid peroxidation by levamisole. *Int J Immunopharmacol*, **1**, 85–91

65. Tarp, U, Overvad, K, Thorling, EB *et al*. (1985). Selenium treatment in rheumatoid arthritis. *Scand J Rheumatol*, **14**, 364–8

66. McCord, JM, Stokes, SH and Wong, K (1979). Superoxide radicals as phagocyte-produced chemical mediators of inflammation. In Weissmann, G (ed) *Advances in Inflammation Research*.(New York: Raven Press), Vol. 1, pp. 273–80

67. Boctor, AM and Pugsley, TA (1986). Effect of CI-922, a potential new antiallergy agent, on arachidonic acid metabolism *in vitro*. *Inflammation*, **10**, 435–41

68. Hope, WC, Welton, AF, Fielder-Nagy, C *et al*. (1983). In vitro inhibition of the biosynthesis of slow-reacting substance of anaphylaxis (SRS-A) and lipoxygenase activity by quercetin. *Biochem Pharmacol*, **32**, 367–71

69. Capasso, F, Tavares, IA, Tsang, R and Bennett, A (1985). Effects of d-penicillamine, levamisole and tiopronin on eicosanoid synthesis by rat gut tissue. *Agents Actions*, **17**, 395–6

70. Lee, TH, Hoover, RL, Williams, JD *et al*. (1985). Effect of dietary enrichment with eicosapentaenoic and docosahexaenoic acids on *in vitro* neutrophil and monocyte leukotriene generation and neutrophil function. *N Engl J Med*, **312**, 1217–24

71. Leslie, CA, Gonnerman, WA, Ullman, MD *et al*. (1985). Dietary fish oil modules macrophage fatty acids and decreases arthritis susceptibility in mice. *J Exp Med*, **162**, 1336–49

72.   Prickett, JD, Trentham, DE and Robinson, DR (1984). Dietary fish oil augments the induction of arthritis in rats immunized with type II collagen. *J Immunol*, **132**, 725–9
73.   Kremer, JM, Bigaouette, J, Michalek, AV *et al.* (1985). Effects of manipulation of dietary fatty acids on clinical manifestations of rheumatoid arthritis. *Lancet*, **1**, 184–7
74.   Kremer, JM, Jubiz, W, Michalek, A *et al.* (1987). Fish-oil fatty acid supplementation in active rheumatoid arthritis. *Ann Intern Med*, **106**, 497–502

# 8
# Gold(I)-thiolates: slow-acting anti-arthritic drugs

**Davin R. Haynes and Michael W. Whitehouse**
Department of Pathology, University of Adelaide, Box 498 Adelaide, South Australia 5001

*It is much easier to write upon a disease than upon a remedy. The former is in the hands of Nature and a faithful observer with an eye of tolerable judgment cannot fail to delineate a likeness. The latter will ever be subject to the whim, the inaccuracies and blunder of mankind.*

William Withering (1741–1799)

## 1. INTRODUCTION

Chrysotherapy, the current use of gold-containing drugs to treat rheumatoid disease, presents many problems - some intriguing, others quite vexing:

- For patients there is the slow action of these drugs and the risk of developing such serious side-effects that all aspects of their well-being must be frequently monitored. So these drugs then become doubly expensive to use, requiring repeated clinical tests to monitor kidney, marrow and other functions likely to be at risk.

- For physicians prescribing chrysotherapy there are few guidelines to assist the selection of rheumatoid patients likely to gain the most benefit with least intoxication, or to identify those non-responders who will only suffer the side-effects. The question of whether chrysotherapy can control other arthritic diseases has still to be resolved[1].

- For pharmacologists and others wanting to know how the clinically effective gold drugs act *in vivo* (other than as non-specific toxins) there is a shortage of consistent and relevant disease models with which to qualify or quantify their anti-arthritic activity. Attempts to side-track

*New Developments in Antirheumatic Therapy.* Rainsford, KD and Velo, GP (eds), Inflammation and Drug Therapy Series, Volume III.

this problem using cellular systems seem only to disclose the ambivalent actions of these gold drugs, that are often very dependent on the precise experimental conditions.

All this is still rather surprising considering the high status and relatively long history of chrysotherapy[1], considerable knowledge of the biological chemistry of gold in either its monovalent or trivalent states[2,3] or the number of studies detailing some properties of gold drugs in various biosystems and accessible from recent reviews[2,4-7].

With the exception of Auranofin, these gold drugs are 'orphans' in the sense that their manufacturers sponsor little or no further research upon them. Is this merely because they are now beyond patent protection? They also attract little research support from other sources, since they show little promise for treating viral infections, cancer or other high-priority diseases. Yet they still hold their own in the market place: there are no obvious successors to render them obsolete in the short term at least. Partly this is attributable to their 'mystique' in containing the most noble element; partly to the widely held belief that they are the drugs most likely to cure (or provide long-term remission) when lesser drugs fail.

This latter assumption often presumes all gold drugs are equal, which is far from the truth. They certainly differ in physical properties, in molecular size, biostability, gross toxicity and mode of administration. It may be a disservice to clinical science to treat them collectively merely on the basis of their unusual chemical composition. This point may not become apparent until Au(I) drugs have been identified with quite different, but useful, pharmacological activities, e.g. CNS-regulant, anti-tumour, etc.

## 2. CHEMISTRY AND BIODISPOSITION OF GOLD(I) DRUGS: SOME PROBLEMS AND UNCERTAINTIES

Gold readily forms stable complexes in its monovalent (aurous, Au(I), or trivalent (auric, Au(III) states. Gold(I) forms linear complexes with two ligands. By contrast, the gold(III) complexes contain four ligands disposed around the gold in a square planar geometry and show some analogy with the cytotoxic platinum(II) complexes, e.g. binding to DNA. However, only the gold(I) complexes formed with various thiols have shown anti-arthritic activity to date (Figure 1).

Gold(I), when it is not stabilized by complexation, readily dismutates yielding metallic gold ($Au^0$) and trivalent gold, an oxidizing agent. So when bioactive gold(I)-thiolates dissociate *in vivo*, there is always the possibility of both $Au^0$ *and* Au(III) being formed *except* when (a) other Au(I) ligands are present either in excess (e.g. other thiols) or these extraneous ligands have a higher affinity for Au(I) (e.g. cyanide), or (b) reducing agents are available to regenerate Au(I) from Au(III).

The pharmacology of Au(I) then becomes quite complicated: the

Au(I)-thiolates given as anti-arthritic agents may in fact only be pro-drugs, generating new Au(I) complexes *in vivo* on the one hand, or metallic gold deposits and/or Au(III) complexes on the other hand, each with a range of drug/toxin action. Nearly all studies of the biodisposition of gold(I) drugs have relied on using either[195]Au (or[198]Au) as a radioactive tracer or spectroscopic analysis for gold in tissues - in effect disclosing the overall distribution of gold and its kinetics but not defining the atomic/molecular species present (by ignoring the ligands, if any, to which it may be bound). Even studies which show a rapid transfer of gold(I) to human serum albumin[8] rarely establish if all the gold that is albumin-bound is still Au(I) and does not include perhaps some Au(III). Transfer of gold to sites of potential toxicity, e.g. kidney, marrow, has been frequently demonstrated but rarely analysed rigorously to determine in which valency state the gold is actually present. While the bulk of the deposited gold may be benign, traces of gold in a second or

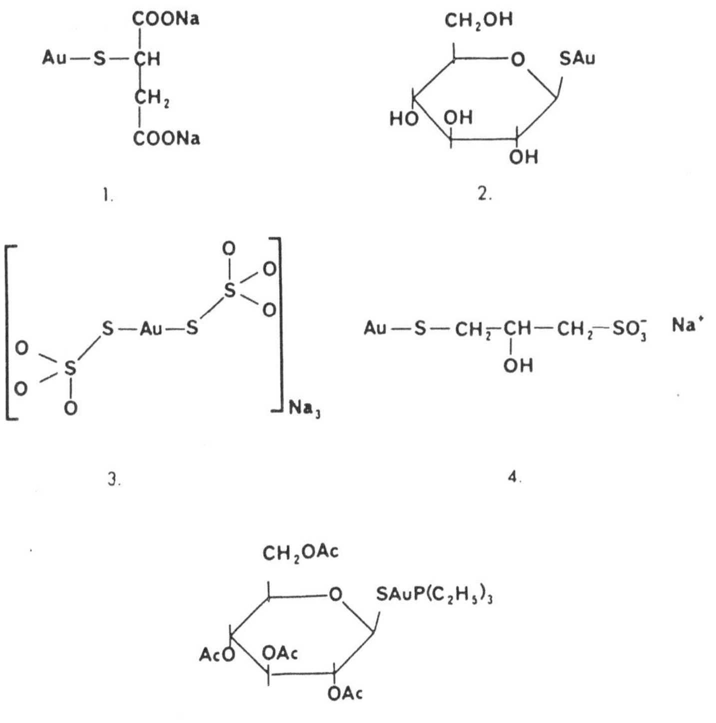

Figure 1 Biologically active gold(I) formulations: (1) gold sodium thiomalate (Myochrisine); (2) gold thioglucose (Solganal); (3) gold sodium thiosulphate (Sanochrysine); (4) gold sodium thiopropanolsulphonate (Allocrysine); (5) S-2,3,4,5-tetraacetyl-1-β-D thioglucose (triethylphosphine) gold(I) (From reference 6 by courtesy of the publishers).

third valency state may be quite toxic if the tissue lacks detoxication mechanisms for these other forms of gold.

The two gold(I)-thiolates that are now most widely used to treat rheumatoid diseases, namely sodium aurothiomalate (ATM) and auranofin (AF), have quite distinctive properties (Table 1) beyond their different chemical constitutions (Figure 1). This means that it is rather improbable that they act by identical means unless they are both pro-drugs which happen to generate the same effector species *in vivo*. Could this perhpas be Au(III), the marker for which might be locally deposited metallic gold? If, however, we invoke specific receptors for their mode(s) of action or toxicity, then *either* these gold receptors must tolerate considerable diversity among the thioligands associated with Au(I) (assuming common receptors), *or* there are distinct receptors for the ultimate pharmacoactive metabolites of ATM and AF respectively. With these present uncertainties it would seem prudent to assume these two types of gold(I) drugs may have *different* pharmacologies that happen to overlap in their common anti-arthritic action, rather than glibly presuming they are two pro-drugs for the one active molecular species.

**Table 1    Aurothiomalate (ATM) and Auranofin (AF) are two quite distinct drugs/pro-drugs**

| Regarding | ATM | AF |
|---|---|---|
| Composition | Thiol ligand only | Also contains a non-thiol ligand (tri-ethylphosphine) |
| | 50.5% Au | 29.0% Au |
| Physical properties | Water-soluble | Lipophilic |
| | Polymer in aqueous solution | Monomer |
| | Highly charged polyanion | Neutral |
| | Not absorbed by intestine | Absorbed, but with possible intestinal detoxification* |
| Biological properties | Needs parenteral administration | Orally effective |
| | Low cytotoxicity | Cytotoxic |
| | — | Mimics phorbol esters(s) |
| Side-effects | Induces nephrosis | Minimal effect on kidney |
| | Minimal effect on intestine | Induces diarrhoea |
| Anti-arthritic dose | 50 mg (weekly) | ≤ 5 mg (daily) |

* See section 7.

210

Other gold(I)-thiolates currently used clinically include anionic complexes formed with thiosulphate or 3-thiopropan-2-ol-sulphonate ions, or the neutral complex formed with 1-thioglucose. These all seem to mimic ATM clinically, being water-soluble, probably oligomeric and in requiring parenteral administration. Since any of these three latter thioligands ('aurophores') will substitute effectively for thiomalate (mercaptosuccinate), it is rather unlikely that ATM is a unique pro-drug in the sense of releasing an active metabolite = thiomalate *in vivo*. There is certainly some attraction in trying to show that the clinical similarity in action between ATM and well-established anti-arthritic thiols (D-penicillamine captopril, alpha-mercaptopropionylglyine, etc.) may be due to ATM and its congeners acting as precursor drugs, in essence supplying free thiomalate/alternative thiols to mimic D-penicillamine, etc., *in vivo*. However, comparisons of the biological effects of thiomalate with ATM (Table 2) would seem *not* to justify this unitary hypothesis, i.e. that ATM and other gold(I)-thiolates are merely cryptic thiol drugs. This being so, we must find out why ATM is in fact active and thiomalate (and even penicillamine) is not, in some animal models of chronic arthritis.

**Table 2   Comparison of aurothiomalate (ATM) with thiomalate (TM)**

|  | *ATM* | *TM* |
|---|---|---|
| Physical properties | Polymer | Monomer |
|  | Relatively stable | Readily oxidizes |
| Biological properties | Anti-arthritic activity in rats | Inactive |
|  | Inhibits lymphocyte proliferation | Inactive |
|  | Modifies rheumatoid arthritis (↓sedimentation rate, ↓rheumatoid factor, etc.) | Questionable clinical activity |

## 3.  CLINICAL RESPONSE TO GOLD DRUGS: IS IT GENETICALLY DETERMINED?

### A.  In animals

Experimental studies have shown that the beneficial effects of gold drugs upon arthritis/inflammation are not always easy to demonstrate in small animals. This is in contrast to so many other drugs that also suppress arthritic inflammation, e.g. NSAIDs or cytotoxic agents which usually manifest the same spectrum of therapeutic activities in different animals and in different laboratories. Gold drugs have suppressed the development in rats of the adjuvant-induced polyarthritis[9] or the type II collagen induced arthritis[10] in some laboratory studies, but not in others. Furthermore, auranofin many not show

211

anti-arthritic activity when aurothiomalate does[10,11], indicating that even when the experimental conditions seem 'right' for demonstrating a therapeutic activity of one gold drug, they are not necessarily sufficient to disclose the activity of another gold drug (or perhaps its active metabolites).

A genetic factor does seem to be involved, inasmuch as two strains of rats housed within the same laboratory and inoculated with the same arthritogen can respond quite differently to a common course of treatment with either parenteral or oral gold drugs[9]. This type of experimentation can identify gold-responsive and gold-resistant rat strains. Cross-breeding experiments have shown that the gold responsiveness may be easily lost, inasmuch as the (R x S) F1 hybrid bred from mating a resistant (R) rat strain with a susceptible (S) rat strain is also gold-resistant.

However, there may be other factors as well, such as the general environment, food and water supply, which ultimately influence the handling of metal drugs *in vivo*. Induction of metal-detoxicant mechanisms by ambient metals (derived from cages, food, water, etc.) could profoundly influence the *in vivo* properties of a gold drug, so that workers in one laboratory using an identical gold-responsive rat may not necessarily duplicate the findings from another laboratory.

These complications, expressed in the following equation:

'Gold responsiveness = function of genes and environment, and?'

at least help us to understand why it has taken so long to learn so little about the mechanisms of action of gold drugs in experimental animals.

## B. In patients

Many rheumatoid patients do not respond well to the parenteral gold drugs. This is not unique, as for example non-responders to sulphasalazine[12] or indomethacin[13] have also been clearly identified. Attempts to predict which patients might respond to gold therapy have so far been largely unsuccessful[14].

The actual proportion of non-responders to chrysotherapy has been variously estimated to be both low (10%) and rather high (> 50%). Some patients who responded well to an initial course of treatment may subsequently prove refractory to a second course. Taken together, these 'erratic' results of chrysotherapy suggest that the drug action is largely conditioned by the patient's pathophysiological status. For example, the destructive components of rheumatoid disease may have matured to a chrysotherapy-resistant stage during the time interval that the first line of therapy was to use NSAIDs.

Other variables within a patient population, such as genetic constitution, diet or environment, may also enable or prevent certain individuals from responding beneficially to gold drugs. This latter aspect has been the subject of many, rather confusing and contradictory, reports which sought to relate predisposition to adverse effects of chrysotherapy with certain genetic markers, particularly the HLA antigens DR3 or B8. Unfortunately this type of analysis has not so far confidently identified the 'non-toxic' groups of patients. Thus in one survey of 29 published reports covering 763 patients carried out in 1985, at least 60% of gold-treated patients exhibiting nephrotoxic reactions were noted to be DR 3-negative[15]. Absence of the HLA-DR4 antigen and presence of HLA-A3 has been suggested as possibly predisposing patients to a successful outcome of gold therapy[14].

It would certainly be helpful to have some type of prognostic indicator for at least two groups of patients: (i) those whose disease is particularly susceptible to gold-regulation, and (ii) those who will most likely suffer intoxication rather than gain therapeutic benefit. Some individuals in this latter group may lack gold-neutralizing mechanisms within the organ at risk (marrow, kidney, skin) but others may be so hypersensitive (immunostimulated?) that it is unlikely that any one biochemical test (e.g. measuring gold-detoxifying proteins such as metallothionein) will serve as a sufficient screen. Again progress is hampered by lack of well-developed animal models with which to probe both the efficacy and toxicity of the gold(I) drugs and enquire how nutrition, genetics and the many different phases of a chronic inflammatory response may actually affect their potency and tolerance.

## 4. THE EFFECT OF GOLD(I) DRUGS ON CELLS BOTH *IN VIVO* AND *IN VITRO*

This survey is primarily restricted to leucocytes, being the dominant cells in mounting the immune and/or inflammatory responses. It is often difficult to compare reports from different clinics and laboratories even when the same cellular properties or functions are being measured, because the actual conditions for stimulating leucocytes may vary quite significantly (e.g. the use of live or killed bacteria for studies of phagocytosis).

### A. Lymphocytes

Large numbers of lymphocytes (Table 3) are often found at sites of both chronic and acute inflammation[46]. These cells are important regulators of immune responses, particularly those involved in inflammation. Lynphocytes isolated from the joints of individuals with active rheumatoid arthritis are known to be in a state of activation, having undergone, or being just about to undergo, cell division[47].

Table 3   Effect of two gold(I) drugs on lymphocytes from the peripheral blood

| Function | Conditions and origin | | Effect | | References |
|---|---|---|---|---|---|
| (i) Antibody responses | In vivo | human | ATM↑ | | 16,17 |
| | In vivo | human | ATM↑ | AF↓ | 18 |
| | In vivo | human | ATM↓ | | 19,20,21 22,23,24 |
| | In vivo | human | ATM→ | | 25 |
| | In vitro | human | ATM↑ | | 26 |
| | In vitro | human | ATM↓ | | 27 |
| | In vivo | rabbit | ATM→ | | 28 |
| | In vivo | mouse | ATM↑ | | 29,30,31 |
| (ii) Mitogen stimulated proliferation | In vitro | human | ATM↓ | | 20,32,33 |
| | In vitro | human | | AF↓ | 37 |
| | In vitro | human | ATM↓ | AF↓ | 38 |
| | In vivo | human | ATM↑ | | 39,40 |
| (iii) Interleukin 1 stimulated proliferation | In vitro | mouse | ATM↓ | AF↓ | 41 |
| (iv) Interleukin 2 production | In vivo | human | ATM↑ | | 42 |
| | In vivo | rat | | AF↑ | 43 |
| | In vitro | mouse | | AF↓ | 44 |
| (v) Cytotoxicity | In vivo | human | ATM↑ | | 39,40 |
| | In vitro | human | ATM↓ | | 42 |
| | In vitro | human | | AF↓ | 45 |
| (vi) T helper cell activity | In vivo | rat | | AF↓ | 44 |
| (vii) T suppressor cell activity | In vitro | rat | ATM→ | AF↓ | 43 |

Abbreviations : ↑ increased activity; ↓ decreased activity; → no effect; ↑ ↓ biphasic response; ATM = aurothiomalate; AF = Auranofin; ATG = aurothioglucose

## (i) Antibody production and lymphoproliferation

Any effects of gold drugs in regulating B-lymphocytes could be particularly important as these are the cells which produce antibodies (and hence the immune complexes and rheumatoid factors seen in rheumatoid disease[10]). Immune complexes can activate macrophages and fix complement, leading to production of chemotactic agents and other mediators which enhance and sustain inflammation. High levels of IgM rheumatoid factor, particularly when it is intra-articular, are generally associated with more severe rheumatoid disease[48].

Despite the large number of studies of the effect of gold drugs on antibody production there is little consistency in the findings. On balance, more studies, particularly those in vitro, have shown a suppression of immuno-

214

globin production. The levels of rheumatoid factor generally decrease in patients who respond to gold treatment. It is suggested that this is a direct effect of gold (and other disease-modifying drug) therapy[49]. Gold drugs may suppress immuglobulin production by affecting accessory cell function (in triggering an immune response) or directly affect the B lymphocyte's ability to proliferate in response to cytokines and other stimuli. We have found both ATM and Af will suppress IL-1-induced lymphocyte proliferation *in vitro* at or below concentrations found in the serum of patients receiving the drugs[41]. These gold compounds will similarly inhibit mitogen-induced lymphoproliferation[19,32,37]. Reduced lymphoproliferation could be responsible for many of the suppressed lymphoid responses. In our hands the *in vitro* suppression of lymphoproliferation by AF seems to be due to its immediate cytotoxicity.

Many lympocyte responses are mediated by cytokines, such as IL-2, BAF, IL-1. etc., which stimulate lymphocyte differentiation and proliferation. IL-2 production by lymphocytes is a prime trigger for further lymphoproliferation and subsequent antibody production *in vitro*. Gold drugs have been shown to inhibit IL-2 production *in vitro* [41,43].

On the other hand *in vivo* studies, where an antigen and ATM were given simultaneously, showed enhanced IgM antibody responses to the antigen[29,30]. Highton and colleagues[39,40] observed increased lymphoproliferative responses in the peripheral blood of patients treated with ATM. Lymphocytes from rats with adjuvant arthritis were found to have reduced IL-2 production (and responses there from) that could be increased to normal levels by *in vitro* treatment with AF[44]. Similarly suppressed IL-2 function in patients with pemphigus vulgaris could be restored to normal levels by ATM treatment[42].

Collectively, these reports seem to offer contradictory statements concerning the effects of gold drugs *in vitro* and *in vivo*. Many studies indicate the immunoreactive activity of lymphoid cells from the peripheral blood of patients and arthritic animals is abnormally low. *In vivo* treatment with gold drugs, instead of further decreasing their responsiveness as often seen *in vitro*, actually increases their response to normal levels.

The body's attempt to control an overactive local immune response, such as that found within the inflamed synovium (behaving like an ectopic lymph node), could result in suppression of distal or systemic immune responses. If gold treatment controls the overactive local response, the associated suppressive factors might no longer be available to affect the distal responses (Figure 2). These systemic responses could then return (increase) to normal levels. Such local→distal effects of a gold drug could affect a variety of lymphocyte responses including antibody production, cytotoxicity to target cells, and cytokine secretion. The *in vitro* studies may therefore be quite significant, despite appearing to contradict some *in vivo* findings, as they may actually disclose the real/local effects of gold therapy upon those cells within sites of inflammation.

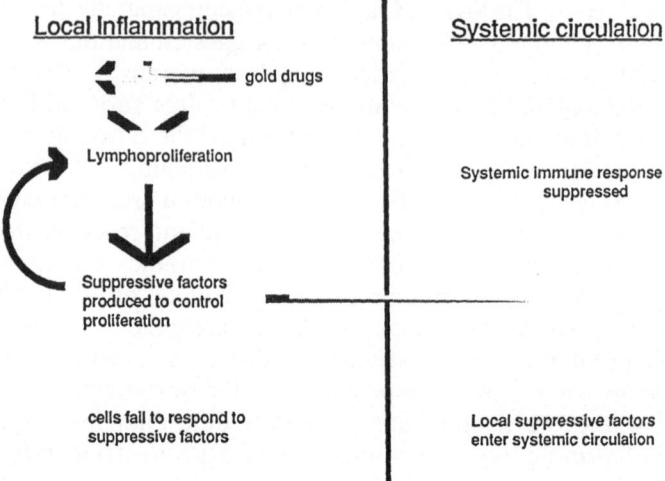

**Figure 2** Suppressive factors produced by an active local immune response may result in suppression of the peripheral (distal) immune response. If so, then gold drugs inhibiting lymphoproliferation would remove systemic suppressant effect (after Highton *et al.*, ref. 39).

### (ii) Helper and suppressor lymphocyte populations

The combined activity of helper and suppressor lymphocytes plays an important role in regulating the onset and duration of an immune response. Although several studies have shown abnormal ratios of helper to suppressor lymphocyte populations (OKT4[+]/T8[+] ratio) in patients with rheumatoid arthritis[50], it is uncertain if this is actually an important factor for maintaining disease. Several studies have shown changes in the ratios of these lymphocyte populations in patients following gold treatment[50,51]. If gold could affect one population more than the other, as suggested[43,44], then the immune response would be tipped in favour of either prolongation or suppression.

### B. Mononuclear phagocytes

Macrophages not only play an important role in local destruction in chronically inflamed tissues but also regulate other cells of the immune system. The idea has long been advanced that the beneficial action of gold drugs in rheumatoid arthritis may result from their capacity to alter the function of the mononuclear phagocytes at the site of inflammation[54,63,70,71]. This is strongly supported by ultrastructural studies which show phagocytes selectively accumulate of gold in the lysosomes of the type A synovial cells and other macrophages of the synovium in patients treated by chrysotherapy[70,72,73]. ATM is also actively taken up by peritoneal macrophages[63] and can alter the morphology of human peripheral blood monocytes (our own observations)[56].

216

Thus because gold accumulates in macrophages, the long-lived leucocytes regulating inflammation, the slow-onset benefits of gold therapy may well be mediated by changes in macrophage function. Enhancement of the mononuclear phagocyte's ability to bind and then remove particulare matter and/or immune complexes could be beneficial in relieving inflammation sustained by these persisting irritants.

Table 4   Effect of some gold(I) drugs on mononuclear phagocytes

| Function | Conditions and origin | | Effect | | References |
|---|---|---|---|---|---|
| (i)  Phagocytosis | In vivo | human | ATM↓ | | 50 |
| | In vivo | rat | ATM↓ | | 51 |
| | In vitro | human | ATM↓ | 52,53,54 | |
| (ii)  Receptor expression | In vitro | rat | ATM↑ | | 55 |
| | In vitro | mouse, | | | |
| | | rat | ATM↑ | AF→ | 56 |
| | In vitro | human | ATM↓ | AF→ | 57 |
| (iii)  Chemotaxis | In vitro | human | ATM↓ | | 58 |
| | In vitro | human | ATM↓ | AF↓ | 59 |
| (iv)  Enzyme production | In vivo | human | ATM↓ | | 60 |
| | In vivo | human | ATM↓ | AF↓ | 60,61,62 |
| (v)  Monokine production | In vitro | mouse | | AF↓ | 44 |
| | In vitro | mouse, | | | |
| | | rat | ATM→ | AF↓ | 45 |
| | In vitro | human | ATM→ | | 63 |
| | In vitro | human | ATG↓ | | 64 |
| | In vitro | human | ATM↓ | | 38 |
| | In vivo | human | ATM↑ | | 42 |
| (vi)  Maturation | In vitro | human | ATM↓ | | 59 |
| (vii)  Prostaglandin formation | In vitro | human | ATM→ | AF→ | 60 |
| | In vitro | mouse, | | | |
| | | rat | ATM↓ | AF→ | 41 |
| (viii)  Intracellular killing of bacteria | In vitro | human | ATM↓ | 65 |
| (ix)  Superoxide production | In vitro | mouse | ATM↓ | | 66,67 |

See Table 3 for explanation of abbreviations

## (i)  Phagocytes and receptor function

Several recent studies have shown elevated Fc receptor function in the peripheral blood of patients with active arthritis[74,75] and rats with adjuvant arthritis[58].

ATM treatment of adjuvant arthritic rats resulted in a decrease in peripheral blood receptor function. Similarly using the skin window technique to study peripheral macrophages, Vernon-Roberts and his co-workers[52,53] observed decreased phagocytosis of carbon particles in patients and rats treated with ATM. However, in adjuvant arthritic rats we have found that gold treatment increases the expression of both Fc and complement receptors on the peritoneal macrophage population. This increase in Fc receptor function could also be induced *in vitro* by ATM treatment of peritoneal macrophage[57,58]. Hence ATM treatment can affect mononuclear phagocytes in different ways depending upon the anatomical site from which they are obtained. Therefore observations of gold-induced changes in the activity of cells drawn from the peripheral blood may not truly reflect crucial changes at the site of inflammation.

### (ii) Monokines and other products secreted by activated macrophages

Inhibition of enzyme production, particularly collagenase[62], can reduce inflammation and tissue damage. Intracellular killing of bacteria by the oxidative burst[61] and macrophage superoxide production[68,69] were also shown to be inhibited by gold drugs. It has been suggested[61] that these particular effects on macrophage function are associated primarily with inhibition of macrophage differentiation and maturation.

Macrophage will release several cytokines capable of stimulating the inflammatory response. Of these the monokine interleukin 1 (IL-1) exhibits a wide range of biological activities. There is considerable evidence that IL-1 might play a central role in many inflammatory disorders including rheumatoid arthritis[77,78]. AF appears to inhibit IL-1 production *in vitro*[44] but this may only reflect the inherent toxicity of AF for the macrophage . By contrast ATM treatment of patients with pemphigus vulgaris has been reported to restore defective IL-1 production[42].

Lipsky and Ziff[33] showed that ATM inhibits *in vitro* macrophage-dependent lymphocyte proliferation. ATM does not seem to affect the production of IL-1 as measured in the LAF assay[79], by normal LPS-stimulated macrophage *in vitro*[41]. Even if gold drugs do not affect IL-1 production, they can affect its function (see Table 3). It is possible that IL-1 is a carboxypeptidase-like molecule, losing its activity when divalent cations are depleted[80], but re-activated when $Zn^{2+}$ is reintroduced[66,81]. This might explain why gold salts are more effective at inhibiting IL-1 lymphoproliferation when the level of thiols is reduced[41].

Other cytokines released by macrophages may be affected by gold treatment. Aurothioglucose and thioglucose were shown to inhibit the *in vitro* elaboration of a human lymphokine, the leucocyte migration inhibitory factor (LIF)[66]. Since thioglucose was equally effective, this particular effect of ATG may not be dependent on the gold moiety. It could be reversed in the presence of equimolar concentrations of $Zn^{2+}$ and other divalent cations.

## C. Polymorphonuclear cells (neutrophils, granulocytes)

Polymorphonuclear cells (PMNs) like mononuclear phagocytes, play an important role in the inflammatory process (Table 5). They are one of the first cells to appear at an inflammatory site and their presence is usually associated with the inflammation. In comparison to mononuclear phagocytes, PMN's are highly active cells which when stimulated elicit an immediate but short-lived response.

**Table 5 Effect of two gold(I) drugs on polymorphonuclear cells**

| Function | Conditions and origin | | Effect | | Reference |
|---|---|---|---|---|---|
| Reactive oxygen species | In vitro | human | ATM↓ | AF↓ | 80,81,82 |
| generation | In vitro | human | | AF↓ | 83 |
| | In vivo | human | ATM↑ | | 84 |
| Chemiluminescene | In vitro | human | | AF↑↓ | 85 |
| | In vivo | human | | AF↑ | 85 |
| | In vivo | human | ATM→ | AF↓ | 86 |
| Enzyme release | In vitro | human, rat | | AF↓ | 87 |
| | In vitro | human | | AF↑↓ | 83,85 |
| | In vitro | human | ATM→ | | 88 |
| Chemotaxis | In vivo | human | | AF↑↓ | 85 |
| | In vivo | rat | | AF→ | 89 |
| | In vitro | rat | | AF→ | 89 |
| | In vitro | human | | AF↓ | 83,90,91,92 |
| | In vitro | human | ATM↓ | | 90,92 |
| Adherence | In vitro | human | | AF↑ | 85 |
| Phagocytosis | In vitro | human | ATM↓ | AF↓ | 86 |
| Bacteria killing | In vivo | human | ATM↑ | | 93 |
| | In vitro | human | | AF↓ | 86 |
| PMN numbers | In vivo | human | ATM↑ | | 84,93,94,95 |

See Table 3 for explanation of abbreviations

Their importance in protecting the host from disease is indicated by the increased susceptibility to infection of individuals with reduced PMN numbers or PMN functions[98]. PMNs may also have an important role in chronic inflammatory disorders.

### (i) Oxygen-derived free radicals

The production of oxy-radicals during the respiratory burst of phagocytic cells plays an essential role in bacterial killing[99]. Many cells, in particular polymorphonuclear cells (PMNs), monocytes and macrophage, will produce oxy-radicals in response to a variety of stimuli such as the immune complexes formed with rheumatoid factors. These radicals injure cells and provoke inflammatory reactions consistent with those seen in inflamed joints[100,101].

Several studies have recently been carried out to evaluate the possible antioxidant effect of gold compounds. The results indicate, AF, in particular, can substantially interfere with *in vitro* oxy-radical production by activated PMNs[82-84,102]. AF will inhibt receptor-mediated stimulation (e.g. by fMLP, PMA). However it does not affect PMN stimulation that is not receptor-mediated (e.g. with calcium ionophores), indicating that the inhibition of oxy-radical generation by AF is probably receptor-mediated[102]. AF also inhibits the production by PMNs of the hydroxyl radical[82]. This radical is an extremely potent tissue toxin[100]. ATM is not as effective as AF at inhibiting cellular production of these oxygen-derived species. In contrast to AF, the levels of ATM which have an antioxidant effect are probably higher than one would expect to find *in vivo* > 100 µg/ml[83].

Gold complexes inhibit a wide variety of other neutrophil functions *in vitro* in a dose-dependent manner. There is some evidence that the *in vitro* effect of AF is biphasic, augmenting some functions at low concentrations but inhibiting them at higher concentrations[87]. Gold drugs inhibit enzyme release from PMNs as they do from mononuclear phagocytes (see previous section). Both AF and ATM inhibit random movement and chemotaxis of PMNs *in vitro*.

### (ii) In vivo enhancement of PMN functions

Once again the results reported from *in vivo* and *in vitro* studies seem to differ. Generally, ATM *in vitro* suppresses many PMN functions; however the few *in vivo* studies suggest it enhances PMN functions[86,87]. Of particular interest is the effect of gold treatment upon Felty's syndrome and leukopenia associated with rheumatoid arthritis. These disorders are characterized by qualitative and quantitative neutrophil defects believed to contribute to the increased incidence of infection seen in these individuals. Gold therapy will actually restore the leucocyte count, decrease fever and reduce the susceptibility to infections[95-97]. A recent study has shown that the defects in neutrophil superoxide generation associated with Felty's syndrome[103] can be reversed after standard gold therapy[86]. There is no evidence for differences in oxy-radical generation by peripheral blood PMNs from RA patients and from normal individuals[103]. As yet the *in vivo* effects of gold drugs on oxy-radical production by neutrophils from RA patients have not been reported. Patients, however, show a marked *increase* in several other neutrophil functions (e.g. bactericidal, migration and chemotaxis) after prolonged AF treatment[87].

It is not known if the enhanced *in vivo* PMN functions are due to the improved clinical status of the patient or the pharmacological effect of the drug. As noted with mononuclear phagocytes, the concentrations and effect of gold on the peripheral blood population may differ markedly from those seen at an inflammatory site. Either directly or indirectly gold therapy can very likely affect PMN *in vivo*, and so possibly contribute to the beneficial therapeutic effects obtained with gold drugs.

## D. Platelets (thrombocytes)

Platelets are known to be involved in acute inflammation. They are thought to accumulate in the inflamed joint[104] and have been detected in the synovial fluid and membrane[105,106]. They contain many inflammatory mediators including histamine and serotonin, as well as being a rich source of prostaglandins[107] and proteolytic enzymes[108].

### (i) Inhibition of platelet function

Recent studies suggest that AF can inhibit both platelet release and aggregation mechanisms which may be relevant to its anti-arthritic activity[109]. It has been suggested AF may block the activity of prostanoids and interfere with thromboxane-mediated release of platelet factors[110].

### (ii) Gold-induced thrombocytopenia

Thrombocytopenia affects 1-3% of the patients undergoing gold therapy[111]. There is evidence for at least two forms of this iatrogenic disease[112]. One form is manifest by a slow decline in platelet numbers over weeks and months that usually occurs late in therapy. Platelet numbers return to normal on cessation of gold therapy. This decline in the number of platelets is usually a part of a general pancytopenia, probably due to cumulative toxicity of gold within the bone marrow. The second form is a more severe thrombocytopenia that occurs rapidly at any time during gold therapy and seems to be a gold-induced autoimmune disease, due to enhanced autoantibody formation. This may not be reversed on ceasing therapy[113]. There is evidence for phagocytosis of platelets in the spleen and the blood may contain antiplatelet antibodies. These autoantibodies will bind to platelets in the absence of gold, indicating complexation with gold does not mediate their binding[114]. The

221

only effective treatment for this form of thrombocytopenia is either corticosteroid treatment or splenectomy. It is interesting to compare these findings
to those already discussed (see section on lymphocytes) where *in vivo* gold
treatment often *enhances* various antibody responses.

## E. Prostaglandin synthesis by leucocytes

There is no need to expand here upon the multifunctional and, in general,
detrimental role that arachidonic metabolites play in inflammation[115]. Inhibition of prostaglandin synthesis by a gold drug may possibly provide
beneficial effects similar to those seen with non-steroidal anti-inflammatory
drug treatments. Some studies have been carried out showing inhibition of
prostaglandin $E_2$ (PGE2) synthesis by ATM and other gold compounds, at
levels of gold found therapeutically[116]. Other studies show little or no effect.
It is difficult to compare all these studies as a number of different cell types
and stimulants are used to promote PGE2 synthesis. Our recent studies of
LPS-stimulated macrophages and those of Parente et al.[117] would indicate
that AF and ATM have no effect on PGE2 synthesis, and so do not behave
like the conventional non-steroidal anti-inflammatory drugs. However other
pathways of arachidonate oxygenation, such as leukotriene production, may
be affected by gold drugs[117,118].

## F. Effect of AF on transmembrane signalling

AF is highly lipid-soluble due to the presence of the triethylphosphine group.
It quickly finds it way into cell membranes in culture and so may affect many
normal membrane functions. Many forms of intercellular communication
(e.g. by cytokines, hormones, etc.) involve transmembrane signalling via cell
surface receptors. When a cytokine binds to its receptor, protein-kinase C
(PKC) is often activated and intracellular $Ca^{2+}$ is mobilized[119]. Recent *in
vitro* studies have indicated AF can modulate functions involving PKC. For
example, AF inhibits platelet aggregation[109] and phorbol-ester induced
superoxide anion release from human neutrophils[102] and blood monocytes[120]. AF, however, does not affect superoxide anion release from monocytes by the $Ca^{2+}$ ionophore, A23187[120], in the same way, suggesting the
drug affects events involving PKC.

AF can also affect receptor expression. For example, it will reduce the
binding of epidermal growth factor to HeLa cells by down-regulating its receptor[121]. Similarly, mouse erythrocyte receptor expression on human
leukemic B cells is reduced in a thiol-dependent manner[122]. It has been suggested that thiols may be involved in the uptake of AF by the cells[123]. Human
B lymphocytes making IgM rheumatoid factor express mouse erythrocyte receptor and its down-regulation may indicate an important mode of action of
AF. In contrast, recent evidence suggests that gold drugs may also act as cell

stimulators (Table 6) by activating cellular transduction pathways[123,124]. In the case of AF it may directly activate PKC[124].

## 5.  EFFECT OF GOLD ON EXTRACELLULAR FUNCTIONS

### A.  Enzymes

There are many enzymes released from a variety of cells that are actively involved in inflammation. PMNs alone release 20 or so hydrolytic enzymes, the most important being acid hydrolases (such as β-glucuronidase and acid phosphatase) and neutral proteases (such as collagenase and elastase). These enzymes not only break down connective tissue, but also produce chemotactic factors. Several authors have reviewed the effect of gold drugs on hydrolytic and other enzymes[2,4,5]. The inhibition of these enzymes is probably due to the interaction of gold with one or more of the free sulphydryl groups, found in the cysteine moieties of the enzyme. Persellin and Ziff[63] showed that after incubation of macrophage with ATM, only those enzymes associated with the lysosomal fractions were inhibited. Gold(I) complexes will also inhibit the release of lysosomal enzymes[5]. This not surprising, as it is known gold selectively accumulates in the lysosomes of macrophages (see section on mononuclear phagocytes). This effectively 'targets' gold(I) to inhibit the action and release of lysosomal enzymes, perhaps thereby reducing inflammation in patients receiving gold therapy. Some of these studies report enzyme inhibition at concentrations of gold actually found in the serum of patients undergoing gold therapy. However, many other enzymes require considerably higher concentrations for an inhibitory effect.

### B. Collagen

Adams[125] and his co-workers have investigated the action of gold on collagen. Collagen fibres from gold-treated rats showed greater resistance to a variety of physical and chemical tests. Electron microphages reveal that gold may accumulate in the collagen of rat fibrils. It was suggested that gold crosslinks the collagen molecules, creating a more stable structure. It was also shown tha the adverse effects of lathyrogenic chemicals and copper deficiency, both of which decrease collage cross-linkages, could be reversed by gold treatment[126]. As yet there is no evidence that gold cross-links occurs in the connective tissue of human patients on gold therapy.

### C. Complement

Immune complexes and complement are both found in the inflamed arthritic joint. Complement activation by immune complexes results in cell lysis and also the production of chemo-attractants. ATM but not TM will inhibit complement-mediated haemolysis at 0.05–1 mM levels[127]. It will also inhibit the alternative pathway of complement activation[128]. As yet, however, there is no correlation between serum gold and serum complement levels in patients undergoing therapy[129].

Table 6    Some biological responses induced by gold(I) drugs

| | Response | Gold drug | References |
|---|---|---|---|
| 1. | Enhanced *In vivo* IgM production (mouse spleen cells) | ATM | 29,30 |
| 2. | Enhanced IL-2 production (spleen cells, adjuvantized arthritic rat) | AF | 43 |
| 3. | Enhanced inflammatory response (biochemical parameters, human) | ATM,AF | 130 |
| 4. | Increased lysosomal enzymes (rat alveolar macrophage) | ATM | 131 |
| 5. | Increased (Cu,Au) metallothionein (cultured rat kidney cells) | ATM | 132 |
| 6. | Increased Fc receptor activity (rat peritoneal macrophage) | ATM | 56 |
| 7. | Increased PMN numbers and function (Felty's syndrome, human) | ATM | Section 4 C(ii) |
| 8. | Induction of platelet auto-antibody (gold induced thrombo-cytopenia, human) | ATM | Section 4 D(ii) |
| 9. | Increased lymphoproliferation (peripheral blood lymphocytes, human) | ATM | 39,40 |
| 10. | Activation of cellular transduction (leucocytes) | ATM, AF | 124 |

Abbreviations: ATM = aurothiomalate; AF = Auranofin; PMN = polymorphonuclear cells

## 6.    DO GOLD(I) DRUGS INDUCE SOME ANTI-ARTHRITIC MECHANISMS?

The original literature contains several suggestions that gold drugs may produce paradoxical effects – mainly an enhanced bioreactivity, where the original working hypothesis was to look for gold-suppressed phenomena. Table 6 lists a few such observations. Since most induced responses require a latent period for the induction phenomenon to occur and then be expressed, the time period for their expression cannot be as rapid as direct inhibitory effects

224

on pre-established biosystems. Perhaps the short time span of much experimentation with gold drugs in model systems has hindered the recognition of some of these apparent induction phenomena. However, the time delay may also indicate non-specificity: perhaps where the gold drug is acting merely as an irritant or toxin, thereby eliciting homeostatic counter-irritant and/or gold-detoxifying mechanisms which happen to have beneficial consequences, e.g. stimulating the adrenal cortex→enhance metallothionein synthesis.

Some of these induction phenomena do make sense if we are prepared to believe, for example, that increased IgG production or increased levels of macrophage lysosomal hydrolases might facilitate eradication of persistant arthritogen(s), rather than just being pathogenic *per se*. Indirect effects on copper and zinc distribution might ensue from Au-induction of raised level of tissue (Cu, Zn)metallothioneins. These thioneins = sulphydryl-rich peptides are also important scavengers of tissue-intoxicating free radicals, such as are produced by inflammatory cells[133].

Other phenomena may not be true examples of induction, but rather the suppression by a gold drug of a natural suppressive factor or cell. One example of this seems to be the effect of auranofon in T-suppressor cells in adjuvant arthritic rat spleens which is manifest experimentally by raised level of IL-2 production[43]. Perhaps it is quibbling to try to distinguish this type of double suppression from a real stimulation wrought by a gold drug.

## 7. CONCLUDING COMMENTS

This review has not addressed several less well-researched areas of possible relevance. For example, these drugs may affect other cells than leucocytes (e.g. fibroblasts, endothelial cells, etc.) which participate in the mounting of, and repair after, an inflammatory event. We know some gold complexes can exert dramatic effects on yet other cells in the body, e.g. aurothioglucose inducing an experimental obesity in mice[134]. Perhaps they can regulate other endocrine actions, in essence regulating the regulators.

A particular difficulty with respect to Auranofin is establishing whether any of the *in situ* effects attributed to this drug (including the mimicking of phorbol esters) are clinically relevant, in the light of one report that Auranofin is extensively hydrolysed (deacetylated) on transit through the intestinal mucosa[135]. This in essence immediately transforms the drug from a highly toxic, lipophilic entity to a more hydrophobic molecule, the pharmacology of which has yet to be disclosed.

We must conclude therefore that our perception of the gold drugs is necessarily clouded because:

(a)   certain hypotheses concerning their actions have not yet been rigorously tested,

(b)   *in vitro* studies may not disclose *veritas*,

(c)    *in vivo* studies using peripheral blood cell populations may not necessarily reflect the drug's action at the site of inflammation,

(d)    the long lag phase for their onset of action has been too often ignored,

(e)    the right animal models are not being sought with enough diligence as yet, and

(f)    interactions with other key regulators, e.g. selenium antoxidants[136], cyanide generation[137,138] and other trace elements[139] may also have to be considered.

## ACKNOWLEDGEMENTS:

Original work described here was supported by the National Health and Medical Research Council of Australia. We are indebted to Prof. B. Vernon-Roberts for his support and encouragement.

## REFERENCES

1.    Kean WF, Forester F, Kassam Y, Buchanan WW and Rooney PJ (1985)  The history of gold therapy in rheumatoid disease. *Sem Arth Rheum*, **14**, 180-6
2.    Shaw CF (1979) The mammalian biochemistry of gold: an inorganic perspective of chrysotherapy. *Inorg Persp Biol Med*, **2**, 287-355
3.    Brown DH and Smith WE (1980) The chemistry of gold drugs used in the treatment of rheumatoid arthritis. *Quart Rev Chem Soc*, **9**, 217-40
4.    Leibfarth JH and Persellin RH (1981) Mechanism of action of gold. *Agents Actions*, **11**, 458-72
5.    Lewis AJ and Waltz DT (1982) Immunopharmacology of gold in G.P.Ellis and G.B.West (eds) pp 1-57 (Elsevier Biomedical Press). *Prog Med Chem*, **19**
6.    Betts WH, Garrett IR and Whitehouse MW (19  Therapy with metal complexes. In: Rainsford KD (ed.) *Anti-inflammatory and Anti-rheumatic Drugs* ( : ), vol. III, pp65-103
7.    Crooke TS, Synder RM, Butt TR, Ecker DJ, Allandeen AS, Monia B and Mirabelli CK (1986) Cellular and Molecular pharmacology of auranofin and related gold complexes. *Biochem Pharmacol*, **35**, 3423-31
8.    Pedersen SM (1986) Binding of sodium aurothiomalate to human serum albumin *in vitro* at physiological conditions. *Ann Rheum Dis*, **45**, 712-17
9.    Garrett IR, Whitehouse MW, Vernon-Roberts B and Brooks PM (1985) Ambivalent properties of gold drugs in adjuvant induced polyarthritis in rats. *J Rheumatol*, **12**, 1078-82
10.    Lewis AJ, Carlson RP, Chang J and Delustro F (1984) Effect of gold salts, D-penicillamine and benoxaprofen and type II collagen induced arthritis in rats. *Agents Actions*, **14**, 705-14
11.    Carlson RP, Datko LJ, O'Neill-Davis L, Blazek EM, Delusto F, Beideman R, Lewis AJ (1985) Comparison of inflammatory changes in established type II collagen - and adjuvant-induced arthritis using outbred Wistor rats. *Int J Immunopharmacol*, **7**, 811-26
12.    Martin L, Sifar OS, Chalmers IM and Hunter T (1985) Sulfasalazine in severe rheumatoid arthritis: a study to assess potential correlates of efficacy and toxicity. *J Rheumatol*, **12**, 270-3
13.    Baber N, Halliday LDC, Van der Heurel WJA, Walker RW, Sibeon R, Kenan T, Lit-

tler T and Orme ML (1979) Indomethacin in rheumatoid arthritis. *Ann Rheum Dis* **38**, 128-37

14.  O'Duffy JK, O'Fallon WM, Hunter GG, McDuffie FC and Moore SB (1984) An attempt to predict the response to gold therapy in rheumatoid arthritis. *Arthritis Rheum* **27**, 1210-27

15.  Dequeker J, De Clerck L and Ceuppens J (1985) Side effects of gold complexes and D-penicillamine: genetic aspects. In: Rainsford KD and Velo GP (ed), *Side-effects of Antiinflammatory Drugs*, (Lancaster: MTP Press), Part 2, pp 185-96

16.  Bretza J, Wells L, Old L and Novey HS (1983) Association of IgE antibodies to sodium aurothiomalate and adverse reactions to chrysotherapy for rheumatoid arthritis. *Am J Med,* **74**, 945-9

17.  Baenkler VHW and Scheiffarth F (1971) Lymphozytransformation und immunglobuline unter goldbehandlung. *Z Rheumatol*, **30**, 236-9

18.  Waltz DT, DiMartino MJ and Griswold DE (1979) Immunopharmacology of auranofin and gold sodium thiomalate: Effects of humoral immunity. *J Rheumatol* (suppl 5), **6**, 78-81

19.  Hanly GH, Hassan J, Whelan A, Feigherg C and Bresniham B (1986) Effects of gold therapy on the synthesis and quantity of serum and synovial fluid IgM, IgG and IgG rheumatoid factors in rheumatoid arthritis patients. *Arthritis Rheum*, **29**, 480-7

20.  Hassan J, Hanly J, Bresnihan B, Fughery C and Whelan CA (1986) The immunological consequences of gold therapy : a prospective study in patients with rheumatoid arthritis. *Clin Exp Immunol*, **63**, 614-20

21.  Alarcon GS, Koopman WJ and Schrohenloher RE (1982) Association of chrysotherapy with diminished in vivo immunoglobulin synthesis *Arthritis Rheum*, (Suppl) 25:S132

22.  Olsen NJ and Jason HE (1984) Decreased poleweed mitogen-induced IgM and IgM rheumatoid factor synthesis in rheumatoid arthritis patients treated with gold sodium thiomalate or penicillamine. *Arthritis Rheum*, **27**, 985-94

23.  Lorber A, Simon T, Leeb J, Peter A and Wilcox S (1978) Chrysotherapy : suppression of immunoglobulin synthesis. *Arthritis Rheum*, **21**, 785-91

24.  Gottleib NL, Kiem IM, Pennys NS and Schultz DR (1975) The influence of chrysotherapy on serum protein and immunoglobulin levels, rheumatoid factor and anti-epithelial antibody titres. *J Lab Clin Med*, **86**, 962-72

25.  Pardo I and Livinson AE (1983) Circulating immunoglobulin-secreting cells in rheumatoid arthritis. *Clin Immunol. Immunopathol*, **29**, 29-34

26.  Patel V, Panayi GS and Unger A (1983) Spontaneous and pokeweed mitogen induced *in vitro* immunoglobulin and IgM rheumatoid factor production by peripheral blood and synovial fluid mononuclear cells in rheumatoid arthritis. *J Rheumatol*, **10**, 364-72

27.  Rosenburg SA and Lipsky PE (1979) Inhibition of pokeweed mitogen-induced immunoglobulin production in humans by gold compounds. *J Rheumatol*, (Suppl.) **5**, 107-11

28.  Persellin RH, Hess EV and Ziff M (1967) Effect of a gold salt on the immune response. *Arthritis Rheum*, **10**, 99-106

29.  Measel JW Jr (1975) Effect of gold on the immune response of mice. *Infect, Immun*, **11**, 350-4

30.  Scheinfforth F, Baenkler HW and Pfister (1971) The influence of gold on the kinetics of plaque-forming cells. *Int Arch Allergy Appl Immunol*, **40**, 117-23

31.  Robinson CJG, Balazs T and Egorov I (1986) Mercuric chloride-gold sodium thiomalate - and D-penicillamine - induced anti-nuclear antibodies in mice. *Toxicol Appl Pharmacol*, **86**(2) 156-69

32.  Harth M, Stiller CR, Sinclair NR, StC, Evans J McGirr D and Zuberi R (1977) Effects of a gold salt on lymphocyte responses. *Clin Exp Immunol*, **27**, 357-64

33. Lipsky PE and Ziff M (1977) Inhibition of antigen and mitogen induced human lymphocyte proliferation by gold compounds. *J Clin Invest*, **59**, 455-66

34. Cahill RNP (1971) Effect of sodium aurothiomalate "Myocrisin" on DNA synthesis in phytohaemagglutination-stimulated cultures of sheep lymphocytes. *Experientia*, **27**, 913-14

35. Cannon GW, Cole BC and Ward JR (1986) Differential effects of *in vitro* gold sodium thiomalate on the stimulation of human peripheral blood mononuclear cells by *Mycoplasma arthritis* T cell mitogen, concanavalin A and phytohaemagglutinin. *J Rheumatol*, **13**, 52-7

36. Hamilton JA and Williams N (1986) *In vitro* inhibition of myelopoiesis by gold salts and D-penicillamine. *J Rheumatol*, **12**, 892-6

37. Salmeron G and Lipsky PE (1982) Modulation of the human immune responsiveness in vitro by Auranofin. *J Rheumatol*, (Suppl. 8), **9**, 25-31

38. Barret ML and Lewis GP (1986) Unique properties of Auranofin as a potential antirheumatic drug. *Agents Actions*, **19**, 109-15

39. Highton J, Panayi GS, Shepherd P, Griffin J and Gibson T (1981) Changes in immune function in patients with rheumatoid arthritis following treatment with sodium aurothiomalate. *Ann Rheum Dis*, **40**, 252-62

40. Highton J, Panayi GS and Griffin J (1980) Cellular aspects of anti-rheumatic agents: improvement in peripheral blood lymphocyte response to concanavalin A pokeweed mitogen during gold treatment of rheumatoid arthritis. *Agents Actions*, **10**, 507-8

41. Haynes DR, Whitehouse MW and Vernon-Roberts B (1987) Effects of some antiarthritic drugs on interleukin-1 (IL-1): Studies using the LAF assay. *Clin Exp Pharmacol Physiol*, **12**, 11-12

42. Blistein-Willinger E (1985) Normalization of defective interleukin 1 and interleukin 2 production in patients with pemphigus vilgaris following chrysotherapy. *Clin Exp Immunol*, **62**, 705-14

43. Lee JC, Rebar L, DeMuth S and Hanna N (1985) Suppressed Il-2 production and response in AA rats : Role of suppressor cells and the effect of auronofin treatment. *J Rheumatol*, **12**, 385-91

44. Griswold DE, Lee JC, Poste G and Hanna N (1985) Modulation of macrophage lymphocyte interactions by the antiarthritic gold compound, auranofin. *J Rheumatol*, **12**, 490-7

45. Lorber A, Simar TM, Leib J, Peter A and Wilcox SA (1979) Effect of chrysotherapy on parameters of the immune response. *J Rheumatol*, **6**, 82-90

46. Harth M, Stiller C, McGirr D, Emens J and Sinclair N (1976) Effects of sodium aurothiomalate (SATM) on lymphocyte responses in normal man and patients with rheumatoid arthritis (RA). *J Rheumatol*, **36**, 216-18

47. Keystone CC, Poplonski L, Miller RG, Corczynski R and Gladman D (1986) *In vivo* activation of lymphocytes in rheumatoid arthritis. *J Rheumatol*, **13**, 694-9

48. Hay FC, Naieham LJ, Perumal R and Roitt IM (1979) Intra-articular and circulating immune complexes and antiglobulins (IgG and IgM) in rheumatoid arthritis : correlation with clinical features. *Ann Rheum Dis*, **38**, 1-7

49. Pritchard MH and Nuki G (1978) Gold and penicillamine : a proposed model of action in rheumatoid arthritis, based on synovial fluid analysis *Ann Rheum Dis* **37**, 493-503

50. Mathieu A, Mereu MC and Pala R (1983) Peripheral T lymphocyte subpopulations defined by monoclonal antiboides in rheumatoid arthritis: distribution in patients untreated and treated by oral gold therapy. *Eur J Rheumatol, Inflamm*, **6**, 182-6

51. Pfreundschuh M, Parino G, Gram N, Brloker A, Gause A and Hunstein W (1983) The influence of chrysotherapy on T-lymphocyte subpopulations in rheumatoid arthritis. *Z Rheumatol*, **42**, 328-31

52. Jessop JD, Vernon-Roberts B and Harris J (1973) Effects of gold salts and prednisolone on inflammatory cells I. The phagocytic activity of macrophage and neutro-

phil polymorphs in inflammatory exudates studies by 'skin-window' technique in rheumatoid and control subjects. *Ann Rheum Dis*, **32**, 294-300

53. Vernon-Roberts B, Jessop JD and Dore J (1973) Effects of gold salts and predniso-lone on inflammatory cells II. Suppression of inflammation and phagacytosis in the rat. *Ann Rheum Dis*, **32**, 301-7

54. Lipsky PE, Ugai K and Ziff M (1979) Alterations in human monocyte structure and function induced by incubation with gold sodium thiomalate. *J Rheumatol* 6 (Suppl.) 107-11

55. Viken KF and Lamvik JO (1976) Effect of aurothiomalate on human mononuclear cells cultured *in vitro. Acta Pathol Microbiol Scand Sect C*, **84**, 419

56. Ugai K, Ziff M and Lipsky PE (1979) Gold induced changes in morphology and func-tional capabilities of human monocyte. *Arthritis Rheum*, **22**, 1352-60

57. McCormack PL, Mayers DB and Palmer DG (1978) Increase in Fc receptor activ-ity of mouse peritoneal macrophages induced by sodium aurothiomalate. *Proc Univ Otago Medical School*, **56**, 17-9

58. Haynes DR, Garret IR and Vernon-Roberts B (1985) The effects of gold complexes on Fc receptor binding by monocytes isolated from rats. *XVI International Congress of Rheumatology Anstracts*, p319

59. Scheinborg MA, Santos LMB and Finkelstein AE (1982) The effect of auranofim and sodium aurothiomalate on peripheral blood monocytes. *J Rheumatol*, **9**(3), 366-9

60. Ho PPK, Young AL and Southard GL (1978) Methyl ester of N-formylmethionyl-leucylphenylalanine: chemotactic responses of human blood monocytes and inhibi-tion of gold compounds. *Arthritis Rheum*, **21**, 133-6

61. Liffman BH and Hall RE (1985) Effects of gold sodium thiomalate on functional correlates of human monocyte maturation. *Arthritis Rheum*, **28**, 1384-92

62. Otha A, Louie JS and Uitto J (1986) Collagenase production by human mononuclear cells in culture : inhibition by gold containing compounds and other antirheumatic agents. *Ann Rheum Dis*, **45**, 996-1003

63. Persellin Rh and Ziff M (1966) The effect of gold salt on lysosomal enzymes of the peritoneal macrophage. *Arthritis Rheum*, **9**, 57-65

64. Moroz LA (1979) Effects of gold sodium thiomalate on fibrinolysis. *J Rheumatol*, **6** (Suppl 5), 149-53

65. Petersen J and Bendtzen K (1982) Involvement of monokines in antigen and lectin-induced human lumphokine production. *Acta Pathol Microbiol Scand Sect C*, **90**, 229

66. Bendtzen K and Mayland L (1982) Role of $Zn^{2+}$ and other divalent metal ions in human lymphokine production in vitro. *Scand J Immunol* **15**, 81-6

67. Pruzanski W, Saito S and DeBoer G (1983) Modulation of phagocytosis and bacter-cidal acttivity of human polymorphonuclear and mononuclear phagocytes by anti-arthritic agents. *J Rheumatol*, **10**, 197-203

68. Sung CP. Mirabelli Ck and Badger J (1984) Effect of gold compounds on phorbol myristic acetate (PMA) activated superoxide ($0_2$) production by mouse peritoneal macrophage. *J Rheumatol*, **11**, 153-7

69. Hafstrom I, Seligman BE, Freidman MM and Gallin JI (1984) Auranofin affects early events in human polymorphonuclear neutrophil activation by receptor-mediated stimuli. *J Immunol*, **132**, 2007-14

70. Vernon-Roberts B, Dore JL, Jessop JD and Hendersen WJ (1976) Selective concen-tration and localization of gold in macrophages of synovial and other tissues during and after chrysotherapy in rheumatoid patients. *Ann Rheum Dis*, **35**, 477-86

71. Ghadially FN, Oryschak AF and Mitchell DM (1976) Ultrastructural changes in rheumatoid synovial membrane by chrysotherpay. *Ann Rheum Dis*, **35**, 67-72

72. Norton WL, Lewis DC and Ziff M (1968) Electron-dense deposits following injec-tion of gold sodium thiomalate and thiomalic acid. *Arthritis Rheum*, **11**, 436-43

73. Nakamura H and Igarashi M (1977) Localization of gold in synovial membrane of

rheumatoid arthritis treated with sodium aurothiomalate : studies by electron micro-scope and electron probe x-ray microanalysis. *Ann Rheum Dis*, **36**, 209-15

74. Carter SD, Bourne JT, Elson CJ, Hutton CW, Czndeck R and Dieppe PA (1984) Mononuclear phagocytes in rheumatoid arthritis: Fc-receptor expression by periph-eral blood monocytes. *Ann Rheum Dis*, **43**, 424-9

75. Katayama S, Chia D, Nasu H and Kutson DW (1981) Increased Fc receptor activity in monocytes from patients with rheumatoid arthritis. A study of monocyte binding and catabolism of soluble aggregate of IgG in vitro. *J Immunol*, **127**, 643-7

76. Dinarello CA (1985) An update on human interleukin-1 from molecular biology to clinical relevance. *J Clin Immunol*, **5**, 287-97

77. Nori AME, Panayi GS and Goodman SM (1984) Cytokines and the chronic inflam-mation of rheumatic disease I. The presence of interleukin-1 in synovial fluids. *Clin Exp Immunol*, **55**, 295-302

78. Bodel PT and Hollingsworth JW (1968) Pyrogen release from human synovial exu-date cells. *Br J Exp Pathol*, **49**, 11-19

79. Gery I, Gersham RK and Waksman BH (1971) Potentiation of cultured mouse thy-mocyte responses by factors released by peripheral leucocytes. *J Immunol*, **107**, 1778-80

80. Pertersen J and Bendtem K (1983) Immunosuppressive action of gold salts. *Scand J Rheumatol*, Suppl 51, 28-35

81. Gillis S, Mochizuki DY, Coulon PJ, Hefeneider SH, Ramthum CA, Gillis AE, Frank MB, Henry CS and Watson JD (1982) Molecular characteristics of interleukin-2. *Im-munol Rev*, **63**, 167-209

82. Miyachi Y, Yoshioka A, Imamura S and Niwa Y (1987) Anti-oxidant effects of gold compounds. *Br J Dermatol*, **116**, 39-46

83. David P and Johnston C (1986) Effects of gold compounds on function of phagocytic cells: comparative inhibition of activated polymorphonuclear leucocytes and mono-cytes from rheumatoid arthritis and control subjects. *Inflammation*, **10**, 311-20

84. Davis P, Johnston C, Miller CL and Wang K 1983) Effects of gold compounds on the function of phagocytic cells. II. Inhibition of superoxide radical generation of tri-peptide activated polymorphonuclear leukocytes. *Arthritis Rheum*, **26**, 82-6

85. Bertouch JV, Johnston C and Davis P (1987) Reversal of depressed neutrophil super-oxide production in Felty's syndrome after gold therapy. *J Rheumatol*, **14**, 52-4

86. Coates RD, Wolach B, Tzeng DY, Higgins C, Baehner RL and Boxer LA (1983) The mechanism of action of the anti-inflammatory agents, dexamethasone and Auranofin in human polymorphonuclear leucocytes. *Blood* **62**, 1070-7

87. Hofstrom I, Voten A and Palmbled J (1983) Modulation of neutrophil functions by Auranofin. *Scand J Rheumatol*, **12**, 97-105

88. Davis P, Miller CL and Russel AS (1982) Effects of gold compounds on the func-tion of phagocytic cells. I Suppresseion of phagocytosis and the generation of chemi-luminesence by polymorphonuclear leucocytes. *J Rheumatol*, **9** (Suppl 8), 18-24

89. Wojtecka-Lukasik E, Sopata I and Maslinski (1986) Auranofin modulates mast cell histamine and polymorphonuclear leukocyte collagenase release. *Agents Actions*, **18**, 68-70

90. Larevic I (1985) Effects of D-penicillamine, diclofenac sodium and gold sodium thio-malate upon the selective release of lysosomal enzymes from human polymorphonu-clear leukocytes to immune complexes. *Agents Actions*, **16**, 407-1

91. Pham Hay D, Roch-Arveiller M, Mutitaner O and Giroud JP (1985) In vitro and in vivo effects of gold salts on chemotaxis and random migration of rat polymorphonu-clear leukocytes. *Agents Actions*, **16**, 363-8

92. Mowak AG (1978) Neutrophil chemotaxis in rheumatoid arthritis: effect of D-peni-cillamine, gold salts and levamisol. *Ann Rheum Dis* **37**, 1-8

93. Turner RA, Johnson JA and Semble EL (1983) Antirheumatic drug effects on neu-

trophil response to chemotactic factors : a comparison of analytical technique. *Proc Soc Exp Biol Med* 173, 200-4

94.    Pecound A, Leimgramber A and Frei PL (1980) Effect of one gold salt, of betamethasome and of aspirin on the chemotaxis of human neutrophils measured in vitro. *Ann Rheum Dis*, 39, 25-30

95.    Luthra HS, Conn DL and Ferguson RH (1981) Felty's syndrome response to parenteral gold. *J Rheumatol*, 8, 902-9

96.    Mastgli GL and Owen ET (1982) A study of the response of the leucopenia of rheumatoid arthritis to gold salt therapy. *J Rheumatol*, 8, 658-60

97.    Hurd ER and Cheatum DE (1976) Depressed spleen size and increased neutrophils in patients with Felty's syndrome : effects of gold sodium thiomalate therapy. *J Am Med Assoc*, 235, 2215-17

98.    Gupta RC, Laforce FM and Mills DM (1983) Polymorphonuclear leukocyte inclusions and impaired bacterial killing in patients with Felty's syndrome. *J Lab Clin Med*, 88, 183-93

99.    Babior MB (1978) Oxygen-dependent microbial killing by phagocytes. *N Engl J Med*, 298, 659

100.   McCord JM (1974) Free radicals and inflammation: protection of synovial fluid by superoxide dismutase. *Science*, 185, 529-31

101.   McCord Jm and Fridovich I (1978) The biology and pathology of oxygen radicals. *Ann Int Med*, 89, 122-7

102.   Hafstrom I, Seiglemann BE, Friedman MM and Gallun JI (1984) Auranofin effects early events in human polymorphonuclear neutrophil activation by receptor-mediated stimuli. *J Immunol*, 132, 2007-14

103.   Chiu PL, Davis P, Wong K and Aasgupta M (1983) Superoxide production in neutrophils of patients with rheumatoid arthritis and Felty's syndrome. *J Rheumatol*, 10, 694-700

104.   Farr M, Scott DL, Constable TJ, Hawker RJ, Hawkins CF and Stuart J (1983) Thrombocytosis of active rheumatoid disease. *Ann Rheum Dis*, 42, 545-

105.   Endressen GKM (1981) Investigation of blood platelets in the synovial fluid from patients with rheumatoid arthritis *Scand J Rheumatol* 10, 204-8

106.   Palmer DG, Hogg N and Revell PA (1986) Lymphocytes, polymorphonuclear leucocytes, macrophages and platelets in synovium involved by rheumatoid arthritis. A study with monoclonal antiboides. *Pathology*, 18, 431-7

107.   Willis AL (1979) Platelet aggregation mechanisms and their implications in haemostasis and inflammatory disease, In: *Handbook of Experimental Pharmacology*, (Berlin: Springer), vol. 50(1), 138

108.   Chesney CM, Harper E and Colman RW (1974) Human platelet collagenase. *J Clin Invest*, 53, 1647-54

109.   Nathan I, Funkelstein AE, Walz DT and Dvilansky (1982) Studies of the effect of Auranofin, a new antiarthric agent, on platelet aggregation. *Inflammation*, 6, 79-85

110.   Gerrard JM and White JG (1978) Prostaglandins and thromboxanes: 'Middle man' modulating platelet function in hemostasis and thrombosis. *Prog Hemostasis Throm* 4, 87-125

111.   Gerber RC and Paulus HE (1975) Gold therapy. *Clin Rheum Dis*, 307-18

112.   Katagl (1976) Mycotoxicity of gold. *Br Med J*, 1, 1266-8

113.   Stanford BT and Crosby WH (1978) Late onset of gold induced throbocytopenia. *J Am Med Assoc*, 239, 50-1

114.   Van Der Borne AEG, Pegels JG, Van der Stadt RJ, Van der Plas-Van Dalen CMC and Helmerhorst FM (1986) Thrombocytopenia associated with gold therapy: a drug induced autoimmune disease. *Br J Haematol*, 63, 509-16

115.   Goodwin JS and Webb DR (1980) Regulation of the immune response by prostaglandin. *Clin Immunol Immunopathol*, 15, 106-22

116. Gordon D and Lewis GP (1984) Effects of piroxicam on mononuclear cells; comparison with other antiarthritic drugs. *Inflammation* 8, S87-102

117. Parente JE, Wong K, Davis P *et al.* (1986) Effect of gold compounds on leukotriene B4, leukotriene C4 and prostaglandin E2 production by polymorphonuclear leukocytes. *J Rheumatol*, 13, 47-51

118. Marone G, Columbo M, Galeone D *et al.* (1986) Modulation of the release of histamine and arachidonic acid metabolites from human basophils and mast cells by Auranofin. *Agents Actions*, 18, 100

119. Nishizuka Y (1984) The role of protein kinase C in cell surface signal transduction and tumour promotion. *Nature,* 308, 396-8

120. Hurst NP, Solank V and Murray AW (1986) Differential effects of auranofin on stimulus responses coupling in human monocytes and platelets - Auranofin enhances protein phosphorylation. *Br J Rheumatol*, 25(A), 106

121. Froscio M, Hurst NP and Murray AW (1987) Inhibition of epidermal growth factor binding to HELA cells by auranofin. *Biochem Pharmacol* 36, 769-72

122. Zalewski PD, Hurst NP, Valente L and Forbes IJ (1987). Modulation of the mouse erythrocyte receptor in human B-cells by Auranofin in a thio dependent manner. *Arthritis Rheum* (in press)

123. Snyder RM, Mirabelli CZ, Ziegler JT *et al.* (1986) Effect of Auranofin and other gold containing compounds on the activities of phospholipase C. *Fed Proc*, 45(A), 1021

124. Parente JE, Wong K and Davis P (1986) The paradox of gold compounds: activators or inhibitors? *J Rheumatol*, 13, 846-8

125. Adams M and Kuhn K (1968) Investigations in the reaction of metals with collagen *in vivo*: comparison of the reaction of gold thiosulphate with collagen *in vivo* and *in vitro*. *Eur J Biochem*, 3, 407-10

126. Deyl Z, Rosmus J and Adam M (1970) Investigation of the reaction of metals with collagen *in vivo*. *Eur J Biochem*, 18, 589-92

127. Bing SG and Eisen V (1981) Effect of gold salts and penicillamine on serum complement. *Arch Int Pharmacolyn Ther*, 249, 126-36

128. Hasselbaker P (1980) The effect of gold sodium thiomalate on activation of the classical and alternative pathways of complement in serum. *Clin Res*, 218, 605A

129. Pritchard MH and Nuki G (1978) Gold and penicillamine: proposed mode of action in rheumatoid arthritis based on synovial fluid analysis. *Ann Rheum Dis*, 37, 493-503

130. Rae JK, MacKay CNN, McNeil CJ, Brown DH, Smith WE, Lewis D and Cappel HA (1986) Early and late changes in sulphydryl groups and copper protein concentrations and activities during drug treatment with aurothiomalate and Auranofin. *Ann Rheum Dis* 45, 839-46

131. Turkall RM, Warr GA and Tsan M (1982) Effect of *in vivo* administration of gold sodium thiomalate on rat macrophage function. *Agents actions*, 12, 489-98

132. Mogilnicka ERM and Webb M (1981) Comparative studies on the distribution of gold, copper and zinc in the livers and kidneys of rats and hamsters after treatment with sodium [$^{125}$Au]aurothiomalate. *J Appl Toxicol*, 1, 287-91

133. Thornally PJ and Vabeck M (1985) Possible role of methallothinein in protection against radiation-induced oxidative stress. *Biochem Biophys Acta*, 827, 36-44

134. Massicot F, Falcou R, Haymans F, Godfroid J and Apfelbaum M (1987) Effects of a new anoretic drug (PM 170) on development of gold thioglucose-induced obesity in mice. *Gen Pharmacol*, 18, 149-52

135. Tepperman K, Finer R, Donovan S, Doi J, Ratcliff D and Ng K (1984) Intestinal uptake and metabolism of Auranofin, a new oral gold based anti-arthritis drug. *Science*, 225, 430-2

136. Dillard CJ and Tappel AL (1986) Are some major in vivo effects of gold related to microenvironments and decreased selenium? *Med Hypothesis*, 20, 407-20

137. Graham GG, Bales JR, Grootveld MC and Sadler PJ (1985) $^1$H, $^{13}$C NMR, and elec-

tronic absorption spectroscopic studies of the interaction of cyanide with aurothio-malate. *J Inorg Biochem*, **25**, 163-73

138.    Graham GG, Haavisto TM, Jones HM and Champion GD (1984) The effect of cyanide on the uptake of gold by red blood cells. *Biochem Pharmacol*, **33(8)**, 1257-62

139.    Sharma RP (1983) Metabolism of intracellular zinc and copper following single and repeated injections of gold sodium thiomalate. *Agents Actions*, **13**, 380-8

# 9

# Do platelet activating factor antagonists have a potential role in the therapy of rheumatoid arthritis?

**C.P. Page and A.J. Coyle**
Department of Pharmacology, King's College, University of London,
Chelsea Campus, Manresa Road, London SW3

## I. INTRODUCTION

Rheumatoid arthritis (RA) is a systemic connective tissue disorder which predominantly affects the synovial joints. RA is characterized pathologically by an extensive accumulation of inflammatory cells in the synovial lining of joints and tendons. In addition, there is collagen and connective tissue degradation, fibrinoid necrosis and deposition of immune complexes on vascular endothelium generating local inflammation and infarction.

At present the aetiology of RA is unclear. It has been proposed that the disorder involves a genetic predisposition in combination with a triggering agent resulting in a self-perpetuating inflammatory reaction. A number of potential mediators have been implicated in the pathogenesis of RA, but to date none have fully explained the underlying pathology or symptoms of this common disease. Recently, platelet activating factor (PAF) has been demonstrated to be a potent pro-inflammatory mediator capable of inducing many of the features observed in inflammatory joint lesions.

This review discusses the properties of PAF that may have relevance to the pathophysiology of RA and the potential of recently identified PAF antagonists in the future therapy of the disorder.

## II. PLATELET ACTIVATING FACTOR

### (1) Historical background

In 1966 Barbaro and Zweifler[1] demonstrated the acute release of histamine following allergen exposure in the sensitised rabbit. It was believed that the histamine release was platelet-derived as it had been previously demonstrated that this blood element was the primary source of histamine in the

*New Developments in Antirheumatic Therapy.* Rainsford, KD and Velo, GP (eds),
Inflammation and Drug Therapy Series, Volume III.

rabbit. It was subsequently demonstrated in 1972 that the release of histamine was a consequence of IgE-dependent basophil activation resulting in the secretion of a material which produced platelet aggregation[2]. Benveniste *et al.* described a method for the preparation of this basophil-derived mediator which was referred to as platelet activating factor (PAF)[2]. Physiochemical analysis of this mediator suggested PAF was a phospholipid[3] and PAF has now been identified by three independent groups as an ether-linked phospholipid, 1-O-alkyl-2-acetyl-sn-glyceryl-3-phosphorylcholine (Figure 1)[4-6], variously referred to as AGEPC[4], APRL[5] or Paf-acether[6]. Total synthesis of this molecule has been achieved[7], and the structural requirements for biological activity are well documented[8].

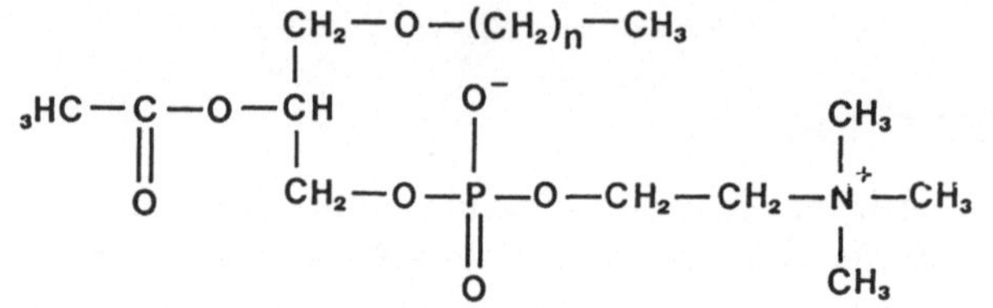

**Figure 1** Structure of platelet activating factor

## (2) Synthesis and metabolism

Activation of a $Ca^{2+}$-dependent phospholipase A2 following either allergic or non-allergic stimuli results in the formation of 1-O-alkyl-glyceryl-3-phosphorylcholine (lyso-PAF)[9]. Lyso-PAF, the precursor of PAF, has similar physiochemical properties to PAF but is devoid of biological activity. In order to synthesize PAF a cytoplasmic acetyltransferase enzyme has to be activated, an enzyme known to be present in a number of inflammatory cell types including macrophages[9,10], platelets[11], neutrophils[12] and eosinophils[13]. This enzyme is known to be the rate-limiting enzyme regulating the synthesis of PAF[14].

A single-step biosynthetic pathway for PAF has also been described in non-inflammatory cell types involving a choline phosphotransferase enzyme[14]. At present the contribution of the two enzymatic routes to PAF formation in vivo is not established, although it appears that in inflammatory cells the two-step pathway involving the rate-limiting acetyltransferase enzyme predominates[15].

PAF is rapidly degraded by a cytosolic acetylhydrolase enzyme which has been identified in the plasma of several mammalian species including man[16]. This enzyme cleaves the acetate moiety at the sn-2 position to form lyso-PAF. Lyso-PAF can then be reincorporated into ether-linked phospholipids by an acyltransferase. Alternatively, lyso-PAF can be further metabolized by removal of the O-alkyl group that is similar to or identical with the well-characterized tetrahydropteridine alkyl mono-oxygenase enzyme

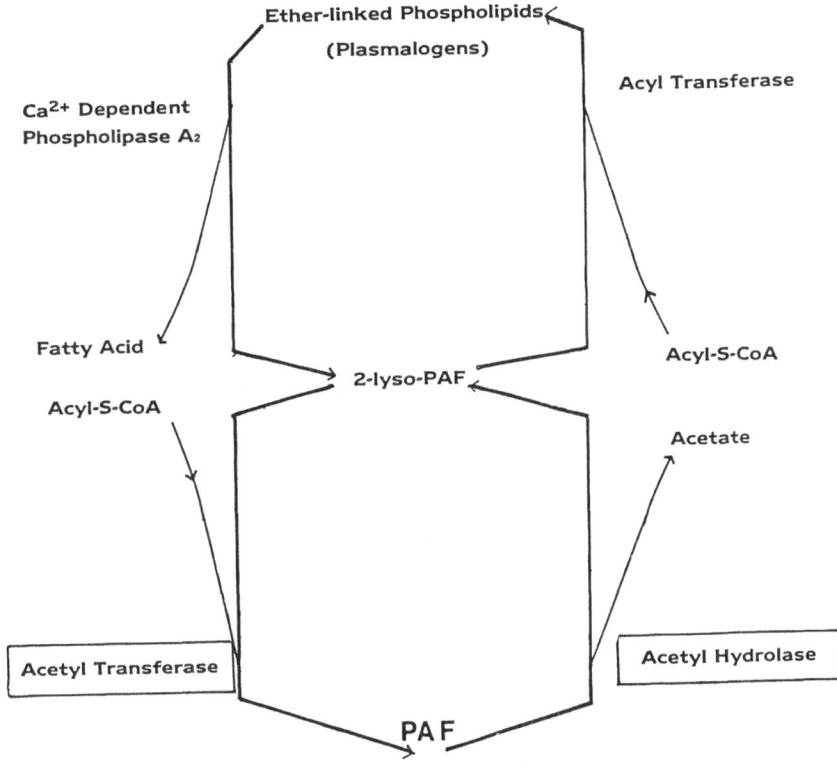

**Figure 2** A schematic representation of the synthesis and metabolism of platelet activating factor

isolated from the rat liver, resulting in the formation of a fatty aldehyde and a glyceryl-3-phosphorylcholine[17] (see Figure 2).

## (3) PAF as mediator of the inflammatory response

In 1910, Dale proposed several criteria for the identification of chemicals as neurotransmitters. A modification of such criteria may be used to assess whether a substance may be considered as a mediator of inflammation.

To date there have been no reports of the effects of PAF administered intra-articularly in experimental animals, hence the basis for the proposal of the hypothesis that PAF may be an important inflammatory mediator in RA is based on data obtained in other experimental models.

### (a) Vasodilation

Both intravenous and oral administration of PAF in a variety of experimental animals produces profound hypotension[18,19]. The ability of PAF to induce such an effect is likely to be mediated by a direct action on vascular smooth muscles, since it is not modified by an array of pharmacological agents including non-steroidal anti-inflammatory drugs and antagonists of histamine, serotonin and beta-adrenoreceptors[20]. Furthermore, PAF-induced hypotension is independent of circulating platelets since it is not abrogated by prior depletion of circulating blood platelets with a selective antiplatelet antiserum[20]. This is reinforced by the observation that PAF will produce hypotension in the rat, a species whose platelets are wholly unresponsive to PAF[20]. Additionally, PAF is known to have an effect on blood flow in a number of organs, and has been studied extensively in the skin where PAF has both vasodilator and vasoconstrictor properties. Intradermal injection of PAF in man produces a wheal (discussed below) and flare response indicative of local vasodilation. The PAF-induced flare response is partly due to released histamine since it can be reduced by pretreatment with H-1 antagonists such as chlorpheniramine[21-23].

### (b)   Increased vascular permeability

Increased vascular permeability is a prominent feature of the inflammatory response. In experimental animals, increased vascular permeability may be investigated by monitoring the accumulation of radiolabelled plasma proteins (e.g. [$^{125}$I]albumin), an increase in deposition of colloidal carbon particles or an increase in the wet to dry ratio of the tissue.

Intradermal administration of picomolar concentrations of PAF to experimental animals elicits an increased plasma protein extravasation (IPPE) indicative of increased vascular permeability[21]. In this respect PAF is more potent than any described mediator, eliciting IPPE with picomolar concentrations in the guinea-pig and being more than 1000 times more potent than histamine in rabbit skin[24]. PAF-induced IPPE is likely to be mediated directly via an effect on the vascular endothelium and is not modified by pretreatment with a variety of pharmacological agents including H-1 and serotonin antagonists and cyclo-oxygenase inhibitors[21-25]. Unlike many other inflammatory mediators such as C5a and LTB$_4$, PAF-induced IPPE is neutrophil-independent, as demonstrated by the inability of cytotoxic drugs such as nitrogen mustard to modify the plasma protein extravasation[25-27]. Furthermore, PAF-induced plasma protein extravasation is independent of platelet activation since both platelet depletion with selective antiplatelet serum and treatment with various antiplatelet drugs fail to modify PAF-induced IPPE[28,29]. In addition, PAF will elicit increased vascular permeability in the skin of the rat[25] and pretreatment with antiplatelet agents such as prostaglandin E$_1$ (PGE$_1$) or analogues of prostacyclin (e.g. ZK36374) actually enhances IPPE[28,30]. This observation is in agreement with the hypothesis that

IPPE is a consequence of an interaction between a vasodilator such as PGE₁ and an agent capable of increasing vascular permeability such as PAF[31].

Intradermal injection of PAF in man elicits acute oedema formation, as assessed by wheal formation which is independent of histamine or cyclo-oxygenase products of arachidonic acid metabolism[21]. Histological examination of tissue removed from the site of PAF injection reveals dilation of the dermal blood vessels associated with expansion of the interstitial spaces characteristic of oedema formation within the first 30 min[32]. The ability of PAF to produce an increase in vascular permeability has been reported in other vascular beds. Thus PAF elicits a dose related increase in [$^{125}$I]fibrinogen deposition in the kidney[33], the bronchial[34] and pulmonary vasculature[35,36] although the effect of PAF on the permeability of the vasculature in the synovial joints is unknown.

PAF receptors have been identified on vascular endothelium[37] and electron microscopic studies have demonstrated the ability of PAF to produce a contraction of the endothelial cell layer associated with the passage of colloidal carbon across the vascular endothelium at the site of PAF administration[38]. Similar results have been obtained with human endothelial cells (HEC) in culture where PAF elicits a reorganization of the microfilaments in HEC and causes the endothelial cells to lose intimate contact with each other[39].

## (c)  Cellular accumulation

The synovial joints of individuals with RA are characterised by an accumulation of activated inflammatory cells. PAF was first identified as a mediator of platelet aggregation[2], but since this initial observation, the ability of PAF to activate many cell types, including neutrophils[40], eosinophils[41] and monocytes[42], has been demonstrated.

(i)  *Platelets.*  Platelets have a well-established role in thrombosis and haemostasis. However, more recent work suggests that platelets have an important role to play in a variety of allergic and non-allergic disorders and may function as inflammatory cells in their own right[43]. Platelets have been observed in the synovial fluid[44] and small platelet thrombi have been detected in acutely inflamed synovial villi of individuals with RA[45]. In addition, radioactively labelled platelets have been demonstrated to accumulate in inflamed joints[45]. Moreover, the number of platelets in the synovial fluid is well correlated with various active markers of synovial inflammation[46]. There is also evidence of the release of platelet-derived substances in the inflamed synovial joints[47].

In response to stimulation, platelets are capable of releasing a variety of intracellular constituents which have potent pro-inflammatory properties. Platelets can release a cationic protein which increases vascular permeability and various mitogenic substances which stimulate smooth muscle proliferation and fibroblast deposition[43]. In addition to releasing many preformed mediators, activated platelets can produce a variety of membrane-derived mediators formed *de novo*, such as thromboxane $A_2$ ($TXA_2$) (a potent vaso-constrictor which stimulates further platelet activation) and 12-lipoxygenase metabolites of arachidonic acid (e.g. 12-HETE which is a chemoattractant for neutrophils)[48].

PAF produces platelet aggregation[20] at concentrations as low as 0.3 nM. In this respect PAF ranks as one of the most potent inducers of platelet aggregation which is reflected as thrombocytopenia when PAF is administered systemically[18,20].

Intradermal or intravenous administration of PAF has been demonstrated to produce an extravascular accumulation of platelets in experimental animals[49]. It is important to stress that such platelet accumulation is distinct from that induced by other platelet agonists such as ADP, since these extravasated platelets are not aggregated into platelet thrombi, but are often present as single platelets that have undergone diapedesis. Such pathological changes are not observed following treatment with other platelet agonists such as ADP, and may be secondary to an effect of PAF on the vascular endothelium.

As well as being a potent mediator of platelet activation PAF itself is released from platelets[11] which could result in further platelet activation and an amplification of the inflammatory response.

Platelets have been demonstrated to express surface receptors for various immunoglobulins including IgE[50], IgG, and IgM[51]. Studies *in vitro* have demonstrated the ability of IgG rheumatoid factor (IgG-RF) to produce platelet aggregation[52] and more recently, Cunningham and co-workers[53] demonstrated the ability of serum factor(s), possibly IgG-RF or IgG containing immune complexes, to mediate platelet activation in rheumatoid vasculitis. The observation of immune complex involvement in RA, coupled with the postulated role of PAF in enhancing immune complex deposition and the ability of PAF antagonists to inhibit immune complex deposition[54], suggests PAF may have a major pathological role to play in the antibody-mediated platelet activation resulting in host tissue damage.

*(ii) Neutrophils.* The role of the neutrophil in inflammation has been discussed as length[55-57]. On activation, the neutrophil secretes its granular enzymes by exocytosis. The granules contain a variety of substances capable of producing damage to host tissue including myeloperoxidases, neutral proteases (cathepsin G, elastase and collagenase), acid hydrolases, lysosomes and cationic proteins. Oxygen radicals are also formed on activation and in conjunction with granule-derived chemicals are potent mediators of tissue destruction[55-57]. PAF is capable of stimulating most of the functions of the neutrophil[56]. Thus PAF induces aggregation and degranulation, promotes neutrophil adhesion to the vascular endothelium, stimulates the generation of superoxide free radicals and lipoxygenase metabolites of the arachidonic acid cascade and enhances C3 receptor expression.

PAF is also a potent chemotactic and chemokinetic agent for neutrophils[40]. This effect is reflected *in vivo* by a transient neutropenia when administered intravenously to both experimental animals and man[18,56]. This neutropenia is associated with a massive sequestration of neutrophil aggregates in capillary beds, primarily in the pulmonary vasculature[38]. Moreover, local administration of PAF to the skin or lungs produces a cellular infiltrate rich in neutrophils, indicating a possible role for PAF as a mediator of neutrophil accumulation[32,38,59].

An interaction between neutrophils and platelets has been reported by several independent groups[60,61] and these cell types have been observed in close proximity to each other in inflammatory reactions following local administration of PAF[38]. Recently it has been demonstrated that PAF-induced $O_2$-generation from human neutrophils was enhanced in the presence of platelets, suggesting that PAF-induced platelet activation may be an important step in superoxide generation from neutrophils during the inflammatory response[61].

*(iii)    Eosinophil*    The role of the eosinophil in RA is unclear. Over 30 years ago Short and co-workers reported a mild elevation in the percentage of circulating eosinophils in individuals with RA[62]. In more recent years attention has been redirected towards the eosinophil following the isolation and characterization of the eosinophil's granular contents such as eosinophil cationic protein (ECP)[63] and major basic protein (MBP)[64]. These proteins have been demonstrated to exhibit cytotoxic properties against several cell types, and it is believed that they play a role in parasitic infections and may mediate host tissue damage in a variety of allergic and non-allergic disorders[64]. Hallergen *et al.* have recently demonstrated a five-fold increase in ECP levels in the synovial fluid of individuals with RA compared to normal individuals[65], although no eosinophils were detected in the synovial fluid. This clinical observation is similar to observations made in asthmatics where large amounts of eosinophil-derived products are often found in the lung associated with tissue-damage, although eosinophils are not always present[66].

One of the most impressive properties of PAF is that it is a potent chemotactic and chemokinetic factor for human eosinophils[41]. Intradermal administration of PAF to atopic individuals has been shown to induce a selective accumulation of eosinophils after 24 hours equivalent to allergen provocation in the same individuals with evidence of eosinophil degranulation[67]. Such inflammatory changes have not been observed in normal individuals where a mixed cellular infiltrate follows intradermal administration[32]. However, to date no studies have been undertaken in individuals with RA.

Nonetheless, PAF-induced eosinophil activation and subsequent release of cytotoxic mediators has been proposed to play a central role in mediating the tissue damage observed in asthmatic individuals[66], and it remains plausible that the eosinophil activation observed in the synovial joints of individuals with RA may contribute to the inflammatory response and tissue damage.

241

*(iv)* *Mononuclear cells* Mononuclear cells are the predominant cell type in inflamed synovial joints. There is considerable evidence of lymphocyte activation in the synovial fluid of individuals with RA, suggesting that these cells may have a central role to play in the aetiology of this disorder[68]. In recent years attention has been focused on the role of monocyte-derived mediators in RA. Interleukin-1 (IL-1) is a polypeptide released from activated macrophages, and is believed to play a pivotal role in the pathogenesis of inflammatory joint disease. IL-1 is present in the synovium[69] and promotes the breakdown of synovial cartilage in culture[70], induces osteoblast proliferation[71] and stimulates osteoblasts to resorb bone[72]. In addition, IL-1 is chemotactic for neutrophils and promotes neutrophil adhesion to the vascular endothelium[73]. Furthermore, intra-articular injection of IL-1 in rabbits produces cellular accumulation and proteoglycan degradation[74].

PAF produces aggregation of mononuclear cells *in vitro* and stimulates the release of other inflammatory mediators[42]. Intradermal administration of PAF, both in experimental animals and man, produces a perivascular accumulation of predominantly lymphocytes and histiocytes at 24-48 hours[32].

It is therefore of considerable interest in the context of RA that PAF stimulates the formation of IL-1 from human adherent macrophages[75]. In addition, it has been demonstrated that IL-1 will in turn stimulate PAF release from human endothelial cells[76]. Such an interaction may therefore be involved in the self-perpetuating inflammatory response observed in the synovial joints.

When activated, lymphocytes are also capable of releasing another polypeptide, interleukin-2 (IL-2)[77]. It is believed that this polypeptide plays a role in regulating the inductive phase of the immune response by stimulating the proliferation of T cells in response to mitogen and by promoting the accumulation of lymphocytes, macrophages and neutrophils at the site of inflammation. Recently, PAF has been demonstrated to enhance IL-2-induced lymphocyte proliferation[78]. Moreover, the effects of IL-2 on lymphocyte mitogenesis were inhibited by selective PAF antagonists[78]. At present there are few reports on the effect of PAF on lymphocyte function *in vivo*. However, PAF antagonists have recently been demonstrated to be effective agents in the prevention of experimental allograft rejection[79,80], a reaction which is believed to be mediated by lymphocyte activation. In this model PAF antagonists have been demonstrated to interact synergistically with glucocorticosteroids and cyclosporin[81].

Thus preliminary data suggest that PAF may modulate lymphocyte function during the inflammatory reponse, and may therefore play an important role in amplification of the inflammatory response and thus contribute to the positive feedback mechanisms that probably lead to chronic inflammation.

## (d) Pain

Individuals with RA frequently report persistent pain at the site of the inflammatory lesion. PAF administration to human volunteers has been reported to elicit algesia[82], although this has not been confirmed in a more detailed study[83]. In rats, subplantar administration of PAF has been demonstrated to produce hyperalgesia[84], although a detailed analysis of this phenomenon has yet to be undertaken.

## (e) Tissue damage

A prominent feature of the synovial joints of individuals with RA is the extensive tissue damage, principally cartilage and connective tissue destruction, associated with oesteoblast proliferation and bone resorption. PAF is capable of inducing widespread tissue damage. Intradermal administration of PAF in experimental animals and man produces vasculitic changes associated, as discussed previously, with widespread endothelial disruption and infiltration of inflammatory cells. The ability of PAF to stimulate a variety of

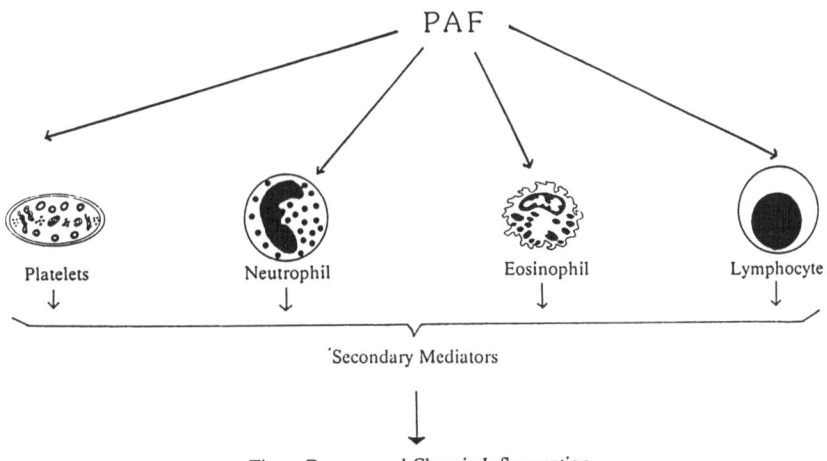

**Figure 3** PAF is capable of inducing activation of a number of inflammatory cell types resulting in the release of secondary mediators (see text for details) which may lead to tisssue damage and chronic inflammation

cell types to release a range of mediators that are capable of inducing host tissue damage suggests that PAF should be considered as a mediator contributing to the synovial tissue destruction observed in individuals with RA (Figure 3).

## (4)   Generation of PAF in the inflammatory response

Detection of PAF in inflammatory lesions has been difficult due to the lack of a suitable assay procedure and the rapid inactivation of PAF by both plasma- and cell-associated acetylhydrolase. However, PAF and its metabolite, lyso-PAF, have been identified in a number of inflammatory reactions both in experimental animals and man. Lyso-PAF release has been demonstrated in carrageenan-induced pleurisy in the rat[85] and PAF release detected during IgE anaphylaxis in the rabbit[86].

PAF has recently been shown to be released in a number of clinical conditions including idiopathic urticaria[87], late-asthmatic reactions[88] and in blister fluid obtained from allergic individuals undergoing late-onset inflammatory responses in the skin[89]. More direct evidence for PAF release in RA is provided by a recent report demonstrating increased levels of PAF in the synovial joints of antigen-induced arthritis in the rabbit[90] and the detection of PAF in the synovial fluid of individuals with RA[91].

## III.   PAF ANTAGONISTS

One of the most interesting developments in the PAF field has been the appearance of a wide range of PAF antagonists. In 1981 an analogue of PAF, CV3988, was described as the first selective PAF antagonist[92] and this compound has been followed by a series of PAF analogues having PAF antagonistic activity. Such compounds include ONO 6240[93], Ro-19370[94] and SRI 63-072[95]. However, despite being potent PAF antagonists it is likely that PAF analogues will be of limited use clinically, as they have poor oral bioavailability in comparison to the other PAF antagonists now available.

The second type of PAF antagonist described was a natural product isolated from a Chinese medicinal herb, *Piper futokadsurae*, belonging to the chemical class of lignans. This material has been named Kadsurenone[96] and related synthetic neo-lignans have now been described including L-652-731[97]. Both Kadsuranone and the related neo-lignans are orally active, and have been demonstrated to inhibit PAF-induced effects selectively *in vitro* and *in vivo*. Very shortly after the discovery of Kadsurenone, another group of naturally occurring PAF antagonists were discovered in the leaves obtained from the *Ginkgo biloba* tree[98], another remedial herb from southern China which has been particularly used in the treatment of inflammation. This compound belongs to the ginkolide family of compounds of which BN 52021 is the most active constituent so far described from this herb. Extracts of the *Ginkgo biloba* tree have been available commercially in various parts of western Europe for the treatment of a number of ailments which has led to the availability of these materials for clinical use. Recently, a gingkolide extract, BN 52063 containing a mixture of three active compounds (BN 52020, BN 52021 and BN 52022), has been demonstrated to have specific PAF antagonist activity in normal healthy volunteers[99]. Oral ingestion of BN

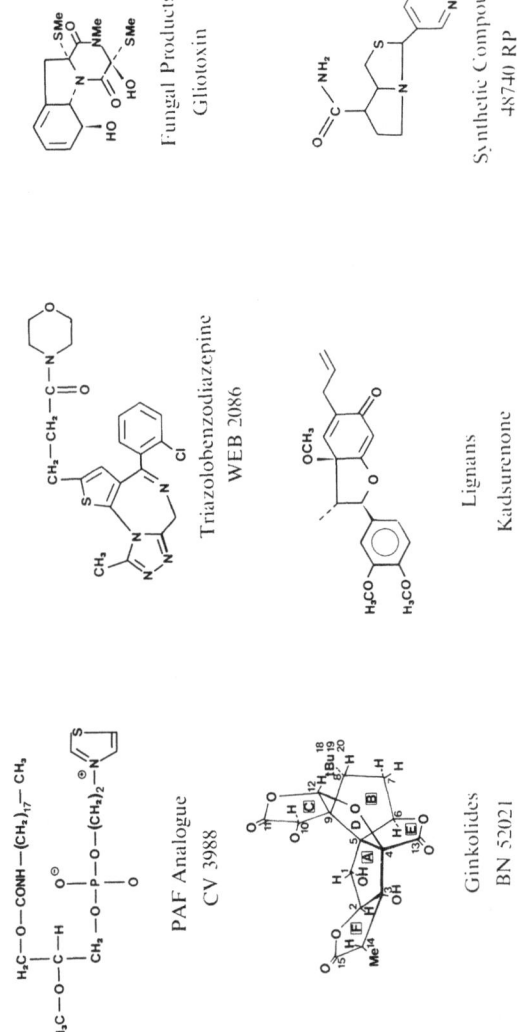

**Figure 4** Structure of some PAF antagonists. A representative example of the major classes

245

52063 results in a dose-related inhibition of PAF-induced wheal-and-flare responses in human skin and *ex vivo* platelet aggregation induced by PAF. No significant inhibitory effect was observed for BN 52063 against histamine-induced wheal-and-flare responses and on ADP-induced platelet aggregation *in vivo*[99]. Studies are currently under way investigating the ability of BN 52063 to inhibit a variety of more complex inflammatory responses in the clinical arena.

Several other classes of PAF antagonist have been described in the literature which have a diverse range of chemical structures. These include drugs previously recognized for some other pharmacological property such as the triazolobenzodiazepines[100] (e.g. alprazolam, triazolam, brotizolam) and newer analogues (WEB 2086)[101]; certain classes of calcium antagonists[102] (e.g. diltiazem) and totally novel synthetic structures such as the thiazole derivative[103] RP-48740. The various classes of PAF antagonist are illustrated in Figure 4 and have been reviewed elsewhere[104].

Although superficially PAF antagonists appear to have a wide range of structures, it has recently been proposed that these structures can be accompanied in the putative structure of the PAF receptor site estimated from structure activity relationships of PAF analogues[8]. To date the PAF antagonists have been demonstrated to inhibit most of the biological properties of PAF, although recent evidence suggests that there may be more than one PAF receptor as some of the currently available PAF antagonists have differential effects on different tissues in the same animal[105].

At present there are few reports of the effects of PAF antagonists in complex experimental models of inflammation of relevance to RA. Nonetheless, some experimental observations have been made which could have a bearing on the potential of this new class of drugs in the future treatment of chronic inflammatory conditions such as RA. Most of the initial work with selective PAF antagonists in models of inflammation has been directed towards anaphylaxis or shock, where a variety of PAF antagonists have been shown to have a protective effect against both antigen and endotoxin-induced pathology[106,107]. However, L-652-731 has been shown to inhibit the arthus response in the skin of rabbits[108], and SRI-63441 has been shown to inhibit immune complex vasculitis[54]. As already reported, a number of PAF antagonists have been demonstrated to retard allograft rejection in rats[79-81], suggesting a possible role for PAF in lymphocyte-driven inflammatory responses which has considerable implications for the possible involvement of PAF in RA. PAF antagonists have been reported to be effective in carrageenan-induced inflammation[109], although the value of this model in our understanding of chronic inflammation may be limited. What effect PAF antagonists have in models such as antigen-induced arthritis has yet to be established, but the availability of specific PAF antagonists for clinical use should prove useful in determining the precise role of this potent mediator in the pathogenesis of RA.

## IV. CONCLUSION

Rheumatoid arthritis is a common, chronic inflammatory disease affecting predominantly the synovial joints. PAF is one of the most potent mediators of inflammation identified to date, and is capable of inducing many of the pathological changes known to occur in the synovial joints of individuals with RA.

At present there are no reports that administration of PAF intra-articularly in experimental animals produces a condition similar to that seen in RA, or that treatment of individuals with RA with PAF antagonists causes an improvement in symptoms. However, as PAF can mimic many of the facets seen in inflammatory joints, be it in other experimental systems, together with the observation that PAF is present in the synovial fluid of individuals with RA[91], the possibility remains that PAF has a role to play in the initiation and/or maintenance of RA.

At present the therapeutic agents available to the clinician for pharmacological intervention are limited. It is generally accepted that the non-steroidal anti-inflammatory drugs provide only symptomatic relief without altering the course of the disease, and those agents that are capable of modifying the disease frequently produce unacceptable toxic side-effects. It is hoped that PAF antagonists may represent a novel class of anti-inflammatory drugs of potential therapeutic benefit in the management of rheumatoid arthritis.

## REFERENCES

1. Barbaro, JF and Zweifler, NJ (1966). Antigen-induced histamine release from platelets in rabbits producing homologous PCA antibody. *Proc Soc Exp Biol Med*, **121**, 1245-7

2. Benveniste, J, Henson, PM and Cochrane, CG (1972). Leucocyte dependent histamine release from rabbit platelets: the role of IgE, basophils and a platelet activating factor. *J Exp Med*, **136**, 1356-77

3. Benveniste, J, Le Couedic, JP, Polonsky, J and Tence, M (1977). Structural analysis of purified platelet activating factor by lipases. *Nature*, **269**, 170-1

4. Demopolous, CA, Pinkard, RN and Hanahan, DJ (1979). Platelet activating factor: evidence for 1-O-alkyl-2-acetyl-sn-glyceryl-3-phosphorylcholine as the active component (a new class of lipid chemical mediators). *J Biol Chem*, **254**, 9355-8

5. Blank, MC, Synder, F, Byers, BC et al. (1979). Antihypertensive activity of an alkyl ether analog of phosphatidylcholine. *Biochem Biophys Res Commun*, **90**, 523-34

6. Benveniste, J, Tence, M, Varenne, P et al. (1979). Semi-synthese et structure proposee du facteur activant les plaquettes (PAF): Paf-acether, un alkyl ether analague de la phosphtidylcholine. *CR Acad Sci (Paris)*, **289**, 1037-40

7. Godfroid, JJ, Heymans, F, Michel, E et al. (1980). Platelet activating factor (Paf-acether): total synthesis of 1-O-octa-decyl-2-O-acetyl-sn-glyceryl-3-phosphorylcholine. *FEBS Lett*, **116**, 161-4

8. Godfroid, JJ and Braquet, P (1986). Paf-acether binding sites: 1. Quantitation of SAR activity of Paf-acether analogues. *Trends Pharmacol Sci*, **7**, 368-70

9. Mencia-Heurta, JM, Ninio, E, Roubin, R and Benveniste, J (1981). Is platelet acti-

vating factor (Paf-acether) synthesis by murine peritoneal cells (Pc) a two step process? *Agents and Actions*, 11, 556-8

10. Mencia-Heurta, JM and Benveniste, J (1981). Platelet activating factor (Paf-acether) and macrophages: Phagocytosis-associated release of Paf-acether from rat peritoneal macrophages. *Cell Immunol*, 57, 281-92

11. Benveniste, J, Chignard, M, Le Couedic, JP and Vargaftig, BB (1982). Biosynthesis of platelet activating factor (Paf-acether) II. Involvement of phospholipase $A_2$ in the formation of Paf-acether and lyso-Paf-acether from rabbit platelets. *Thromb Res*, 25, 556-8

12. Jouvin-Marche, E, Ninio, E, Beurain, G and Benveniste, J (1984). Biosynthesis of platelet activating factor (Paf-acether) Vii. Precursors of Paf-acether and acetyltransferase activity in human leukocytes. *J Immunol*, 133, 892-8

13. Lee, TC, Lenihan, DJ, Malone, B et al. (1984). Increased biosynthesis of platelet activating factor in activated human eosinophils. *J Biol Chem*, 259, 5526-30

14. Synder, F (1985). Chemical and biochemical aspects of platelet activating factor: a novel class of acetylated ether-linked choline phospholipids. *Med Res Rev*, 5, 107-40

15. Synder, F (1987). The significance of dual pathways for the biosynthesis of platelet activating factor: 1-alkyl-2-lyso-sn-glycero-3-phosphate as a branchpoint. In Lee, ML and Winslow, CM (eds) *New Horizons in Platelet Activating Factor Research*, pp.13-26. (New York: John Wiley)

16. Farr, RS, Cox, CP, Wardlow, ML and Jorenson, R (1980). Preliminary studies of an acid labile factor (ALF) in human sera that inactivates platelet activating factor (PAF). *Clin Immunol Immunopathol*, 15, 318-30

17. Lee, TC, Blank, MC, Fitzgerald, V and Synder, F (1981). Substrate specificity in the biocleavage of the 1-alkyl-2-acetyl-sn-glyceryl-3-phosphorylcholine (a hypotensive platelet activating lipid) and its metabolites. *Arch Biochem Biophys*, 208, 353-7

18. Demopoulos, CA, Tsaikibalis, GE and Kapoulas, VM (1981). Intravascular pathobiology of acetylglyceryl ether phosphorylcholine (ACEGPC), a synthetic platelet activating factor (PAF). Intravenous infusion in guinea pigs. *Immunol Lett*, 3, 133-5

19. Caillard, CG, Monod, S, Zundel, JL and Julou, L (1982). Hypotensive activity of PAF-acether in rats. *Agents Actions*, 12, 5725-30

20. Vargaftig, BB, Chignard, M, Benveniste, J et al. (1981). Background and present status on research on platelet activating factor, (Paf-acether). *Ann NY Acad Sci*, 370, 119-37

21. Archer, CB, MacDonald, DM, Morley, J et al. (1985). Effects of serum albumin, indomethacin and histamine H1 antagonists on Paf-acether-induced inflammatory responses in the skin of experimental animals and man. *Br J Pharmacol*, 85, 109-13

22. Fjellner, B and Hagermark, O (1985). Experimental pruitis evoked by platelet activating factor (Paf-acether) in human skin. *Acta Dermatol Venereol*, 65, 409-13

23. Sciberras, DG, Drake, K, Dyer, T et al. (1987). Effects of H1-antagonism on the inflammatory responses to Paf-acether and histamine. *Br J Clin Pharmacol*, (In press)

24. Humphrey, DM, McManus, LM, Satouchi, K et al. (1982). Vasoactive properties of acetyl glyeryl ether phosphorylcholine and analogues. *Lab Invest*, 46, 422-7

25. Pirotzky, E, Page, CP, Roubin, R et al. (1984). Paf-acether induced plasma exudation in rat skin is independent of platelets and neutrophils. *Micro Endo Lymph*, 1, 107-22

26. Wedmore, CV and Williams, TJ (1981). Platelet activating factor (PAF), a secretory product of polymorphonuclear leucocytes, increases vascular permeability in rabbit skin. *Br J Pharmacol*, 71, 916-17P

27. Bjork, J and Smedegaard, G (1983). Acute microvascular effects of Paf-acether, as studied by intravital microscopy. *Eur J Pharmacol*, 96, 87-94

28. Morley, J, Page, CP and Paul, W (1983). Inflammatory actions of platelet activating factor (paf-acether) in guinea-pig skin. *Br J Pharmacol*, 80, 503-9

29.   Paul, W, Page, CP, Cunningham, FM and Morley, J (1985). The PPE responses to Paf-acether is independent of platelet accumulation. *Agents Actions*, **15**, 80-2

30.   Archer, CB, Frohlich, W, Page, CP *et al.* (1984). Synergestic interaction between prostaglandins and Paf-acether in experimental animals and man. *Prostaglandins*, **27**, 495-500

31.   Williams, TJ and Peck, MJ (1977). Role of prostaglandin mediated vasodilation in inflammation. *Nature*, **270**, 530-2

32.   Archer, CB, Page, CP, Morley, J and MacDonald, DM (1985). Accumulation of inflammatory cells in response to intracutaneous platelet activating factor (Paf-acether) in man. *Br J Dermatol*, **112**, 285-90

33.   Pirotzky, E, Page, CP, Morley J *et al.* (1985). Vascular permeability induced by Paf-acether (platelet activating factor) in the perfused rat kidney. *Agents Actions*, **16**, 17-18

34.   Barnes, PJ, Chung, KF, Evans, TW and Rodgers, DS (1986). Increased airway vascular permeability induced by platelet activating factor: effect of specific antagonists and platelet depletion. *Br J Pharmacol*, **89**, 764P

35.   Heffner, JE, Shoemaker, SA, Canham, EM *et al.* (1983). Acetyl glyceryl ether phosphorylcholine stimulated human platelets cause pulmonary hypertension and oedema in isolated rabbit lungs. *J Clin Invest*, **71**, 351-7

36.   Mojarad, M, Hamasaki, Y and Said, SI (1983). Platelet activating factor increases pulmonary microvascular permeability and induces pulmonary oedma. *Bull Eur Physiopathol Resp*, **104**, 253-7

37.   Bussolino, F, Aglietta, M, Sanavio, F *et al.* (1985). Alkyl-ether phosphoglycerides induce calcium fluxes into human endothelial cells. *J Immunol*, **135**, 2748-53

38.   Dewar, A, Archer, CB, Paul, W *et al.* (1984) Cutaneous and pulmonary histopathological responses to platelet activating factor in the guinea-pig. *J Pathol*, **144**, 25-30

39.   Bussolini, F, Camussi, G, Aglietta, M *et al.* (1986). PAF induces a re-organisation of the microfilaments in human endothelial cells. Abstract presented to the *Second International Conference on Platelet Activating Factor and Structurally Related Alkyl Ether Lipids.* Gatlinburg, TN, USA, October

40.   Czarnetzki, BM and Benveniste, J (1981). Effect of synthetic Paf-acether on human neutrophil function. *Agents and Actions*, **11**, 549-53

41.   Wardlow, AJ, Moqbel, R, Cromwell, O and Kay, AB (1986). Platelet activating factor: a potent chemotactic and chemokinetic factor for human eosinophils. *J Clin Invest*, **78**, 1701-6

42.   Yasaka, T, Boxer, LA and Baehner, RL (1982). Monocyte aggregation and superoxide anion response to formyl-methionyl-leucyl-phenylanaline (FMLP), and platelet activating factor. *J Immunol*, **128**, 1939-44

43.   Nachmann, RL (1980). The platelet as an inflammatory cell. In De Gaetano, G and Garatini, S (eds) *Platelets: A Multidisciplinary Approach.* p. 199. (New York: Raven Press)

44.   Farr, M, Wainwright, A, Salmon, M *et al.* (1984). Platelets in the synovial fluid of patients with rheumatoid arthritis. *Rheumatol Int*, **4**, 13-17

45.   Simmling-Annefield, M and Fassbender, HG (1979). Transformation of the capillary wall elements in synovial tissue in rheumatoid arthritis. *Z Rheumatol*, **38**, 153-62

46.   Farr, M, Scott, DC, Constable, T *et al.* (1981). Platelets and rheumatoid vasculitis. *Ann Rheum Dis*, **40**, 617

47.   Zeller, J, Weissbarn, E, Banith, B *et al.* (1983). Serotonin content of platelets in inflammed rheumatic disease. *Arthritis Rheum*, **26**, 532-40

48.   Turner, SR, Tainer, JA and Lynn, WS (1975). Biogenesis of chemotactic molecules by the arachidonate lipoxygenase system of platelets. *Nature*, **257**, 680-2

49.   Lellouch-Tubiana, A, Lefort, J, Pirotzky, E *et al..* (1985). Ultrastructural evidence for extravascular platelet recruitment in the lung upon intravenous injection of platelet activating factor (PAF-acether) to guinea-pigs. *Br J Exp Pathol*, **66**, 345-55

50.   Joseph, M, Auriault, C, Capron, A et al. (1984). A new function for platelets: IgE-dependent killing of Schistosomes. Nature, 303, 310-12
51.   Henson, PM and Ginsberg, MH (1981). Immunological reactions of platelets. In: Gordon, JL (ed) Platelets in Biology and Pathology. Vol. 2, pp. 265-308. (Amsterdam: Elsevier/North Holland)
52.   Fink, PC, Piercing, V, Friche, M and Diecher, H (1979). Platelet aggregation and aggregation inhibition by differential antiglobulins and antiglobulin complexes from sera of patients with rheumatoid arthritis. Arthritis Rheum, 22, 896-903
53.   Cunningham, T, Medcalf, RL, Mathews, JD and Muirden, KD (1986). Platelet releasing activity in sera of patients with rheumatoid vasculitis. Ann Rheum Dis, 45, 15-20
54.   Camussi, G, Pawlowski, I, Saunders, R et al. (1987). A receptor antagonist of platelet activating factor inhibits inflammatory injury by in situ formation of immune complexes in renal glomeruli and in skin. J Lab Clin Med, 110, 196-206
55.   Henson, PM (1981). Neutrophil secretion: mechanisms and consequences in inflammation. In Venge, P and Lindblom, A (eds) The Inflammatory Process - An Introduction to the Study of Cellular and Humoral Mechanisms. pp. 161-82. (Stockholm: Almquist Wiskell)
56.   Poitevin, B, Mencia-Heurta, JM, Roubin, R and Benveniste, J (1985). Role of Paf-acether (platelet activating factor) in neutrophil activation. In Said, SI (ed) The Pulmonary Circulation and Acute Lung Injury. pp. 357-73. (Mount Kisco, NY: Futura)
57.   Henson, PM (1981). Platelet activating factor as a mediator of neutrophil platelet interactions in inflammation. In Russo-Marie, F et al. (ed) Pharmacology of Inflammation and Allergy. Vol. 100, pp. 63-81. (Paris: INSERM)
58.   Cammussi, G, Tetta, L and Bussolini, F (1981). Mediators of immune complex induced aggregation of polymorphonuclear neutrophils. 11. Platelet activating factor as the effector substance of immune induced aggregation. Int Arch Allergy Appl Immunol, 64, 25-41
59.   Cammussi, G, Pawlowski, I, Tetta, C et al. (1983). Acute lung inflammation induced in the rabbit by local instillation of 1-O-octadecyl-2-acetyl-sn-glyceryl-3-phosphocholine or native platelet activating factor. Am J Pathol, 112, 78-88
60.   Coeffier, E, Chignard, M, Delautier, D and Benveniste, J (1984). Co-operation between platelets and neutrophils for Paf-acether formation. Fed Proc, 43, 2900
61.   Moon, DG, Weston, LK, Kaplan, JE and Malik, AB (1986). Platelet-neutrophil interaction: platelet activating factor induced superoxide anion production. Abstract presented to the Second International Conference on Platelet Activating Factor and Structurally Related Alkyl Ether Lipids. Gatlinburg, TN, USA, October
62.   Short, CC, Bauer, W and Reynolds, WE (1957). Rheumatoid Arthritis. p. 3352. (Cambridge, Mass.: Harvard Press)
63.   Venge, P, Dahl, R, Fredens, K et al. (1983). Eosinophil cationic proteins, (ECP and ECX) in health and disease. In Yoshida, T and Torisu, M (eds) Immunobiology of the Eosinophil. p. 163. (New York, Oxford, Amsterdam: Elsevier)
64.   Ackermann, S, Durack, DT and Gleich, GJ (1982). Eosinophil effector mechanisms in health and disease. In Gallin, J and Fauci, AS (eds) Host Defense Mechanisms. Vol. 1, p. 269. (New York: Raven Press)
65.   Hallergen, R, Feltelius, N, Karin, S and Venge, P (1985). Eosinophil involvement in rheumatoid arthritis as reflected as elevated serum levels of eosinophil cationic protein. Clin Exp Immunol, 59, 539-46
66.   Frigas, E and Gleich, GJ (1986). The eosinophil in the pathophysiology of asthma. J Allergy Clin Immunol, 77, 527-37
67.   Henocq, E and Vargaftig, BB (1986). Accumulation of eosinophils in response to intracutaneous Paf-acether and allergens in man. Lancet, ii, 1378-9
68.   Janossy, G, Panayi, GS, Duke, O et al. (1981). Rheumatoid arthritis: a disease of T-lymphocyte/macrophage immunoregulation. Lancet, ii, 839-42

69. Wood, DD, Ihrie, EJ, Dinarello, CA and Cohen, PC (1983). Isolation of an interleukin-1-like substance from human joint effusions. *Arthritis Rheum*, **26**, 975-82
70. Saklatvala, J and Dingle, JJ (1981). Identification of catabolin, a protein from synovium which induces degradation of a cartilage in organ culture. *Biochem Biophys Res Commun*, **96**, 1225-31
71. Gowen, M, Wood, DD and Ihrie, EJ (1983). An Interleukin-1 like factor stimulates bone resorption in vitro. *Nature*, **306**, 378-80
72. Rifa, SL, Shen, F, Mitchell, K and Peck, WA (1984). Macrophage-derived growth factor for oesteoblast-like cells. *Proc Natl Acad Sci*, **81**, 4558-62
73. Granstein, MD, Margalis, R and Mizel, SB (1985). In Kluger, MJ *et al.* (ed) *Physiologic, Metabolic and Immunologic Actions of Interleukin 1.* (New York: Alan R Liss)
74. Pettipher, R, Higgs, GA and Henderson, B (1986). Interleukin 1 induces leucocyte infiltration and proteoglycan degradation in the synovial joints. *Proc Natl Acad Sci USA*, **83**, 8749-53
75. Barrett, ML, Lewis, GP, Ward, S and Westwick, J (1987). Platelet activating factor induces interleukin 1 production from human adherent macrophages. *Br J Pharmacol*, **90**, 113P
76. Bussolini, F, Breviario, F, Tetta, C *et al.* (1986). Interleukin-1 stimulates platelet activating factor production from human cultured endothelial cells. *Pharmacol Res Commun*, **18**, 133-7
77. Gillis, S, Fern, MM, Ou, W and Smith, KAA (1978). T-cell growth. Parameters for production and a quantitative microassay for activity. *J Immunol*, **120**, 2027-34
78. Braquet, P and Rola-Pleszczynski, M (1987), The role of PAF in the immune response. *Immunol. Today*, **8**, 345-350
79. Foegh, ML, Alijani, MR, Helfrich, GB *et al.* (1985). Prolongation of cardiac allograft survival with the PAF antagonist BN52021 and with the thromboxane receptor antagonists L640035 and L636499. *Advances in Prostaglandin, Thromboxane and Leukotriene Research*. Vol. 15, p. 38. (New York: Raven Press)
80. Foegh, ML, Khirabadi, BS, Rowles, JR *et al.* (1986). Prolongation of cardiac allograft survival with BN52021, a specific antagonist of platelet activating factor. *Transplant Proc*, **42**, 86-8
81. Foegh, ML, Bijans, S, Khirabadi, BS *et al.* (1987). Synergistic effect of a PAF antagonist with azathioprine and cyclosporin in allograft survival. In Winslow, CM and Lee, M (eds) *New Horizons in Platelet Activating Factor*. p. 343-6. (New York: John Wiley)
82. Basran, GS, Page, CP, Paul, W and Morley, J (1984). Platelet activating factor: a possible mediator of the dual response to allergen? *Clin Allergy*, **14**, 75-9
83. Scibberas, DGJ, Fox, J, James, I and Baber, NS (1987). The intradermal responses to injection of platelet activating factor (PAF) in man. *Br J Clin Pharmacol*, **23**, 116P
84. Bonnet, J, Loiseau, AM, Orvoen, M and Bessin, P (1981). Platelet activating factor (Paf-acether) involvement in acute inflammatory and pain processes. *Agents Actions*, **11**, 559-62
85. Parente, L and Flower, RJ (1985). The generation of lyso-PAF in experimental inflammation. In Higgs, GA and Williams, TJ (eds) *Inflammatory Mediators*. pp. 65-72. (London: MacMillan)
86. Henson, PM and Pinkard, RN (1977). Basophil derived platelet activating factor (PAF) as an in vivo mediator of acute allergic reactions: demonstration of specific desensitization of platelets to PAF during IgE-induced anaphylaxis in the rabbit. *J Immunol*, **119**, 2179-84
87. Grandel, KE, Farr, RS, Wanderer, AA *et al.* (1985). Association of platelet activating factor with primary acquired cold urticaria. *N Engl J Med*, **313**, 405-9
88. Nakamura, T, Morita, Y, Kuriyama, M *et al.* (1987). Platelet activating factor in late asthmatic responses. *Int Arch Allergy Appl Immunol*, **82**, 57-61

89.     Valone, F, Shalit, M, Atkins, P et al. (1987). Platelet activating factor release in aller-
        gic skin sites in humans. J Allergy Clin Immunol, 79, A494
90.     Fitzgerald, MF, Henderson, GA, Higgs, GA et al. (1985). The levels of PAF and lyso-
        PAF in the joint fluids of rabbits with antigen induced-arthritis. Br J Pharmacol, 86,
        422P
91.     Pickett, WC and Ramesha, CS (1986). Distribution of PAF molecular species in sy-
        novial fluid of patients with Rheumatoid Arthritis. Abstract presented to the Second
        International Conference of Platelet Activating Factor and Structurally Related Alkyl
        Ether Lipids. Gatlinburg, TN, USA, October
92.     Terashita, Z, Tseshima, S, Yoshioka, Y et al. (1983). CV3988, a specific antagonist
        of platelet activating factor (PAF). Life Sci, 32 (17), 1975-82
93.     Miyamoto, T, Ohno, H, Yano, T et al. (1985). ONO-6240: a new potent antagonist of
        platelet activating factor. In Hayahiri, O and Yamamoto, S (eds) Advances in Pros-
        taglandin, Thromboxane and Leukotriene Res. Vol. 15, pp.719-720. (New York: Raven
        Press)
94.     Burri, K, Burner, R, Cassal, JM et al. (1985). Platelet activating factor: from agonist
        to antagonist by synthesis. Prostaglandins, 30, 691
95.     Winslow, CM, Anderson, RC, D'Aries, FJ et al.. (1987). Towards understanding the
        mechanism of action of PAF receptor antagonists. In Lee, ML and Winslow, CM
        (eds) New Horizons in Platelet Activating Factor Research. pp. 153-64. (New York:
        John Wiley)
96.     Shen, TY, Hwang, SB, Chang, MN et al. (1985). Characterization of a platelet acti-
        vating factor antagonist isolated from haifenteng (Piper futokadsura): specific inhibi-
        tion of in vitro and in vivo platelet activating factor induced effects. Proc Natl Acad
        Sci USA, 83, 672-6
97.     Hwang, SB, Lam, MH, Biftu, T et al. (1985). Trans-2,5-dis-(3,4,5-trimethoxyphe-
        nyl)tetrahydrofuran. An orally active specific and competitive receptor antagonist of
        platelet activating factor. J Biol Chem, 260, 15639-45
98.     Braquet, P, Spinnewyn, B, Braquet, M et al. (1985). BN 52021 and related com-
        pounds: a new series of highly specific Paf-acether receptor antagonists isolated from
        Ginko biloba. Blood Vessels, 16, 559-72
99.     Chung, KF, Dent, G, McCusker, M et al. (1987). Effects of a ginkolide mixture
        (BN52063) in antagonising skin and platelet responses to platelet activating factor in
        man. Lancet, i, 248-50
100.    Kornecki, E, Erlich, YH and Lennox, RH (1984). Platelet activating factor-induced
        aggregation of human platelets specifically inhibited by triazolobenzodiezepines.
        Science, 226, 1454-6
101.    Casals-Stenzel, J (1987). Protective effect of WEB 2086, a novel antagonist of PAF
        in endotoxin shock. J Pharmacol Exp Ther, 135, 117-21
102.    Westwick, J, Marks, G, Powling, MJ and Kakkar, VV (1983). Diltiazem, the cardiac
        slow calcium antagonist, is a potent, selective and competitive inhibitor of platelet
        activating factor (PAF) on human platelets. J Pharmacol (Paris), 14, 62
103.    Sedivy, P, Weber, S, Gregoire, J et al.. (1987). 48740 RP inhibits PAF-induced pla-
        telet aggregation and thromboxanes B2 generation ex-vivo in volunteers. Clin Exp
        Physiol Pharmacol, (in press)
104.    Braquet, P and Godfroid, JJ (1986). Paf-acether specific binding sites: 2. Design of
        specific antagonists. Trends Pharmacol Sci, 7, 397-403
105.    Voekel, NF, Chang, SW, Pfeffer, KD et al.. (1987). PAF antagonists: Different ef-
        fects on platelets, neutrophils, guinea-pig ileum and PAF-induced vasodilatation in
        isolated rat lung. Prostaglandins, 32, 359-72
106.    Villian, B, Lagente, V, Touvay, C et al. (1986). Pharmacological control of the in vivo
        passive anaphylactic shock by Paf-acether antagonist compound BN 52021. Pharma-
        col Res Commun, 18, Suppl., 119-26

107.　Terashita, ZI, Imura, Y, Nishikawa, K and Sumida, S (1985). Is platelet activating factor a mediator of endotoxin shock? *Eur J Pharmacol*, **109**, 257-61

108.　Hellewell, PG and Williams, TJ (1986). A specific antagonist of platelet activating factor suppresses oedema formation in an arthus reaction but not oedema formation induced by leukocyte chemoattractants in rabbits. *J Immunol*, **137**, 302-7

109.　Cordeiro, RSB, Henriques, MG, Weg, VB and Vargaftig, BB (1986). Effectiveness of the Paf-acether antagonist BN 52021 and 48740 RP against carrageenin-induced mice paw and pleurisy; comparison with cyclo-oxygenase inhibitors. Abstract presented to the *Second International Conference on Platelet Activating Factor and Structurally Related Alkyl Ether Lipids*. Gatlinburg, TN, USA, October

# 10
# Interleukin 1: past, present, future

**Michael C. Powanda\* and Elizabeth D. Moyer\*\***
\*Letterman Army Institute of Research, Presidio of San Francisco, CA 94129, USA
\*\*KabiVitrum, Inc., 1311 Harbor Bay Parkway, Alameda, CA 94501, USA

## I. INTRODUCTION

Like all historical events, the stages of development of our knowledge and understanding of the family of proteins presently called interleukin-1 (IL-1) can be assigned conveniently to one of three phases: past, present and future. We suggest, however, the key discriminant in the transition from one phase to another is not so much a discrete moment in time, but rather a shift in perspective, which has a temporal component. Thus we have chosen to define the past as beginning with the discovery of an endogenous pyrogen (EP) by Beeson[1] and ending with the demonstration by several research groups that leucocytic endogenous mediator (LEM), which is capable of eliciting a multiplicity of metabolic alterations, is similar to, if not identical with, endogenous pyrogen. The present began with the realization that EP = LEM = IL-1, thus EP became a mediator of immunological consequence as well as a potent physiological and metabolic stimulus. The present also encompasses the growing awareness that IL-1 is not only a monokine released in response to an inflammatory stimulus, but is also a cytokine, arising constitutively from non-phagocytic cells such as kertatinocytes. Though IL-1 was initially discovered during disease states, it may also be a key factor in growth, development and homeostatis in health. The present presages the future in that efforts are already being made to elucidate the regulation of IL-1 production, release and action, the role(s) IL-1 play(s) not only in inflammation, disease and injury but in health; the therapeutic potential of IL-1 and the modulation of IL-1 activity. Let us now explore these phases of our knowledge and understanding of IL-1 in more detail.

The opinions or assertions contained herein are the private views of the authors and are not to be construed as official or as reflecting the views of the Department of the Army, the Department of Defense (AR360-5), or of KabiVitrum, Inc

*New Developments in Antirheumatic Therapy.* Rainsford, KD and Velo, GP (eds), Inflammation and Drug Therapy Series, Volume III.

By our definition, the past begins with Beeson's demonstration that saline extracts of peritoneal exudate cells were pyrogenic[1], but we could have justifiably begun with Metchnikoff and his phagocytic theory of immunity[2] as a reminder that IL-1 is not merely a family of molecules, but rather is an integral part of the process of our interaction with environmental stimuli and stresses, fundamental to our survival. The evolution of the concept of IL-1 being a component of host survival has been articulately presented by Atkins[3].

Noting that acute hypoferraemia in man and animals accompanies fever of various aetiologies, Kampschmidt and Upchurch[4] presented evidence that extracts of leucocytes which caused fever in rabbits produced hypoferraemia, in both rabbits and rats even in endotoxin-tolerant rats. Subsequently, a series of papers appeared which gave evidence that this leucocytic extract, now entitled leucocytic endogenous mediator, not only engendered fever in recipients, but also affected the hepatic uptake of amino acids[5], elicited the tissue distribution of zinc and iron[6], elevated serum copper and caeruloplasmin levels[7], stimulated the release of neutrophils from bone marrow[8] and increased serum $\alpha$-acute phase globulins[8,9]. These studies were carried out using LEM preparations of varying purity, but in the main indicated strongly that LEM was similar to, if not identical with, EP. The question of the identity of LEM and EP continued to be pursued, slowed primarily by the difficulties in purifying and identifying these potent polypeptides[10]. With the exception of some as yet unexplained data indicating that there may be a differential effect of potassium ion concentration on the production and/or release of fever-inducing material versus mediators of amino acid, neutrophil and trace metal alterations[11], the rest of the data strongly supported the hypothesis that EP = LEM[12,13]. Moreover, when it became clear that macrophages were capable of secreting two biochemically and immunologically distinct EPs[14] with differing isoelectric points not attributable to glycosylation[15], retesting of the hypothesis provided confirmatory data, but reintroduced the concept that there are species differences in response to heterologous EP/LEMs[16], particularly with regard to those forms having isoelectric points between 4.5 and 5.0[17].

Concomitantly, other researchers sought to expand the repertoire of EP/LEM. Data which showed that LEM from rabbit peritoneal leucocytes injected 24 hours prior to a usually fatal dose of *S. typhimurium* protected 40 of 46 rats from death[18] provided the first indication that EP/LEM might be of benefit to the host, at least in some instances. Impure rabbit LEM was shown to augment conversion of arachidonic acid to prostaglandins by the cerebral prostaglandin-synthetase system[19], to increase both plasma insulin and glucagon levels in rats in a dose-dependent manner[20], to increase hepatic RNA synthesis as well as acute-phase protein production[21] and to stimulate the intestinal absorption of zinc[22]. Massive doses of crude rabbit LEM also produced transient alterations in the heart rate, blood pressure and total peripheral resistance in Rhesus monkey[23] akin to those seen following severe injury or during acute stages of infection. Highly purified human EP/LEM induced neurtophils to selectively release granulocyte-associated proteins, lysozyme and lactoferrin[24], and to increase superoxide production and hexose monophosphate shunt activity[25]. The discovery of new activities for EP/LEM continues afoot, and will be discussed in more detail in the following section.

## II. PRESENT

The present phase of our knowledge began with two sets of findings indicating that EP may be IL-1. The first was that a purified preparation of human EP was able to partially replace intact peritoneal exudate cells in the T-cell proliferation in response to antigen[26]. The second provided good evidence that two forms of rabbit EP with different isoelectric points (pI 4.6 and 7.3) had lymphocytic activating factor activity, and that antibody to pI 7.3 EP incubated with it blocked both fever and lymphocyte activation[27]. Despite these and subsequent data substantiating that EP = IL-1, there is evidence *in vivo* and *in vitro* that it is possible to separate pyrogenicity from lymphocyte activation using various analogues of muramyl dipeptide[28]. Whether the latter data refute the theories that EP always equals IL-1, or merely confirm that both fever and immunocompetence are of such value to the host that redundant systems exist to mediate these responses, has yet to be established.

At this point the long-held belief that EP was derived from granulocytes was thoroughly examined and appeared to be invalid, for neutrophils, obtained from either the peripheral cavity or blood and purified on Percoll gradients, failed to produce EP or IL-1 when confronted with a variety of stimuli which usually elicit these activities[29,30]. Nonetheless, more recent data suggest that indeed neutrophils not only can produce IL-1[31] but also an IL-1 inhibitor[32], indicating that we still have much to learn about the factors which regulate IL-1 production and release.

More attention began to be paid to the possible sources of IL-1. At first it seemed reasonable that only granulocytes and cells of the mononuclear phagocytic system could give rise to IL-1, and when these and other cell types such as fibroblasts were confronted with a particulate stimulus such as killed bacteria or latex particles, this belief appeared valid[33]. But subsequent studies indicated that there are many sites and cell sources for IL-1 within and on the surface of the body to include not only macrophages, monocytes, neutrophils, and Kupffer cells, but also astrocytes[34], corneal epithelial cells[35], dendritic cells[36], endothelial cells[37], fibroblasts[38], Langerhans cells[39], lymphocytes[40-43], mesangial cells[44,45], microglias[46], smooth muscle cells[47] and the stratum corneum[48-50]. Moreover, in some instances IL-1 appears to be produced constitutively rather than only in response to an inflammatory stimulus. It is quite likely that, under the appropriate conditions, production of IL-1 will be found to be an inherent property of all but a few, highly specialized, cell types.

During the past few years, not only have new sources and forms of IL-1 been found, but additional activities were attributed to these already multi-potent polypeptides. Severe infection is usually accompanied by muscle wasting, lethargy and anorexia. Incubation of rat soleus or extensor digitorum longus muscles with highly purified human IL-1 resulted in increased muscle protein degradation, purportedly mediated by prostaglandins[51]. Whether it is IL-1 itself or a 4.2 kiloDalton (kD) cleavage product (termed proteolysis-inducing factor)[52] which is the major inducer of muscle protein degradation is not readily apparent, since the IL-1 used had a tendency to fragment into a 4 kD peptide[53], but it might also be due to the presence of a contaminant. These data need to be re-examined, since there is some question as to the role prostaglandins play in muscle degradation *in vivo*, since neither indomethacin[54] nor ibuprofen[55] appears to significantly reduce muscle degradation during sepsis or induced by IL-1 infusion[56]. Human IL-1 infused into the lateral cerebral ventricles of rabbits increased slow-wave sleep in a dose-dependent manner[57,58]. Both human and murine recombinant IL-1 reduced food intake in rats[59]. Since it was previously shown that fever was not necessary to produce anorexia[60], suppressed food intake thus could be a direct effect of IL-1.

The initiation of inflammation is generally associated with an infiltration of neutrophils. Consistent with a role for IL-1 in the initiation of inflammation, epidermal cell-derived IL-1 was shown to be chemotactic for neutophils *in vitro* [61]. Subsequent studies demonstrated that murine cell line-derived IL-1 injected intradermally into rabbits stimulated neutrophil accumulation at the injection site and could mediate the local Shwartzman reaction[62]. Human monocyte-derived IL-1 has been shown to be chemotactic for both B and T lymphocytes[63], while epidermally derived IL-1 tested positive as a T cell attractant[64].

Vascular endothelial cells constitute the boundary between the bloodstream and the tissues, controlling access of circulatory cells and fluid to the extravascular spaces; thus endothelial cells are potential modulators of the inflammatory response. Therefore, it is not surprising that IL-1 elicits a number of inflammation-associated responses from endothelial cells. IL-1 induces synthesis and expression of procoagulant activity in human vascular endothelial cells *in vitro* [65], with a peak response between 3 and 6 hours followed by a refractory period. When IL-1 is injected intravenously into rabbits it not only increases endothelial cell procoagulant activity many-fold, it also decreases thrombin-mediated protein C activation and protein C-S complex formation, thereby shifting the balance of procoagulant/anticoagulant reactions to favour clot formation[66]. IL-1 also induces endothelial cell synthesis of prostacyclin (PGI$_2$), a potent inhibitor of platelet aggregation and a vasodilator; induction of PGI$_2$ synthesis requires relatively long exposure ( > 6 hours) of the cells to IL-1[67]. IL-1 promotes the adhesiveness of the neutrophils and monocytes to endothelial cells, again with a maximal response at approximately 4 hours[68]. Under the same conditions, IL-1 did not increase dermal fibroblast adhesivity for leucocytes. Additionally, IL-1 induces endothelial cell synthesis of plasminogen activator inhibitor *in vitro* [69] and *in vivo* [70], most of which is apparently released, and of platelet activating factor[71], which remains primarily cell-associated, and also stimulates the release of granulocyte macrophage-colony stimulating activity[72].

Fibroblasts appear to be another primary cell target for IL-1 release and actions. Considering the evidence for macrophage-fibroblast interactions during wound healing/tissue remodelling[73], again, this is not surprising. IL-1 is capable of stimulating not only fibroblast proliferation[74,75], but also fibroblast production of both collagenase[76] and a collagenase inhibitor[77], of an intracellular adhesion molecule which facilitates the binding of lymphoid cells to fibroblasts[78], as well as of granulocyte-macrophage colony-stimulating activity[79] and prostaglandin E$_2$.

As can be seen, the effects of IL-1 on cells can be complex, manifold and not only concentration- but tissue-dependent. The situation becomes more involved when assessing the role of IL-1 in the development of a multifaceted disease such as arthritis. IL-1 activity was found in the synovial fluid of 17/20 patients with rheumatoid arthritis, but in only 1/16 patients with osteoarthritis[80], indicating that IL-1 might not be involved in the latter disease process. However, a subsequent report found IL-1 activity in joint fluids from patients with osteoarthritis, Reiter's syndrome, gout, psoriatic and traumatic arthritis[81]. The authors suggest that the difference between these and the preceding results may be due to the presence of IL-1 inhibitor(s) which were reduced or eliminated in the second study by gel filtration.

There are a number of *in vitro* studies which indicate the role(s) IL-1 may play in degenerative bone and joint diseases. Human mononuclear cell factors were found to mediate the degradation of matrix proteoglycan and collagen in cartilage explants through chondrocyte activation[82]. Human mononuclear cells also produce factors which stimulate bone resorption and inhibit proline incorporation into collagen, while partially purified human IL-1 was found to inhibit the production of osteocalcin, believed to be a bone-specific protein[83]. IL-1-$\alpha$ from pig leucocytes not only induces proteoglycan breakdown in cartilage explants, but also stimulates production of PGE$_2$ and latent collagenase by fibroblasts and chondrocytes as well as increasing calcium release from calvarial explants[84]. The pig IL-1-$\alpha$ can produce a 4-fold loss in proteoglycan from cartilage in 4 days; removal of IL-1 stopped the further loss of proteoglycan[85]. Partially purified human IL-1 was found capable of stimulating chondrocytes to produce prostaglandins, plasminogen activator and proteoglycanase, of enhancing synovial cell proliferation and of stimulating cartilage resorption[86]. Partially purified human IL-1 can stimulate procollagenase synthesis by rheumatoid synovial fibroblasts as much as 12-14-fold[87]. Purified IL-1 has been shown to increase chondrocyte-associated phospholipase A$_2$ (PLA$_2$) followed by a time- and dose-related release of PLA$_2$ and PGE$_2$ into the medium[88].

Not all of IL-1 effects on joints and joint cells are perforce catabolic; for example, IL-1 enhances synovial cell[89] and chondrocyte[90] hyaluronate synthesis. Mononuclear cell factor, thought to be identical with IL-1, not only promotes synovial cell collagenase and $PGE_2$ production but also stimulates the synthesis of Types I and III procollagen and fibronectin by these cells; indomethacin augments the effect of IL-1 on procollagen and fibronectin synthesis[91]. With regard to bone resorption, the consequence of IL-1 vary, depending not only on dose, but also with regard to exposure. Low doses of IL-1 ($\leq 1$ U/mL) for short periods ($\leq 24$ hours) cause increases in both collagen and non-collagen protein synthesis in fetal rat calvariae, while higher doses of IL-1 and longer incubation periods reduce collagen synthesis, but either have no effect or slightly stimulate non-collagen protein synthesis[92].

When one attempts to elucidate the pathogenesis of a disease, injury or inflammation, one often focuses on the localized tissue responses that are pathognomonic, and IL-1 is indeed a likely mediator of these local events. However, systemic alterations in metabolism and physiology accompany virtually all such pathological conditions, and IL-1 also seems to be directly or indirectly involved in mediating these systemic manifestations.

Considering the increases in glucagon and insulin that IL-1 appears to elicit in rats[20], it is not entirely surprising that mice given IL-1 exhibit hypoglycaemia[93], nor on the other hand is it totally unexpected that hepatocytes derived from rats given IL-1 not only display increased uptake of alanine, but also enhanced glucose production from alanine[94]. What is surprising is that in culture, IL-1, specifically the 17.5 kD, pI 7 form, and only that form, appears to be cytotoxic for islets of Langerhans, reducing insulin secretion as well as insulin and glucagon content[95]. Do these seemingly contradictory data reflect the differences in dose, duration of exposure, and species responses to IL-1, or are they an example of the hazards of relating tissue culture studies to whole animal experiments?

IL-1 and glucocorticoids appear interrelated. Corticosteroids can reduce IL-1 production/release *in vitro*[96] and *in vivo*[97], while a dose of IL-1, which produces hypozincaemia and increases liver metallothionein content in rats, reduces serum corticosterone levels almost 60%[98]. In contrast, there is a report that IL-1 could stimulate release of adrenocorticotrophic hormone (ACTH) from cultured mouse adrenal tumour cells[99]. Consistent with the latter report are the data indicating that IL-1 injected into mice and rats produced increases in both ACTH and corticosterone[100]. However, the amount of IL-1 injected was insufficient to produce fever under the experimental conditions, and no other manifestation of IL-1 activity was measured.

IL-1 can clearly affect hepatocyte protein synthesis directly, causing increases in acute phase proteins and decreases in albumin and some enzymes[101-103] similar to those observed during infection and inflammation. If the hepatic synthesis of serum amyloid P-component is typical of the pattern of acute-phase protein synthesis in response to inflammation, then there is not only an increased synthesis of these proteins by some hepatocytes, but a recruitment of additional hepatocytes. However, it appears that IL-1 increases the amount of acute-phase protein produced per hepatocyte, not the number of hepatocytes synthesizing these proteins[104]. Other macrophage-derived factors appear to be involved in hepatocyte recruitment.

Some of the activities attributed to IL-1 can have positive as well as negative effects, e.g. IL-1 induction of ornithine decarboxylase (the rate-limiting enzyme of polyamine synthesis), in the liver and spleens of mice[105] could as well lead to tissue repair and immune competence as disease, since polyamines can stimulate replication, transcription, and translation processes. IL-1-enhanced production of type IV collagen by epithelial cells[106] may be essential to growth, differentiation and wound healing. Other apparently beneficial effects of IL-1 are its ability to enhance secondary antibody responses of mice to protein antigen in vivo [107], its cytostatic[108] and cytotoxic[109] effects on some tumour cell lines and its role in providing radioprotection to mice[110].

Though increases in circulating IL-1 or its degradation products are usually associated with the presence of disease[52,80,81,111], there are data to indicate that alterations in IL-1 concentration are part of normal physiological processes such as sleep[112], exercise[113], ovulation[114], and perhaps even pregnancy[115]. The effect of exercise on plasma IL-1 was affected by the degree of training of the subjects. Thus, untrained men had lower pre-exercise levels of IL-1 than trained men, and exercise significantly increased plasma IL-1 in untrained men, but generally not in trained men[116].

Due to the difficulties in purifying sufficient IL-1 to allow characterization, many of the studies of IL-1 action until recently have used material usually designated by an apparent molecular weight and/or isoelectric point. In the last few years, however, sufficient progress has been made to allow us to more fully characterize the family of molecules called IL-1. IL-1 derived from human cells appear to exist in a multiplicity of molecular weight and isoelectric forms, the presence of which may depend both on cell incubation conditions and purification procedures. Endotoxin-stimulated monocytes cultured in 1% fetal calf serum give rise to at least four forms:a 15,000-17,000 Dalton (pI 7), a 15,000-17,500 Dalton (pI 5.5), a 35,000 Dalton (pI 7) and a 35,000 (pI 5.5) form, all of which could act as mitogens and comitogens for thymocytes, induce IL-1, activate B cells, stimulate chondrocytes and synoviocytes, and induce serum amyloid A protein in mice[117]. Antibody to the low molecular weight pI 7 form neutralized the 35 kD pI 7 form, but neither of the pI 5.5 forms[118]. The 35 kD form does not appear to be an aggregate of lower molecular weight material, since it is stable even in urea[119]. Monocytes stimulated with endotoxin and cultured in 5% human serum produce extracellular IL-1 in the 15-17 kD range, about 60% of which has an isoelectric point of 6.7, and 40% pI 5.5; the intracellular IL-1 is 90% pI 5.5, but has molecular weights of 15, 26, 45, and > 70 kD[120]. Some of the higher molecular weight forms appear to be aggregates of the 15 kD form[119,120]. The presence of a membrane-associated form of IL-1 which is induced earlier and persists longer than IL-1 secretion[121], and explains why IL-1 secretion is not required for T cell proliferation[122].

The neutral (IL-1 β)[123] and anionic (IL-1 α)[124] forms of IL-1 have been purified, and the amino acid sequence data agree with that predicted from the complimentary DNA and indicate that there are at least two human genes coding for molecules possessing IL-1 activity. The gene which gives rise to the neutral IL-1 (IL-1 β) appears to be on the long arm[125] of human chromosome 2. The complementary DNAs code for a 269 amino acid precursor in the case of IL-1 β and a 271 amino acid precursor in the case of IL-1 α with a molecular weight of ≈ 31,000 which is cleaved to form a 17,500 Dalton polypeptide[126,127]. The recombinant human IL-1 α has been shown to be capable of stimulating T cell and fibroblast proliferation and inducing fibroblast collagenase and prostaglandin production[128]. The recombinant human IL-1 β can produce fever in rabbits and endotoxin-resistant mice, replace monocytes in stimulating T cell blastogenesis and IL-2 production and induce dermal fibroblast $E_2$ production[129], as well as stimulate synovial cell collagenase and $PGE_2$ production[130]. Murine recombinant IL-1 which exhibits a high degree of sequence homology with human IL-1 α has also been cloned and expressed[131], and has been found capable of eliciting fever, hypozincaemia and neutrophilia in rats[132]. Though acute-phase protein levels were not altered in this study after a single injection of IL-1, an earlier study did demonstrate that murine recombinant IL-1 elicits a dose-dependent increase in serum amyloid A messenger RNA and in serum amyloid A plasma protein concentration[133]. Though many more of the activities attributed to native IL-1 still have to be tested for, both *in vivo* and *in vitro*, it does appear that the recombinant IL-1 elicit a number of responses similar to the native molecules. Thus it may be possible to discover why the body produces two distinct very potent molecules with a panoply of physiological, metabolic and immunological actions.

Despite 20 years of research, all of the factors which regulate IL-1 production/release by cells of the reticuloendothelial system have yet to be discovered, never mind the factors for control of IL-1 synthesis and secretion by cells such as keratinocytes and fibroblasts. What has been discovered so far is consistent with the complex set of circumstances which would attend production of a mediator which orchestrates the host's physiological, metabolic and immunological responses to stimuli such as micro-organisms and injury, as well as participates in the integration of processes of growth, development and repair. Bacteria and endotoxin, a product of Gram-negative bacteria, can stimulate leucocytes to synthesize IL-1[134] while sublethal doses of UV radiation can perturb both macrophages[135] and keratinocytes[49] to produce and release Il-1. Tumour necrosis factor[136], a mediator of endotoxin shock[137], leukotrienes[138] generated during tissue damage[139], interferon γ[140-142], a product of stimulated T lymphocytes, as well as hyaluronic acid[143], a constituent of connective tissue, and serum amyloid P component[144], an acute phase reactant, can all potentiate IL-1 production, perhaps through a calcium-mediated event[145,146]. Production, processing and release of IL-1 may also be promoted by various cellular and plasma enzymes such as trypsin, plasmin/plasminogen[147] and pepsin/pepsinogen[148].

Since IL-1 can also induce the synthesis of some of these stimuli, such as hyaluronic acid[89,90] and serum amyloid P component[104], one might expect that once an infection, injury or inflammation reached a certain severity, a biological chain reaction would occur which was likely to lead to multiple organ failure and death. Thus there must be both local and systemic feedback mechanisms to reduce the likelihood of this happening. And indeed there appear to be such negative feedback systems. For example, prostaglandins, the synthesis of which can often be affected by the same stimuli which induce IL-1, can suppress IL-1 production[149]. This action is believed to be the result of a post-transcriptional effect via cyclic AMP[150]. Mononuclear cells not only synthesize IL-1, but also produce a 5-9 kD inhibitor which opposes IL-1 action on thymocytes, but not on peripheral (mature) T cells[151]. Neutrophils, which recently have been shown to be a source of IL-1[31,152], also give rise to inhibitors of IL-1-induced thymocyte proliferation; these inhibitors have molecular weights of 45-70 kD and greater than 160 kD[32]. The submandibular glands of the rat produce factors, one of which has an apparent molecular weight of 54 kD, that inhibit the mitogenic and co-stimulatory effects of IL-1 on thymocytes[153]. Uromodulin, an immunosuppressive 85 kD protein, originally derived from pregnancy urine, is a very potent inhibitor of IL-1-induced thymocyte proliferation[154], effective at concentrations between $10^{-9}$ and $10^{-11}$ M, and is in fact an effective ligand for IL-1[155]. This gives rise to the speculation that uromodulin may be a soluble form of the IL-1 receptor. Recently uromodulin has been shown to be similar to, if not identical with, the Tamm-Horsfall urinary glycoprotein, which is primarily synthesized by the kidney and appears in abundance even in normal urine[156]. It thus should be possible to determine if uromodulin is a soluble form of the IL-1 receptor; otherwise it is not clear what role it might play *in vivo* in modulating IL-1 action, since most circulating IL-1 appears not to be cleared by the kidney[157].

Not a great deal is known about the mode of action of IL-1. Nonetheless, it speaks to the complexity of the problem that leukotrienes which can augment IL-1 synthesis also may play a role in the IL-1 induction of IL-2[158], while PGE2 and cyclic AMP which suppress IL-1 production may be involved in IL-1 stimulation of synovial cell synthesis of plasminogen activator[159].

Recently, a considerable amount of information has accumulated concerning membrane receptors for IL-1 in cultured cells. The receptors recognize both the α and β forms of IL-1 and generally range from 100 to 11,000 sites per cell with a dissociation constant[160-163] approximately equal to $10^{-10}$ M, though human fibroblasts bind native IL-1 with a $K_d$ of $10^{-11}$ M for the β form and $5 \times 10^{-11}$ M for the α form[164]. The molecular weight of the receptors appears to be about 80 kD[163], though a 60 kD form has been found on Epstein-Barr virus-transformed B lymphocytes[170]. The IL-1 receptors appear to recognize both forms of IL-1 from different species but not IL-2, IFN $\gamma$, TNF $\alpha$, bovine acidic fibroblast growth factor, epidermal growth factor or nerve growth factor[161]. Prolonged exposure of cells to low levels of IL-1 appear to downregulate expression of receptors and the IL-1 which is bound is internalized[165]. This downregulation of receptors by IL-1 may explain the large variation in receptor numbers found in some experiments. Despite the apparent similarity in receptors and binding constants, different cell types can vary in their responsiveness to IL-1 by several orders of magnitude[166].

The foregoing has been but a partial enumeration of the actions, modes of action, positive and negative regulators of IL-1. Nonetheless, this brief overview indicates some of the attributes that form our present understanding of IL-1's role in disease and perhaps in health. Let us now look into the future.

## III. FUTURE

The future is already upon us. Progress to date in our understanding of IL-1 has been nonlinear, generating almost as many questions as answers. These questions must be answered before we can intelligently manipulate IL-1 in health and disease.

First and foremost, assays must be developed that identify and quantify the various forms of IL-1 in body fluids and tissue samples, even in the presence of inhibitors and with minimal interassay variation. Though an antibody to human IL-1 has been available for 10 years[167] and a radioimmunoassay was developed based on this antibody[168], detection of IL-1 in body fluids is still based on various bioassays, such as alterations in plasma zinc and amino acid fluxes[111, 169], the induction of fever[113, 170], and an array of acute-phase protein responses in test animals[7-9, 171] or in vitro [101, 172], or variations of the lymphocyte proliferation assay[173-175]. For the last to give a true measure of IL-1 activity in plasma, interfering factors must be removed, usually be means of column chromatography[81, 114, 173]. Unfortunately, none of these assays differentiates amongst the various forms of IL-1 ($\alpha$, $\beta$; 31, 22, 4.2 kD; membrane-bound). Moreover, the bioassays may not be measuring the IL-1 content of a sample, but rather the presence of substances such as TNF, which induces the production of IL-1[176]. Until highly sensitive, form-specific assays are developed, it will be exceedingly difficult to elucidate the roles IL-1 plays in growth, development, and wound repair, as well as disease resistance, and to detect diurnal changes in local as well as systemic concentrations of the various forms of IL-1, which may be either cause or effect of a diverse array of circadian variations in metabolism and physiology in healthy individuals[177,178].

More needs to be learned of the factors which regulate IL-1 synthesis, processing and secretion in both phagocytic and non-phagocytic cells, in situ as well as in vitro. There is evidence that the pattern of IL-1 production in monocytes is influenced by the nature of the stimulus[179,180], as well as the cell source and cell maturity[181]. Is there also an effect of the environment on the IL-1-producing cell? For example, is it coincidence that monocytes produce a form of IL-1 with a pI near neutral which will operate in a near-neutral pH environment, blood, while keratinocytes produce primarily IL-1 α which is likely to find itself in the anaerobic and acid environs of a wound? Would the binding constant for, and array of effects of, IL-1 α differ significantly if assayed in a more acid environment? Is the distribution of forms of IL-1 related to their relative stability, IL-1 α being less heat-labile and less likely to be inactivated by oxidants than IL-1 β and thus more suitable as a 'surface' form of IL-1 exposed to the atmosphere? Why also does epidermis contain 200-900 times more preformed IL-1 than internal organs such as liver, spleen, and thymus[182]? Is this merely a reflection of the variety of stimuli to which skin is chronically exposed: micro-organisms, UV radiation, mechanical stresses, abrasion, and injury?

Much more needs to be learned of the interactions of IL-1 with other cytokines, such as tumour necrosis factor, colony-stimulating factors, hepatocyte-stimulating factor and the various interferons. For example, how much of the hepatic acute-phase protein synthesis in response to infection or injury is due to IL-1, and how much is due to hepatocyte-stimulating factor (HSF)[183] or tumour necrosis factor (TNF)[184], or must all three of these factors be present to obtain maximal effect? Do these seemingly different factors work on different hepatocyte populations? Does either HSF or TNF recruit additional cells to synthesize these proteins; IL-1 appears not to[104], or are there still more macrophage-derived factors to be discovered which mediate hepatic acute-phase protein synthesis?

In point of fact, it may be essential to re-examine the media from macrophages, and other IL-1-producing cell types, which have been exposed to one or more stimuli such as endotoxin, silica, bacteria or UV radiation. These conditioned media would then be compared with highly purified forms of IL-1, as well as recombinant IL-1, in their ability to elicit from cells, organs and whole animals the array of responses attributed to IL-1 when less purified preparations were tested.

Since endotoxin elicits both TNF and IL-1 *in vivo*, to what extent are the physiological and metabolic sequelae of endotoxaemia the result of IL-1 or of TNF? Antibody to TNF protects mice from the lethal effects of TNF[185], but does it also ablate the physiological and metabolic changes? One wonders how many of the deleterious effects attributed to IL-1 based on *in vitro* measurements are the result of using 'pharmacological' doses of IL-1 or are actually mediated by TNF, or at least require the presence and cooperation of TNF or other cytokines *in vivo*?

Since there is some evidence that the results of exposure to IL-1 can be influenced by duration of exposure as well as concentration, what are the consequences of the increased levels of IL-1 found in the plasma of trained athletes? Certainly this could explain the modest acute-phase response found in such individuals, but does it also account for the adverse effects in women that appear to attend intensive running? Would cells from highly trained runners display fewer receptors than those from untrained, non-exercising individuals, since IL-1 can down-regulate receptor expression? Would a different pattern of response be seen in weightlifters or swimmers? Could this information be used to facililtate recovery of muscle function and tone after severe injury, elective surgery, enforced bed rest, or long periods of weightlessness? Could low doses of IL-1 be given to low birthweight infants to hasten growth?

Does the inhibitory effect of prostaglandins on IL-1 induction of lymphocyte activation account for the normally transient anergy seen following injury, when copious quantities of prostaglandins are released at the site of the injury? Also could this transient anergy be designed to prevent the development of autoimmunity to ordinarily occult antigens such as collagen and nucleic acids which are uncovered by tissue damage? What does IL-1 have to do with the so-called 'primacy of the wound', and can IL-1 be used, perhaps topically, to facilitate wound healing?

To intelligently manipulate and/or use IL-1 in treatment, some fundamental information as to the role(s) IL-1 plays in maintaining health, as well as in illness and injury, is still required. To attain these data it will be necessary not only to be able to measure the local and systemic concentrations and activity of IL-1, but also to control IL-1's effects. $\alpha$-Melanocyte stimulating hormone ($\alpha$MSH) acts as an antipyretic when peripherally[186] or centrally[187] administered, and can inhibit IL-1-induced thymocyte proliferation and fibroblast prostaglandin production *in vitro* [188] as well as fever, neutrophilia and serum amyloid P synthesis *in vivo* [189]. Thus it would be of great interest to assess the long-term as well as short-term consequences of infusion of $\alpha$MSH on animals that have been exposed to a variety of non-lethal and lethal viruses and bacteria, and to various forms of injury, internal as well as external. In addition to the questions of survival and the rate of wound healing, it would be important to test animals which survived infection for the development of an effective immune response against subsequent infection with the same micro-organisms, and to test animals which survived injury for the presence of antibodies to collagen and DNA as well as to assess the effect of a subsequent injury.

Finally, in order to manipulate IL-1 intelligently, it will also be necessary to know more of the pathogenesis of each disease, and the process of tissue injury and its repair, to be able to tailor the treatment, so as to ameliorate rather than exacerbate the disease. For example, since prostaglandins inhibit IL-1 production, there may be stages of a disease (such as the early phase of a granuloma formation in response to a parasite) when soluble IL-1 is recruiting leucocytes, and more IL-1 would likely result in a larger granuloma, that administration of prostaglandin inhibitors may be inappropriate. Again, during the early anergic period following injury, prostaglandin synthesis inhibitors might increase the chances of subsequent autoimmunity developing; however, after the first few days they may help to reduce susceptibility to infection, and to facilitate wound healing.

To recapitulate, it was not our intent to encompass all that is known of IL-1, but rather to direct attention to some of the findings that we believe caused IL-1 to be looked at in new and different ways. We also attempted to indicate the multitude of questions about IL-1 that still need to be answered if we are to intelligently manipulate IL-1 in health and disease.

## REFERENCES

### Past

1. Beeson, PB (1948). Temperature-elevating effect of a substance obtained from poly-morphonuclear leukocytes. *J Clin Invest*, **27**, 524
2. Metchnikoff, E (1905). *Immunity in Infective Diseases*. (Boston: Cambridge University Press)
3. Atkins, E (1984). Fever: the old and the new. *J Infect Dis*, **149**, 339-48
4. Kampschmidt, RF and Upchurch, H (1969). Lowering of plasma iron concentration in the rat with leukocytic extracts. *Am J Physiol*, **216**, 1287-91
5. Wannemacher, RW, Pekarek, RS and Beisel, WR (1972). Mediator of hepatic amino acid flux in infected rats. *Proc Soc Exp Biol Med*, **139**, 128-32
6. Pekarek, RS, Wannemacher, RW and Beisel, WR (1972). The effect of leukocytic endogenous mediator (LEM) on the tissue distribution of zinc and iron. *Proc Soc Exp Biol Med*, **140**, 685-8
7. Pekarek, RS, Powanda, MC and Wannemacher, RW (1972). The effect of leukocytic endogenous mediator (LEM) on serum copper and ceruloplasmin concentrations in the rat. *Proc Soc Exp Biol Med*, **141**, 1029-31
8. Kampschmidt, RF, Upchurch, HF, Eddington, CL and Pulliam, LA (1973). Multiple biological activities of a partially purified leukocytic endogenous mediator. *Am J Physiol*, **224**, 530-3
9. Wannemacher, RW, Pekarek, RS, Thompson, WL *et al.* (1975). A protein from poly-morphonuclear leukocytes (LEM) which affects the rate of hepatic amino acid transport and synthesis of acute-phase globulins. *Endocrinology*, **96**, 651-61
10. Murphy, PA, Chesney, PJ and Wood, WB (1974). Further purification of rabbit leukocyte pyrogen. *J Lab Clin Med*, **83**, 310-22
11. Mapes, CA and Sobocinski, PZ (1977). Differentation between endogenous pyrogen and leukocytic endogenous mediator. *Am J Physiol*, **232**, C15-22
12. Merriman, CR, Pulliam, LA and Kampschmidt, RF (1977). Comparison of leukocytic pyrogen and leukocytic endogenous mediator. *Proc Soc Exp Biol Med*, **154**, 224-7
13. Kampschmidt, RF, Pulliam, LA and Merriman, CR (1978). Further similarities of endogenous pyrogen and leukocytic endogenous mediator. *Am J Physiol*, **235**, C118-21
14. Murphy, PA, Cebula, TA, Levin, J and Windle, BE (1981). Rabbit macrophages secrete two biochemically and immunologically distinct endogenous pyrogens. *Infect Immun*, **34**, 177-83
15. Murphy, PA, Cebula, TA and Windle, BE (1981). Heterogeneity of rabbit endogenous pyrogens is not attributable to glycosylated variants of a single polypeptide chain. *Infect Immun*, **34**, 184-91
16. Pekarek, RS, Wannemacher, RW, Chapple, FE *et al.* (1972). Further characterization and species specificity of leukocytic endogenous mediator (LEM). *Proc Soc Exp Biol Med*, **141**, 643-8

17.    Kampschmidt, RF, Upchurch, HF and Worthington, ML (1983). Further comparisons of endogenous pyrogens and leukocytic endogenous mediators. *Infect Immun*, **41**, 6-10

18.    Kampschmidt, RF and Pulliam, LA (1975). Stimulation of antimicrobial activity in the rat with leukocytic endogenous mediator. *J Reticuloendothel Soc*, **17**, 162-9

19.    Ziel, R and Krupp, P (1976). Influence of endogenous pyrogen on the cerebral prostaglandin-synthetase system. *Experientia*, **32**, 1451-3

20.    George, DT, Abeles, FB, Mapes, CA *et al.* (1977). Effect of leukocytic endogenous mediators on endocrine pancreas secretory responses. *Am J Physiol*, **233**, E240-5

21.    Thompson, WL, Abeles, FB, Beall, FA *et al.* (1976). Influence of the adrenal glucocorticoids on the stimulation of synthesis of hepatic ribonucleic acid and plasma acute-phase globulins by leucocytic endogenous mediator. *J Biochem*, **156**, 25-32

22.    Pekarek, RS and Evans, GW (1976). Effect of leukocytic endogenous mediator (LEM) on zinc absorption in the rat. *Proc Soc Exp Biol Med*, **152**, 573-5

23.    Liu, CT, Sanders, RP, Hadick, CL and Sobocinski, PZ (1979). Effects of intravenous injection of leukocytic endogenous mediator on cardiohepatic functions in Rhesus Macaques. *Am J Vet Res*, **40**, 1035-9

24.    Klempner, MS, Dinarello, CA and Gallin, JI (1978). Human leukocytic pyrogen induces release of specific granule contents from human neutrophils. *J Clin Invest*, **61**, 1330-6

25.    Klempner, MS, Dinarello, CA, Henderson, WR and Gallin, JI (1979). Stimulation of neutrophil oxygen-dependent metabolism by human leukocytic pyrogen. *J Clin Invest*, **64**, 996-1002

## Present

26.    Rosenwasser, LJ and Dinarello, CA (1981). Ability of human leukocytic pyrogen to enhance phytohemagglutinin induced murine thymocyte proliferation. *Cell Immunol*, **63**, 134-42

27.    Murphy, PA, Simon, PL and Willoughby, WF (1980). Endogenous pyrogens made by rabbit peritoneal exudate cells are identical with lymphocyte-activating factors made by rabbit alveolar macrophages. *J Immunol*, **124**, 2498-501

28.    Damais, C, Riveau, G, Parant, M *et al.* (1982). Production of lymphocyte activating factor in the absence of endogenous pyrogen by rabbit or human leukocytes stimulated by a muramyl dipeptide derivative. *Int J Immunopharmacol*, **4**, 451-62

29.    Hanson, DF, Murphy, PA and Windle, BE (1980). Failure of rabbit neutrophils to secrete endogenous pyrogen when stimulated with Staphylococci. *J Exp Med*, **151**, 1360-71

30.    Windle, BE, Murphy, PA and Cooperman, S (1983). Rabbit polymorphonuclear leukocytes do not secrete endogenous pyrogens or interleukin 1 when stimulated by endotoxin, polyinosine:polycytosine, or muramyl dipeptide. *Infect Immun*, **39**, 1142-6

31.    Tiku, K, Tiku, ML and Skosey, JL (1986). Interleukin 1 production by human polymorphonuclear neutrophils. *J Immunol*, **136**, 3677-85

32.    Tiku, K, Tiku, ML, Liu, S and Skosey, JL (1986). Normal human neutrophils are a source of a specific interleukin 1 inhibitor. *J Immunol*, **136**, 3686-92

33.    Bodel, P and Miller, H (1977). Differences in pyrogen production by mononuclear phagocytes and by fibroblasts or HeLa cells. *J Exp Med*, **145**, 607-17

34.    Fontana, A, Kristensen, F, Dubs,R *et al.* (1982). Production of prostaglandin E and an interleukin-1 like factor by cultured astrocytes and C6 glioma cells. *J Immunol*, **129**, 2413-19

35.    Grabner, G, Luger, TA, Smolin, G and Oppenheim, JJ (1982). Corneal epithelial cell-derived thymocyte-activating factor (CETAF). *Invest Ophthalmol Vis Sci*, **23**, 757-63

36. Waalen, K, Duff, GW, Dickens, E *et al.* (1985). Interleukin 1 (IL1) in rheumatoid arthritis: Synovial and blood dendritic cell production of IL-1. In Kluger, MJ, Oppenheim, JJ and Powanda, MC (eds) *The Physiologic, Metabolic and Immunologic Actions of Interleukin-1*, pp. 359-64. (New York: Alan R Liss)

37. Miossec, P, Cavender, D and Ziff, M (1986). Production of interleukin 1 by human endothelial cells. *J Immunol*, **136**, 2486-91

38. Iribe, H, Koga, T, Kotani, S *et al.* (1983). Stimulating effect of MDP and its adjuvant-active analogues on guinea pig fibroblasts for the production of thymocyte activating factor. *J Exp Med*, **157**, 2190-5

39. Rasanen, L, Lehto, M, Jansen, C *et al.* (1986). Human epidermal Langerhans cells and peripheral blood monocytes. *Scand J Immunol*, **24**, 503-8

40. Matsushima, K, Procopio, A, Abe, H *et al.* (1985). Production of interleukin 1 activity by normal human peripheral blood B lymphocytes. *J Immunol*, **135**, 1132-6

41. Rimsky, L, Wakasugi, H, Ferrara, P *et al.* (1986). Purification to homogeneity and $NH_2$-terminal amino acid sequence of a novel interleukin 1 species derived from a human B cell line. *J Immunol*, **136**, 3304-10

42. Pistoia, V, Cozzolino, F, Rubartelli, A *et al.* (1986). In vitro production of interleukin 1 by normal and malignant human B lymphocytes. *J Immunol*, **136**, 1688-92

43. Abo, T, Sugawara, S, Amenomori, A *et al.* (1986). Selective phagocytosis of gram-positive bacteria and interleukin 1-like factor production by a subpopulation of large granular lymphocytes. *J Immunol*, **136**, 3189-97

44. Lovett, DH, Sterzel, RB, Ryan, JL and Atkins, E (1985). Production of an endogenous pyrogen by glomerular mesangial cells. *J Immunol*, **134**, 670-2

45. Lovett, DH, Szamel, M, Ryan, JL *et al.* (1986). Interleukin 1 and the glomerular mesangium. I. Purification and characterization of a mesangial cell-derived autogrowth factor. *J Immunol*, **136**, 3700-5

46. Giulian, D, Baker, TJ, Young, DG *et al.* (1985). In Kluger, MJ, Oppenheim, JJ and Powanda, MC (eds) *The Physiologic, Metabolic and Immunologic Actions of Interleukin-1*, pp. 133-42. (New York: Alan R Liss)

47. Libby, P, Ordovas, JM, Birinyi, LK *et al.* (1986). Inducible interleukin-1 gene expression in human vascular smooth muscle cells. *J Clin Invest*, **78**, 1432-8

48. Gahring, LC, Buckley, A and Daynes, RA (1985). Presence of epidermal-derived thymocyte activating factor/interleukin 1 in normal human stratum corneum. *J Clin Invest*, **76**, 1585-91

49. Ansel, JC, Luger, TA and Green, I (1983). The effect of in vitro and in vivo UV irradiation on the production of ETAF activity by human and murine keratinocytes. *J Invest Dermatol*, **81**, 519-23

50. Hauser, C, Saurat, J-H, Schmitt, A *et al.* (1986). Interleukin 1 is present in normal human epidermis. *J Immunol*, **136**, 3317-23

51. Baracos, V, Rodemann, HP, Dinarello, CA and Goldberg, AL (1983). Stimulation of muscle protein degradation and prostaglandin $E_2$ release by leukocytic pyrogen (interleukin-1): a mechanism for the increased degradation of muscle proteins during fever. *N Engl J Med*, **308**, 553-8

52. Clowes, GHA, George, BC, Villee, CA and Saravis, CA (1983). Muscle proteolysis induced by a circulating peptide in patients with sepsis or trauma. *N Engl J Med*, **308**, 545-52

53. Dinarello, CA, Clowes, GHA, Gordon, AH *et al.* (1984). Cleavage of human interleukin 1: Isolation of a peptide fragment from plasma of febrile humans and activated monocytes. *J Immunol*, **133**, 1332-8

54. Hasselgren, P-O, Talamini, M, LaFrance, R *et al.* (1985). Effect of indomethacin on proteolysis in septic muscle. *Ann Surg*, **202**, 557-62

55. Hulton, NR, Johnson, DJ and Wilmore, DW (1985). Limited effects of prostaglandin inhibitors in Escherichia coli sepsis. *Surgery*, **98**, 291-297

56. Sobrado, J, Moldawer, LL, Bistrian, BR *et al.* (1983). Effect of ibuprofen on fever and metabolic changes induced by continuous infusion of leukocytic pyrogen (interleukin 1) on endotoxin. *Infect Immun*, **42**, 997-1005

57. Kreuger, JM, Walter, J, Dinarello, CA *et al.* (1984). Sleep-promoting effects of endogenous pyrogen (interleukin-1). *Am J Physiol*, **246**, R994-9

58. Walter, J, Davenne, D, Shoham, S *et al.* (1986). Brain temperature changes coupled to sleep states persist during interleukin 1-enhanced sleep. *Am J Physiol*, **250**, R96-103

59. McCarthy, DO, Kluger, MJ and Vander, AJ (1985). Suppression of food intake during infection: is interleukin-1 involved? *Am J Clin Nutr*, **42**, 1179-82

60. McCarthy, DO, Kluger, MJ and Vander, AJ (1984). The role of fever in appetite suppression after endotoxin administration. *Am J Clin Nutr*, **40**, 310-16

61. Sauder, DN, Mounessa, NL Katz, SI *et al.* (1984). Chemotactic cytokines: the role of leukocytic pyrogen and epidermal cell thymocyte-activating factor in neutrophil chemotaxis. *J Immunol*, **132**, 828-32

62. Beck, G, Habicht, GS, Benach, JL and Miller, F (1986). Interleukin 1: a common endogenous mediator of inflammation and the local Shwartzman reaction. *J Immunol*, **136**, 3025-31

63. Miossec, P, Yu, C-L and Ziff, M (1984). Lymphocyte chemotactic activity of human interleukin 1. *J Immunol*, **133**, 2007-11

64. Sauder, DN, Monick, MM and Hunninghake, GW (1985). Epidermal cell-derived thymocyte activating factor (ETAF) is a potent T-cell chemoattractant. *J Invest Dermatol*, **85**, 431-3

65. Bevilacqua, MP, Pober, JS, Majeau, GR *et al.* (1984). Interleukin 1 (IL-1) induces biosynthesis and cell surface expression of procoagulant activity in human vascular endothelial cells. *J Exp Med*, **160**, 618-23

66. Nawroth, PP, Handley, DA, Esmon, CT and Stern, DM (1986). Interleukin 1 induces endothelial cell procoagulant while suppressing cell-surface anticoagulant activity. *Proc Natl Acad Sci USA*, **83**, 3460-4

67. Rossi, V, Breviario, F, Ghezzi, P *et al.* (1985). Prostacyclin synthesis induced in vascular cells by interleukin-1. *Science*, **229**, 174-6

68. Bevilacqua, MP, Pober, JS, Wheeler, ME *et al.* (1985). Interleukin 1 acts on cultured human vascular endothelium to increase the adhesion of polymorphonuclear leukocytes, monocytes, and related leukocyte cell lines. *J Clin Invest*, **76**, 2003-11

69. Nachman, RL, Hajjar, KA, Silverstein, RL and Dinarello, CA (1986). Interleukin 1 induces endothelial cell synthesis of plasminogen activator inhibitor. *J Exp Med*, **163**, 1595-1600

70. Emeis, JJ and Kooistra, T (1986). Interleukin 1 and lipopolysaccharide induce an inhibitor of tissue-type plasminogen activator in vivo and in cultured endothelial cells. *J Exp Med*, **163**, 1260-6

71. Bussolino, F, Breviario, F, Tetta, C *et al.* (1986). Interleukin 1 stimulates platelet-activating factor production in cultured human endothelial cells. *J Clin Invest*, **77**, 2027-33

72. Bagby, GC, Dinarello, CA, Wallace, P *et al.* (1986). Interleukin 1 stimulates granulocyte macrophage colony-stimulating activity release by vascular endothelial cells. *J Clin Invest*, **78**, 1316-23

73. Leibovich, SJ and Ross, R (1975). The role of the macrophage in wound repair: a study with hydrocortisone and antimacrophage serum. *Am J Pathol*, **78**, 71-100

74. Schmidt, JA, Oliver, CN, Lepe-Zuniga, JL *et al.* (1984). Silica-stimulated monocytes release fibroblast proliferation factors identical to interleukin 1: a potential role for interleukin 1 in the pathogenesis of silicosis. *J Clin Invest*, **73**, 1462-72

75. Postlethwaite, AE, Lachman, LB and Kang, AH (1984). Induction of fibroblast proliferation by interleukin-1 derived from human monocytic leukemia cells. *Arthritis Rheum*, **27**, 995-1001

76. Postlethwaite, AE, Lachman, LB, Mainardi, CL and Kang, AH (1983). Interleukin 1 stimulation of collagenase production by cultured fibroblasts. *J Exp Med*, **157**, 801-6

77. Murphy, G, Reynolds, JJ and Werb, Z (1985). Biosynthesis of tissue inhibitor of metalloproteinases by human fibroblasts in culture. *J Biol Chem*, **260**, 3079-83

78. Dustin, ML, Rothlein, R, Bhan, AK *et al.* (1986). Induction by IL 1 and interferon-γ: tissue distribution, biochemistry, and function of a natural adherence molecule (ICAM-1). *J Immunol*, **137**, 245-54

79. Zucali, JR, Dinarello, CA, Oblon, DJ *et al.* (1986). Interleukin 1 stimulates fibroblasts to produce granulocyte-macrophage colony-stimulating activity and prostaglandin E₂. *J Clin Invest*, **77**, 1857-63

80. Fontana, A, Hengartner, H, Weber, E *et al.* (1982). Interleukin 1 activity in the synovial fluid of patients with rheumatoid arthritis. *Rheumatol Int*, **2**, 49-53

81. Wood, DD, Ihrie, EJ, Dinarello, CA and Cohen, PL (1983). Isolation of an interleukin-1-like factor from human joint effusions. *Arthritis Rhuem*, **26**, 975-83

82. Jasin, HE and Dingle, JT (1981). Human mononuclear cell factors mediate cartilage matrix degradation through chondrocyte activation. *J Clin Invest*, **68**, 571-81

83. Beresford, JN, Gallagher, JA, Gowan, M *et al.* (1984). The effects of monocyte-conditioned medium and interleukin 1 on the synthesis of collagenous and non-collagenous proteins by mouse bone and human bone cell in vitro. *Biochim Biophys Acta*, **801**, 58-65

84. Saklatvala, J, Pilsworth, LMC, Sarsfield, SJ *et al.* (1984). Pig catabolin is a form of interleukin 1: cartilage and bone resorb, fibroblasts make prostaglandin and collagenase, and thymocyte proliferation is augmented in response to one protein. *Biochem J*, **224**, 461-6

85. Tyler, JA (1985). Chondrocyte-mediated depletion of articular cartilage proteoglycans in vitro. *Biochem J*, **225**, 493-507

86. Richardson, HJ, Elford, PR, Sharrard, RM *et al.* (1985). Modulation of connective tissue metabolism by partially purified human interleukin 1. *Cell Immunol*, **90**, 41-51

87. McCroskery, PA, Arai, S, Amento, EP and Krane, SM (1985). Stimultion of procollagenase synthesis in human rheumatoid synovial fibroblasts by mononuclear cell factor/interleukin 1. *FEBS Lett*, **191**, 7-12

88. Chang, J, Gilman, SC and Lewis, AJ (1986). Interleukin 1 activates phospholipase A₂ in rabbit chondrocytes: A possible signal for IL 1 action. *J Immunol*, **136**, 1283-7

89. Hamerman, D and Wood, DD (1984). Interleukin 1 enhances synovial cell hyaluronate synthesis. *Proc Soc Exp Biol Med*, **177**, 205-10

90. Bocquet, J, Daireaux, M, Langris, M *et al.* (1986). Effect of an interleukin-1 like factor (mononuclear cell factor) on proteoglycan synthesis in cultured human articular chondrocytes. *Biochem Biophys Res Commun*, **134**, 539-49

91. Krane, SM, Dayer, J-M, Simon, LS and Byrne, MS (1985). Mononuclear cell-conditioned medium containing mononuclear cell factor (MCF), homologous with interleukin 1, stimulates collagen and fibronectin synthesis by adherent rheumatoid synovial cells: Effects of prostaglandin E₂ and indomethacin. *Collagen Rel Res*, **5**, 99-117

92. Canalis, E (1986). Interleukin-1 has independent effects on deoxyribonucleic acid and collagen synthesis in cultures of rat calvariae. *Endocrinology*, **118**, 74-81

93. Endo, Y, Suzuki, R and Kumagai, K (1985). Interleukin 1-like factors can accumulate 5-hydroxytryptamine in the liver of mice and can induce hypoglycaemia. *Biochim Biophys Acta*, **840**, 37-42

94. Roh, MS, Moldawer, LL, Ekman, LG *et al.* (1986). Stimulatory effect of interleukin-1 upon hepatic metabolism. *Metabolism*, **35**, 419-24

95. Bendtzen, K, Mandrup-Poulsen, T, Nerup, J *et al.* (1986). Cytotoxicity of human pI 7 interleukin-1 for pancreatic islets of Langerhans. *Science*, **232**, 1545-7

96.     Snyder, DS and Unanue, ER (1982). Corticosteroids inhibit murine macrophage Ia expression and interleukin 1 production. *J Immunol*, **129**, 1803-5

97.     Staruch, MJ and Wood, DD (1985). Reduction of serum interleukin-1-like activity after treatment with dexamethasone. *J Leukocyte Biol*, **37**, 193-207

98.     DiSilvestro, RA and Cousins, RJ (1984). Glucocorticoid independent mediation of interleukin-1 induced changes in serum zinc and liver metallothionein levels. *Life Sci*, **35**, 2113-18

99.     Woloski, BMRNJ, Smith, EM, Meyer, WJ *et al*. (1985). Corticotropin-releasing activity of monokines. *Science*, **230**, 1035-7

100.    Besedovsky, H, Del Rey, A, Sorkin, E and Dinarello, CA (1986). Immunoregulatory feedback between interleukin-1 and glucocorticoid hormones. *Science*, **233**, 652-4

101.    Gauldie,J, Sauder, DN, McAdam, KPWJ and Dinarello, CA (1983). Purified human monocyte IL-1 stimulates hepatocyte secretion of multiple acute phase proteins in vitro. In Kluger, MJ, Oppenheim, JJ and Powanda, MC (eds) *The Physiologic, Metabolic and Immunologic Actions of Interleukin-1*, pp.221-9 (New York: Alan R Liss)

102.    Bauer, J, Weber, W, Tran-Thi, T-A *et al*. (1985). Murine interleukin 1 stimulates $\alpha_2$-macroglobulin synthesis in rat hepatocyte primary cultures. *FEBS Lett*, **190**, 271-4

103.    Ghezzi, P, Saccardo, B, Villa, P *et al*. (1986). Role of interleukin-1 in the depression of liver drug metabolism by endotoxin. *Infect Immun*, **54**, 837-40

104.    Le, PT and Mortensen, RF (1986). Induction and regulation by monokines of hepatic synthesis of the mouse serum amyloid P-component (SAP). *J Immunol*, **136**, 2526-33

105.    Endo, Y, Suzuki, R and Kumagai, K (1985). Induction of ornithine decarboxylase in the liver and spleen of mice by interleukin 1-like factors produced from a macrophage cell line. *Biochim Biophys Acta*, **838**, 343-50

106.    Matsushima, K, Bano, M, Kidwell, WR and Oppenheim, JJ (1985). Interleukin 1 increases collagen type IV production by murine mammary epithelial cells. *J Immunol*, **134**, 904-9

107.    Staruch, MJ and Wood, DD (1983). The adjuvanticity of interleukin 1 in vivo. *J Immunol*, **130**, 2191-4

108.    Lovett, D, Kozan, B, Hadam, M *et al*. (1986). Macrophage cytotoxicity: interleukin 1 as a mediator of tumor cytostasis. *J Immunol*, **136**, 340-7

109.    Onozaki, K, Matsushima, K, Aggarwal, BB and Oppenheim, JJ (1985). Human interleukin 1 is a cytocidal factor for several tumor cell lines. *J Immunol*, **135**, 3962-8

110.    Neta, R, Douches, S and Oppenheim, JJ (1986). Interleukin 1 is a radioprotector. *J Immunol*, **136**, 2483-5

111.    Wannemacher, RW, Pekarek, RS, Klainer, AS *et al*. (1975). Detection of a leukocytic endogenous mediator-like mediator of serum amino acid and zinc depression during various infectious illnesses. *Infect Immun*, **11**, 873-5

112.    Moldofsky, H, Lue, FA, Eisen, J *et al*. (1986). The relationship of interleukin 1 and immune functions to sleep in humans. *Psychosom Med*, **48**, 309-18

113.    Cannon, JG and Kluger, MJ (1983). Endogenous pyrogen activity in human plasma after exercise. *Science*, **220**, 617-19

114.    Cannon, JG and Dinarello, CA (1985). Increased plasma interleukin-1 activity in women after ovulation. *Science*, **227**, 1247-9

115.    Flynn, A (1982). Estrogen modulation of blood copper and other essential metal concentrations. In Sorenson, JRJ (ed) *Inflammatory Diseases and Copper*, pp. 17-30. (Clifton, NJ: Human Press)

116.    Evans, WJ, Meredith, CN, Cannon, JG *et al*. (1986). Metabolic changes following eccentric exercise in trained and untrained men. *J Appl Physiol*, **61**. 1864-8

117.    Wood, DD, Bayne, EK, Goldring, MB *et al*. (1985). The four biochemically distinct species of human interleukin 1 all exhibit similar biologic activities. *J Immunol*, **134**, 895-903

118. Kimball, ES, Simon, PL, Saklatvala, J et al. (1986). Serological characterization of acidic (pI 5.5) and neutral (pI 7.1) forms of 17kD and 35kD interleukin-1. *Lymphokine Res*, **5**, 119-25

119. Ihrie, EJ and Wood, DD (1985). Biochemical heterogeneity of human interleukin-1. *Lymphokine Res*, **4**, 169-81

120. Lepe-Zuniga, JL, Zigler, JS, Zimmerman, ML and Gery, I (1985). Difference between intra- and extracellular interleukin-1. *Mol Immunol*, **22**, 1387-92

121. Kurt-Jones, EA, Bellar, DI, Mizel, SB and Unanue, ER (1985). Identification of a membrane-associated interleukin 1 in macrophages. *Proc Natl Acad Sci USA*, **82**, 1204-8

122. Haq, AU, Mayernik, DG, Orosz, C and Rinehart, JJ (1984). Interleukin 1 secretion is not required for human macrophage support of T-cell proliferation. *Cell Immunol*, **87**, 517-27

123. Cameron, P, Limjuco, G, Rodkey, J et al. (1985). Amino acid sequence analysis of human interleukin 1 (IL-1): evidence for biochemically distinct forms of IL-1. *J Exp Med*, **162**, 790-801

124. Cameron, PM, Limjuco, GA, Chin, J et al. (1986). Purification to homogeneity and amino acid sequence analysis of two anionic species of human interleukin 1. *J Exp Med*, **164**, 237-50

125. Webb, AC, Collins, KL, Auron, PE et al. (1986). Interleukin-1 gene (IL1) assigned to long arm of human chromosome 2. *Lymphokine Res*, **5**, 77-85

126. Auron, PE, Webb, AC, Rosenwasser, LJ et al. (1984). Nucleotide sequence of human monocyte interleukin 1 precursor cDNA. *Proc Natl Acad Sci USA*, **81**, 7907-11

127. March, CJ, Mosley, B, Larsen, A et al. (1985). Cloning, sequence and expression of two distinct human interleukin-1 complementary DNAs. *Nature*, **315**, 641-7

128. Gubler, U, Chua, AO, Stern, AS et al. (1986). Recombinant human interleukin 1 α: Purification and biological characterization. *J Immunol*, **136**, 2492-7

129. Dinarello, CA, Cannon, JG, Mier JW et al. (1986). Multiple biological activities of human recombinant interleukin 1. *J Clin Invest*, **77**, 1734-9

130. Dayer, J-M, de Rochemonteix, B, Burrus, B et al. (1986). Human recombinant interleukin 1 stimulates collagenase and prostaglandin E2 production by human synovial cells. *J Clin Invest*, **77**, 645-8

131. Lomedico, PT, Gubler, U, Hellmann, CP et al. (1984). Cloning and expression of murine interleukin-1 cDNA in Escherichia coli. *Nature*, **312**, 458-62

132. Tocco-Bradley, R, Moldawer, LL, Jones, CT et al. (1986). The biological activity in vivo of recombinant murine interleukin 1 in the rat. *Proc Soc Exp Biol Med*, **182**, 263-71

133. Ramadori, G, Sipe, JD, Dinarello, CA et al. (1985). Pretranslational modulation of acute phase hepatic protein synthesis by murine recombinant interleukin 1 (IL-1) and purified human IL-1. *J Exp Med*, **162**, 930-42

134. Moore, DM, Murphy, PA, Chesney, PJ and Wood, WB (1973). Synthesis of endogenous pyrogen by rabbit leukocytes. *J Exp Med*, **137**, 1263-74

135. Ansel, J, Luger, TA, Kock, A et al. (1984). The effect of in vitro UV irradiation on the production of IL-1 by murine macrophage and P388D1 cells. *J Immunol*, **133**, 1350-5

136. Bachwich, PR, Chensue, SW, Larrick, JW and Kunkel, SL (1986). Tumor necrosis factor stimulates interleukin-1 and prostaglandin E2 production in resting macrophages. *Biochem Biophys Res Commun*, **136**, 94-101

137. Tracey, KJ, Beutler, B, Lowry, SF et al. (1986). Shock and tissue injury induced by recombinant human cachectin. *Science*, **234**, 470-4

138. Rola-Pleszczynski, M and Lemaire, I (1985). Leukotrienes augment interleukin 1 production by human monocytes. *J Immunol*, **135**, 3958-61

139. Denzlinger, C, Rapp, S, Hagmann, W and Keppler, D (1985). Leukotrienes as mediators in tissue trauma. *Science*, **230**, 330-2

273

140. Boraschi, D, Censini, S and Tagliabue, A (1984). Interferon-γ reduces macrophage-suppressive activity by inhibiting prostaglandin $E_2$ release and inducing interleukin 1 production. *J Immunol*, **133**, 764-8

141. Arenzana-Seisdedos, F, Virelizier, JL and Fiers, W (1985). Interferons as macrophage-activating factors. III. Preferential effects of interferon-γ on the interleukin 1 secretory potential of fresh or aged human monocytes. *J Immunol*, **134**, 2444-8

142. Collart, MA, Belin, D, Vassalli, J-D *et al.* (1986). γ Interferon enhances macrophage transcription of the tumor necrosis factor/cachectin, interleukin 1, and urokinase genes, which are controlled by short-lived repressors. J Exp Med, **164**, 2113-18

143. Hiro, D, Ito, A, Matsuta, K and Mori, Y 91986). Hyaluronic acid is an endogenous inducer of interleukin-1 production by human monocytes and rabbit macrophages. *Biochem Biophys Res Commun*, **140**, 715-22

144. Sarlo, KT and Mortensen, RF (1985). Enhanced interleukin 1 (IL-1) production mediated by mouse serum amyloid P component. *Cell Immunol*, **93**, 398-405

145. Simon, PL (1984). Calcium mediates one of the signals required for interleukin 1 and 2 production by murine cell lines. *Cell Immunol*, **87**, 720-6

146. Matsushima, K and Oppenheim, JJ (1985). Calcium ionophore (A23187) increases interleukin 1 (IL-1) production by human peripheral blood monocytes and interacts synergistically with IL-1 to augment concanavalin A stimulated thymocyte proliferation. *Cell Immunol*, **90**, 226-33

147. Matsushima, K, Taguchi, M, Kovacs, EJ *et al.* (1986). Intracellular localization of human monocyte associated interleukin 1 (IL 1) activity and release of biologically active IL 1 from monocytes by trypsin and plasmin. *J Immunol*, **136**, 2883-91

148. Lyte, M (1986). Regulation of interleukin-1 production in murine macrophages and human monocytes by a normal physiological constituent. *Life Sci*, **38**, 1163-70

149. Kunkel, SL, Chensue, SW and Phan, SH (1986). Prostaglandins as endogenous mediators of interleukin 1 production. *J Immunol*, **136**, 186-92

150. Knudsen, PJ, Dinarello, CA and Strom, TB (1986). Prostaglandins posttranscriptionally inhibit monocyte expression of interleukin 1 activity by increasing intracellular cyclic adenosine monophosphate. *J Immunol*, **137**, 3189-94

151. Berman, MA, Sandborg, CI, Calabia, BS *et al.* (1986). Studies of an interleukin 1 inhibitor: Characterization and clinical significance. *Clin Exp Immunol*, **64**, 136-45

152. Yoshinaga, M, Goto, F, Goto, K *et al.* (1985). Biosynthesis and purification of il 1-like factor from polymorphonuclear leukocytes of rabbits with tumor-induced granulocytosis. In Kluger, MJ, Oppenheim, JJ and Powanda, MC (eds) *The Physiologic, Metabolic and Immunologic Actions of Interleukin-1, pp. 385-98. (New York: Alan R Liss)*

153. Kemp, A, Mellow, L and Sabbadini, E (1986). Inhibition of interleukin 1 activity by a factor in submandibular glands of rats. *J Immunol*, **137**, 2245-51

154. Brown, KM, Muchmore, AV and Rosenstreich, DL (1986). Uromodulin, an immunosuppressive protein derived from pregnancy urine, is an inhibitor of interleukin 1. *Proc Natl Acad Sci, USA*, **83**, 9119-23

155. Muchmore, AV and Decker, JM (1986). Uromodulin: an immunosuppressive 85-kilodalton glycoprotein isolated from human pregnancy urine is a high affinity ligand for recombinant interleukin 1α. *J Biol Chem*, **261**, 13404-7

156. Pennica, D, Kohr, WJ, Kuang, W-J *et al.* (1987). Identification of human uromodulin as the Tamm-Horsfall urinary glycoprotein. *Science*, **236**, 83-8

157. Kampschmidt, RF and Jones, T (1985). Rate of clearance of interleukin-1 from the blood of normal and nephrectomized rats. *Proc Soc Exp Biol Med*, **180**, 170-3

158. Farrar, WL and Humes, JL (1985). The role of arachidonic acid metabolism in the activities of interleukin 1 and 2. *J Immunol*, **135**, 1153-9

159. Mochan, E, Uhl, J and Newton, R (1986). Evidence that interleukin-1 induction of synovial cell plasminogen activator is mediated via prostaglandin $E_2$ and cAMP. *Arthritis Rheum*, **29**, 1078-84

160. Matsushima, K, Akahoshi, T, Yamada, M *et al.* (1986). Properties of a specific interleukin 1 (IL 1) receptor on human Epstein Barr virus-transformed B lymphocytes: Identity of the receptor for IL 1-α and IL 1-β. *J Immunol*, **136**, 4496-502

161. Kilian, PL, Kaffka, KL, Stern, AS *et al.* (1986). Interleukin 1α and interleukin 1β bind to the same receptor on T cells. *J Immunol*, **136**, 4509-14

162. Bird, TA and Saklatvala, J (1986). Identification of a common class of high affinity receptors for both types of porcine interleukin-1 on connective tissue cells. *Nature*, **324**, 263-6

163. Dower, SK, Kronheim, SR, Hopp, TP *et al.* (1986). The cell surface receptors for interleukin-1α and interleukin-1β are identical. *Nature*, **324**, 266-8

164. Chin, J, Cameron, PM, Rupp, E and Schmidt, JA (1987). Identification of a high-affinity receptor for native human interleukin 1 β and interleukin 1 α on normal human lung fibroblasts. *J Exp Med*, **165**, 70-86

165. Matsushima, K, Yodoi, J, Tagaya, Y and Oppenheim, JJ (1986). Down-regulation of interleukin 1 (IL 1) receptor expression by IL 1 and fate of internalized [125]I-labelled Il 1 β in a human large granular lymphocyte cell line. *J Immunol*, **137**, 3183-8

166. Dower, SK, Call, SM, Gillis, S and Urdal, DL (1986). Similarity between the interleukin 1 receptors on a murine T-lymphoma cell line and on a murine fibroblast cell line. *Proc Natl Acad Sci USA*, **83**, 1060-4

# Future

167. Dinarello, CA, Renfer, L and Wolff, SM (1977). The production of antibody against human leukocytic pyrogen. *J Clin Invest*, **60**, 465-72

168. Dinarello, CA, Renfer, L and Wolff, SM (1977). Human leukocytic pyrogen: Purification and development of a radioimmunoassay. *Proc Natl Acad Sci USA*, **74**, 4624-7

169. Powanda, MC, Cockerell, GL, Moe, JB *et al.* (1975). Induced metabolic sequelae of tularemia in the rat: Correlation with tissue damage. *Am J Physiol*, **229**, 479-83

170. Critz, WJ (1981). Intracerebroventricular injection of rats: A sensitive assay method for endogenous pyrogen circulating in rats. *Proc Soc Exp Biol Med*, **166**, 6-11

171. Bailey, PT, Abeles, FB, Hauer, EC and Mapes, CA (1976). Intracerebroventricular administration of leukocytic endogenous mediators (LEM) in the rat. *Proc Soc Exp Biol Med*, **153**, 419-23

172. Ritchie, DG and Fuller, GM (1981). An in vitro bioassay for leukocytic endogenous mediator(s) using cultured rat hepatocytes. *Inflammation*, **5**, 275-87

173. Cannon, JG, Evans, WJ, Hughes, VA *et al.* (1986). Physiological mechanisms contributing to increased interleukin-1 secretion. *J Appl Physiol*, **61**, 1869-74

174. Conlon, PJ (1983). A rapid biologic assay for the detection of interleukin 1. *J Immunol*, **131**, 1280-2

175. Larrick, JW, Brindley, L and Doyle, MV (1985). An improved assay for the detection of interleukin 1. *J Immunol Methods*, **79**, 39-45

176. Dinarello, CA, Cannon, JG, Wolff, SM *et al.* (1986). Tumor necrosis factor (cachectin) is an endogenous pyrogen and induces production of interleukin 1. *J Exp Med*, **163**, 1433-50

177. Moore-Ede, MC, Czeisler, CA and Richardson, GS (1983). Circadian timekeeping in health and disease: Part 1. Basic properties of circadian pacemakers. *N Engl J Med*, **309**, 469-76

178. Moore-Ede, MC, Czeisler, CA and Richardson, GS (1983). Circadian timekeeping in health and disease: Part 2. Clinical implications of circadian rhythmicity. *N Engl J Med*, **309**, 530-6

179. Gery, I, Davies, P, Derr, J *et al.* (1981). Relationship between production and release of lymphocyte-activating factor (interleukin 1) by murine macrophages. *Cell Immunol*, **64**, 293-303

180. Kurt-Jones, EA, Virgin, HW and Unanue, ER (1986). In vivo and in vitro expression of macrophage membrane interleukin 1 in response to soluble and particulate stimuli. *J Immunol*, **137**, 10-14

181. Elias, JA, Schreiber, AD, Gustilo, K *et al.* (1985). Differential interleukin 1 elaboration by infractionated and density fractionated human alveolar macrophages and blood monocytes: Relationship to cell maturity. *J Immunol*, **135**, 3198-204

182. Schmitt, A, Hauser, C, Jaunin, F *et al.* (1986). Normal epidermis contains high amounts of natural tissue IL 1 biochemical analysis by HPLC identifies a MW 17 Kd form with a PI 5.7 and a MW 30 Kd form. *Lymphokine Res*, **5**, 105-18

183. Baumann, H, Hill, RE, Sauder, DN and Jahreis, GP (1986). Regulation of major acute-phase plasma proteins by hepatocyte-stimulating factors of human squamous carcinoma cells. *J Cell Biol*, **102**, 370-83

184. Perimutter, DH, Dinarello, CA, Punsal, PI and Colten, HR (1986). Cachectin/tumor necrosis factor regulates hepatic acute-phase gene expression. *J Clin Invest*, **78**, 1349-54

185. Beutler, B and Cerami, A (1986). Cachectin and tumour necrosis factor as two sides of the same biological coin. *Nature*, **320**, 584-8

186. Murphy, MT and Lipton, JM (1982). Peripheral administration of α-MSH reduces fever in older and younger rabbits. *Peptides*, **3**, 775-9

187. Murphy, MT, Richards, DB and Lipton, JM (1983). Antipyretic potency of centrally administered α-melanocyte stimulating hormone. *Science*, **221**, 192-3

188. Cannon, JG, Tatro, JB, Reichlin, S and Dinarello, CA (1986). α Melanocyte stimulating hormone inhibits immunostimulatory and inflammatory actions of interleukin 1. *J Immunol*, **137**, 2232-6

189. Robertson, BA, Gahring, LC and Daynes, RA (1986). Neuropeptide regulation of interleukin-1 activities: capacity of α-melanocyte stimulating hormone to inhibit interleukin-1-inducible responses in vivo and in vitro exhibits target cell selectivity. *Inflammation*, **10**, 371-85

# 11
# The T cell as a therapeutic target

**Ivan G Otterness and Marcia L Bliven**
Department of Immunology and Infectious Diseases
Pfizer Central Research
Groton, CT 06340, USA

## I. INTRODUCTION

There is a constellation of diseases whose pathology is a direct consequence of the immune response. Since there has been a failure to identify either an infectious aetiology or a pathognomonic immune abnormality, these diseases are characterized as being autoimmune. Rheumatoid arthritis, systemic lupus erythematosus, myasthenia gravis and multiple sclerosis are all well-known examples. An important therapeutic approach to these diseases is the selective inhibition of immune activity.

The pathological manifestations of the immune response can be inhibited in a variety of ways. Single key mechanisms can be targeted with therapeutically important results so long as that mechanism plays an important role in the disease. Thus inhibition of a single pathway such as prostaglandin biosynthesis has been found to be of great utility in ameliorating pain and inflammation of arthritis even though it leaves multiple aspects of arthritic disease untreated. The utility of interfering with other mechanisms of tissue damage such as cell infiltration, enzyme release, antibody formation, immune complex deposition, etc., or other mediators such as interleukin 1 (IL-1), superoxide, leukotrienes, tumour necrosis factor or $\gamma$-interferon, needs to be determined. In contrast, the T cell plays a central role in the overall orchestration of the immune response. It provides factors which are necessary for its full development, for its targeting and regulation. Its central role makes it a suitable therapeutic target for control of diseases characterized by multiple immune mechanisms.

The central role of the T cell in autoimmunity has been strongly supported by studies in animal models. For example, it has been shown that autoimmune diseases can be established in normal animals by the transfer of T cells from diseased animals. This means, first, that T cells must carry the molecular information which determines disease occurrence; second, T cells must have the ability to recruit sufficient effector cells to cause tissue damage; and, finally, they must have sufficient intrinsic replicative capacity to sus-

*New Developments in Antirheumatic Therapy.* Rainsford, KD and Velo, GP (eds), Inflammation and Drug Therapy Series, Volume III.

tain chronic disease. Thus T cell-targeted therapy should be useful for the treatment of chronic autoimmune disease.

## II. AN OVERVIEW OF THE T CELL

The T cell is composed of lymphocytes characterized by the expression of the T cell antigen receptor-CD3 complex on their surface[1]. The T cell antigen receptor (TcAR) is composed of a disulphide-linked 90 kD heterodimer in which there is an α and a β chain. The TcAR is a member of the immunoglobulin supergene family and confers specificity to the T cell in its reactions. After the TcAR reacts with antigen, the CD3 complex is believed to transmit a signal to the cell interior. A second TcAR has also been identified and designated as a γ, δ heterodimer[2,3]. Both TcAR and CD3 must be present to have a functional T cell.

The T cell is not a single, uniform, functionally homogeneous cell. The identification and characterization of functionally distinct subsets of CD3 T cells has been made possible by monoclonal antibodies and by the production of T cell clones. Monoclonal antibodies have allowed the identification and purification of T cells on the basis of cell surface antigens. T cell clones have enabled the study of the biological activities of a single homogeneous T cell phenotype. These two techniques have led to the subdivision of T cells into two major classes called CD4 and CD8 (formerly T4 and T8) in human cells and L3T4 and Lyt 2 in murine T cells respectively. CD4 T cells are characterized by a requirement to interact with antigen in the context of major histocompatibility complex (MHC) type II antigens, i.e. the immune response gene products such as DR, DP and DQ in man, Ia and Ie in the mouse, often generally referred to as IA. It is important to note that many autoimmune diseases show genetic linkage to the immune response genes. Since immunogenic peptides which induce T cell-mediated immunity have been shown to bind to the immune response gene products[4,5], it has been speculated that the genetic linkage of disease with the immune response genes comes through their antigen presentation properties[6,7]. CD8 T cells, by contrast, react with antigen in context with MHC class I gene products, i.e. the classical HLA transplantation antigens in man and the H-2 transplantation antigens in the mouse. It is believed that both CD4 and CD8 molecules augment T cell avidity for antigens by binding to the respective antigen binding class II or I MHC molecules[8].

The major functional activity of CD4 T cells is the synthesis of factors to help B cells to produce antibodies (i.e. IL-4 and IL-5) and to help T cells to expand, proliferate, and mature (i.e. IL-2, IL-4, IL-5) to carry out their functions. CD4 T cells also produce other important factors such as γ-interferon and lymphotoxin. Gamma-interferon, for example, may have a significant role in autoimmunity by inducing increased expression of IA molecules on other cell types. Increased IA increases the presentation of autoantigens to immune cells and may, thereby, increase the occurrence of autoimmune

278

disease[9,10]. Recently, it has been shown that CD4 cells can be further sub-divided by function into two classes, TH1 and TH2[11,12]. The TH1 cells can be distinguished by the presence of the T200 antigen (CD45R) which is also designated as OX22 in rats[13] and as 2H4 in man[14]. The TH1 cells produce IL-2, $\gamma$-interferon and lymphotoxin, and they require IL-2 for autocrine growth. They are involved in delayed hypersensitivity and the transfer of autoimmune disease to naïve recipients. TH2 cells, by contrast, are involved in helper functions. Thus they synthesize IL-4 and IL-5, both of which are major helper factors for antibody production, and require both IL-1 and IL-4 for autocrine growth[15].

T cells bearing CD8 demonstrate two functional characteristics. First they have the ability to lyse target cells such as virus-infected cells and thus act as antigen-specific effector cells. The lytic activity of CD8 cells appears to require the synthesis of IL-4 to induce T cell activation for killing and synthesis of protease[16]. It is not clear whether the killing activity of T cells plays a major role in tissue damage in autoimmune disease, although it has been implicated in experimental autoimmunity. CD8 T cells also can act to down-regulate T cell activity and, when carrying out that function, have been called T suppressor cells. Suppressor cell regulation may play a significant role in preventing the occurrence of autoimmune disease.

While this brief listing of T cell activities is by no means com-prehensive, it illustrates two major roles which the T cell may play in auto-immune disease: (i) they provide factors which recruit, activate and help other cell types to carry on immune activities in an antigen-specific fashion; and (ii) they regulate the overall immune activity in both an antigen-specific and non-specific manner.

## (1) Evidence for a role of T cells in autoimmune disease

The importance of T cells in autoimmune disease has been established by three principal methodologies: the study of pathological tissues, the study of susceptibility of animals with defined genetic constitutions to autoimmune disease, and the examination of the conditions under which disease can be transferred from affected animals into normal animals. The study of tissues from affected patients or animals allows the identification and characteriza-tion of T cells in pathological lesions as has been done in rheumatoid arth-ritis[17-19]. In man, an apparent deficiency has been shown for the suppressor-inducer (CD4+, 2H4+) T cell subset in multiple sclerosis[20], sys-temic lupus erythematosus[21], juvenile arthritis[22] and rheumatoid arth-ritis[23,24]. The reproducible diminution of this T cell subset in these autoimmune diseases is suggestive of pathological significance. Similarly in the diabetes-prone BB/W rat, the loss of the RT6.1+ T cell is correlated with disease[25,26]. In collagen-induced arthritis in animals, the appearance of acti-vated CD4+ T cells is one of the earliest pathological changes[27-29]. In ex-perimental allergic encephalomyelitis (EAE) brain lesions, 49% of infiltrating cells are positive for the Lyt 1 marker and 9% for the Lyt 2 marker[30]. In murine models of systemic lupus, i.e. the NZB/W mouse, developmental abnormalities in the thymus and in T cell differentiation are found[31]. A role for T cells has also been deduced in streptococcal arthritis by the failure to induce chronic autoimmune disease in animals in which T cell reactivity is compromised either by the use of genetically T deficient animals[32,33] or by the use of cyclosporin A to inhibit T cell activity[34]. In other induced models of autoimmune disease, adjuvant arthritis for example, T cells cloned from diseased animals have been shown to transfer the disease to naive animals[35]. Those T cells have recently been shown to have antigenic cross-reactivity between a component of *Mycobacterium* and the proteoglycan core protein of the rat[36]. In collagen arthritis[37-39], experimental thyroiditis[40] and experimental allergic encephalomyelitis[41], T cells from an affected animal similarly transfer disease into normal animals. These T cells also bear antigen-specific reactivity to collagen, thyroglobulin or myelin basic protein, respectively. Moreover, T cell clones derived from diseased animals bearing specificity for the autoantigen can transfer disease to naïve recipients[42,43]. T cell transfer of disease also occurs in chemically induced autoimmunity[44]. Taken together, these data suggest that the T cell is a carrier of key information critical to the onset and perpetuation of autoimmune disease. Actual tissue damage is not necessarily T cell-mediated, but may be[45]; other cell types may be recruited and effector molecules of non-T cell origin may cause the pathological changes. Tissue damage by infectious insult[46,47] or antibody[39,48] may be required for full expression of disease.

## (2) Effectiveness of T cell-targeted therapy: animal studies

Several approaches have been taken to demonstrate that suppression of T cell function can lead to amelioration of autoimmune disease. Perhaps the most direct way to explore T cell-targeted therapy is to alter the function or to specifically delete selected T cells. This has been done effectively in animals with the use of antibodies, toxins and drugs directed to various components of the T cell system. Although none of the therapeutic approaches can unambiguously be shown to act on T cells without affecting other additional immune pathways, taken together they form an impressive body of evidence suggesting T cell therapy may be of benefit in autoimmune disease.

### (a) Anti-T cell therapy

Therapy directed towards the removal and suppression of all T cell function is effective in many autoimmune conditions. Such broadly based therapy also inhibits essentially all facets of the immune response critical for a successful response to an infectious insult. Rat anti-Thy 1.2 has been successfully used to treat spontaneous murine lupus in the MRL/lpr mouse[49]. While it was successful in the MRL/lpr mouse, it was without beneficial effect in the NZB/W mouse, where the development of antibody against the rat anti-Thy 1.2 antibody may have augmented the nephritis by increasing deposition of immune complexes in the kidney. In BXSB mice at 3 months of age, a single injection of anti-Thy 1.2 retarded many signs of autoimmunity such as anti-DNA antibody, but failed to prolong life[50]. Furthermore, continuous treatment with the rat anti-Thy 1.2 antibody led to fatal anaphylaxis. The presence of anaphylactic reactions and immune complex disease suggests limits on the continuous administration of heterologous antibodies, but does not limit use for one time for amelioration of acute immune crises. However, in animals with spontaneous autoimmune disease such as the NZB/W mouse where T cell function may be already seriously compromised pan-T cell therapy may not be as therapeutically useful as a selective T cell therapy targeting a specific functional imbalance. In this case, more general non-specific immunosuppressives such as cyclophosphamide may be advantageous since they block B cell function as well.

## (b) Anti-CD4 therapy

Treatment of mice with anti-CD4 antibody (Gk1.5 anti-L3T4 antibody) prior to immunization with autoantigen leads to the inhibition of disease in collagen arthritis[51], EAE[51-54] experimental myasthenia gravis[55], diabetes in the non-obese mouse (NOD)[56] and NZB/W lupus nephritis[57]. If anti-T cell therapy can be administered before the onset of disease, it can be effective in suppressing the autoimmune response with a short course of therapy. This is, of course, a general immunosuppressive regimen and demonstrates that CD4$^+$ T cells are required for a full immune response. As CD8$^+$ T suppressor cells are not affected, it is possible that antigenic stimulation in the presence of anti-CD4 antibody might shift the CD4/CD8 balance to a more tolerogenic signal. Unlike anti-IL-2R antibody (see below), anti-CD4 antibody does not appear to require the lytic activity of complement in order to be effective, since, for example, it still prevents the influx of T cells into delayed hypersensitivity lesions in C5-deficient mice. The CD4 molecule enhances the efficiency of antigen presentation with IA bearing cells and thus plays an important role in antigen recognition[12]. Further it has also been shown that in systems which bypass the CD4 requirement for binding to antigen presenting cells, anti-CD4 antibodies still suppress the induction of a proliferative response[58,59] suggesting a further possible action of these antibodies. Alternatively, FcR or C3b interaction directed by anti-L3T4 antibody may be sufficient to inhibit T cell function. Thus it is an open question if, in the NZB/W mouse where anti-T cell therapy is less effective, anti-L3T4 acts because it suppresses L3T4 cell function, or whether, by suppression of L3T4 function, it allows the activity of Lyt 2$^+$ cells to be dominant.

The effectiveness of this therapy depends, in fact, upon the isotype of anti-CD4 antibody used[60]. The fluorescence-activated cell sorter was used to select variant anti-CD4 (W3/25) isotypes IgG1, IgG2b, and IgG2a all from the same clone, and all therefore with apparently identical binding specificities for CD4. Both IgG1 and IgG2a were superior to IgG2b antibodies in preventing EAE. They found it was sufficient simply to bind the antibodies to the CD4 receptor; frank depletion of CD4 cells was not necessary for a therapeutic effect[61]. This is consistent with work using anti-CD4 (OX35) antibody Fab fragments in EAE of the rat[62] and using anti-L3T4 Fab fragments in the mouse to induce long-term tolerance[63]. This suggests that the mechanism of anti-L3T4 is most consistent with interference with antigen presentation. That function alone is effectively carried out by Fab anti-L3T4 antibodies.

The use of anti-L3T4 antibodies appears to circumvent one of the major problems of using monoclonal antibodies. Whereas anti-Thy 1.2 therapy elicited a strong immune response with anaphylaxis and death in the BXSB strain, this did not occur with anti L3T4. The strength of the suppressive and tolerogenic signal given by anti-L3T4 antibodies may prevent an immune response to the antibody. Finally, use of this reagent suggests that even if immune pathways other than T cells play a major role in autoimmune disease, those pathways must be directly dependent upon the CD4 T cell for expression of their activity.

## (c) Anti-CD8 therapy

Although the evidence presented above on CD4 therapy suggests its general usefulness, some reservations must be stated based upon the nature of the disease being treated. For example, if viral infection may be important for the continuation of the disease or viral infection may be a side-effect of therapy as in transplantation (see below under anti-CD3), the removal of CD4 cells may exacerbate disease. Thus, in Theiler's virus-induced demyelination[64], treatment with anti-L3T4 around the time of viral inoculation leads to increased demyelination, encephalitis and death in the majority of animals tested. No effect was noted on established disease. By contrast, treatment with anti-Lyt 2.2 (CD8) antibody led to decreased demyelinating lesions irrespective of whether the therapy was administered early or after the disease was established, suggesting that the CD8 T cell was in some manner directly involved in demyelination. While these results are not applicable to all autoimmune diseases, they do emphasize that autoimmune diseases should not be put into a single category for therapeutic treatment, and that caution must be used in extrapolating from one autoimmune disease to another.

## (d) Anti-IA therapy

Antigens must be presented to T cells in the context of IA in order for them to respond. Moreover, in many autoimmune diseases, disease susceptibility is genetically linked to the IA phenotype. Therefore blocking or removal of the specific IA antigen by use of anti-IA antibody might be a method for selective immunosuppression and therefore a candidate for blocking autoimmune disease. In EAE, where disease induction is regulated by the H-$2^s$ gene, the use of specific anti-IA$^s$ antibody prior to immunization with myelin basic protein inhibits onset of clinical disease[65]. Although clinical disease was inhibited, the induction of disease as measured histologically was not prevented, although its severity was much less. Thus T cells were found to have been autoimmunized to myelin basic protein (MBP), and the T cells were shown histologically to have gained entry to the CNS. Moreover, when mice were treated with anti-IA antibody on the first signs of acute paralysis, a dramatic reversal of paralytic signs occurred, sometimes in as short a time as a few hours[66]. These results are not consistent with a primary effect on the induction of the immune response. They suggest an alternative mechanism such as inhibition of endothelial expression of IA with inhibition of cell migration or induction of suppressor T cell activity[67]. Administration of anti-IA$^s$ antibody prior to administration of $^{51}$Cr-labelled MBP-primed T cells clearly diminished the migration of the T cells into the CNS tissue[68]. Anti-IA therapy was also effective in blocking chronic relapsing EAE in mice. Weekly therapy with the antibody started after the first attack of paralysis diminished the number of attacks of paralysis, and eliminated the mortality over a 4 1/2 month treatment period. Similarly in $F_1$ animals (H-$2^s$xH-$2^d$) where disease is dominantly linked to the H-$2^s$ gene, only H-$2^s$ antibody effectively protects against disease induced by passive transfer of T cells. However, antibody against the weaker disease linkage haplotype is also effective in preventing disease induction upon immunization with myelin basic protein[69]. In a spontaneous model of lupus, the NZB/W mouse, treatment of the mice with anti-IA$^z$ was associated with protection from renal disease. That anti-IA$^d$ was effective, but much less so, suggested perhaps a tighter linkage of IA$^z$ with disease[70]. In both of these $F_1$ cases, no absolute linkage of one haplotype with disease was found. In experimental models such as in the response to (HG)-A-L where a non-responder was crossed with a responder to form a $F_1$ hybrid, complete haplotype-specific suppression by anti-IA was found[71]. This should be the case in which disease is tightly IA-linked. If immunization was carried out in complete Freund's adjuvant, haplotype-specific suppression in this system was lost. Anti-IA therapy was also found to be effective in autoimmune thyroiditis[72], collagen arthritis[73] and acetylcholine receptor disease[74] in animals. These results suggest that haplotype-specific suppression of autoimmunity is possible if there is a close disease linkage, but it may be more anti-inflammatory than immunosuppressive in its effects. These results also suggest that anti-IA therapy with antibody is not fully effective in preventing immunization with antigen, perhaps because, unlike anti-CD4 therapy, there is no tolerogenic signal or direct suppression of T cell function. Thus any lack of complete suppression of the response to antigen response or escape of IA from blockage finds the immune system fully capable of responding to antigen.

### (e)   T cell line therapy

Antigen-specific T cell lines have been developed which will transfer autoimmune disease to naïve recipients. Thus, as noted above, T cell lines against type II collagen wil transfer collagen arthritis, *Mycobacterium*-specific T cell lines will transfer adjuvant arthritis, thyroglobulin-specific T cell lines will transfer thyroiditis, and myelin basic protein-specific T cell lines will transfer EAE. These T cell lines can be altered by treatment to render them able to tolerize against disease induction. Thus, after irradiation, a myelin basic protein reactive T cell line which normally transfers disease can be administered to naïve animals, and they are rendered tolerant to disease induction by subsequent administration of myelin basic protein in adjuvant[75]. Using cyclosporin A, suppressor cell lines could be developed from recovered EAE rats. These suppressor lines (CD4+) could also be used to protect against EAE in naïve animals[76]. Similar results have been obtained for adjuvant arthritis[35], thyroiditis[77] and collagen arthritis[78,79]. In adjuvant arthritis, high-pressure treatment has been used to alter T cell lines which normally transmit adjuvant arthritis into T cell lines able to vaccinate against the induction of adjuvant arthritis after exposure to complete Freund's adjuvant. The tolerance mechanism is not immediately clear, but studies of tolerance induced by administration of neuraminidase-treated allogeneic cells suggest the procedure may lead to the elimination or functional compromise of responding T cell clones[80]. Perhaps not surprisingly, tolerance is elicited only to antigen exposure. These T cell lines do not tolerize to the administration of other disease-inducing T cell lines of the same specificity.

The applicability of therapy based upon vaccination with T cell lines appears problematical at this time. First, T cell vaccination appears most effective when given before disease onset. Therefore the likely place to target therapy would be early treatment of genetically susceptible individuals. Even if such a population could be defined with assurance, the next step, producing appropriate T cell clones, would need to be undertaken.

### (f)   Antibody against the T cell antigen receptor (TcAR)

Anti-idiotypic antibody therapy has been undertaken in a number of experimental autoimmune diseases to block production of a dominant autoimmune antibody. This has been attempted, for example, against the anti-DNA antibody of NZB/W lupus[81], the anti-myelin basic protein antibody of

284

EAE[82], and the anti-acetylcholine receptor antibody of experimental auto-immune myasthenia gravis[83]. Although favourable results have been obtained, the overall success with passive anti-idiotypic therapy has been limited, perhaps because of the induction of additional pathogenic antibodies which express other idiotypes, or because the single idiotype may make only a small contribution to the total disease. Thus, for example, in NZB/W nephritis, treatment with antibody against the dominant idiotype of anti-double-stranded DNA (dsDNA) antibody suppressed the dominant dsDNA idiotype. That idiotype was, however, quickly replaced by another idiotype. Nonetheless, therapeutic effects have been obtained in cases where the primary idiotype has been used as an immunogen[84]. These results suggest that a limited autoantibody repertoire should exist before anti-idiotypic antibody can be fully effective. Moreover, even in cases where there is extremely strong evidence for a primary antibody mediation of disease, i.e. in experimental autoimmune myasthenia gravis (anti-acetylcholine receptor disease), there is good evidence that T cell involvement is required in disease because of both the IA linkage[85] and because of the demonstrated requirement for T cell help in antibody formation[86,87]. This raises the possibility that anti-TcAR idiotype antibodies might be a better approach to modifying autoimmune disease: first, because the TcAR appears to have a much more limited repertoire than antibody; second, because it appears to be the T cell which contributes to the chronicity of the disease; and third, because the possibility that manipulation of the TcAR-stimulated T cell will result in a tolerogenic signal.

Some evidence has been elicited which suggests that such an approach may have validity. It has been observed that immunization using T cell lines reactive with autoimmune antigen could protect against subsequent disease upon exposure to specific antigen. This suggests direct use of the TcAR in the protection against autoimmunity. Use of anti-idiotype antibodies against the TcAR might give similar results. For example, immunization of Brown Norway rats with syngeneic T lymphoblasts reactive with renal tubular antigen led to an anti-Id antibody (TB-anti-Id)[88] which was competitively cross-reactive with anti-idiotype antibody prepared against renal eluate antibody (RE-anti-Id). The RE-anti-Id could also react with the tubular antigen-specific lymphoblasts[89]. Both antibodies were also inhibited by tubular antigen, suggesting that the binding was to regions of the antigen-binding variable region of both the anti-tubular antigen antibody and the TcAR. Both antibodies gave partial inhibition of renal tubular disease. Since, in this disease, Lyt 2 cells cause renal injury, inhibition of disease is likely to be due in part to inhibition of nephrogenic Lyt 2 cells via the TcAR.

As greater evidence of T cell antigen receptor specificity and structure is developed, and evidence is produced of limited variable region repertoires in diseases such as arthritis[90], anti-idiotypic therapy directed against the TcAR may become a new therapeutic possibility.

## (g) Factors to shift Ts/Th activity balance

To the extent that T suppressor cells regulate the expression of autoimmunity, and T helper cells facilitate the expression of autoimmune disease, factors which shift the balance from T help to T suppressor activity may be useful in disease treatment. Anti-L3T4 (see above) and cyclosporin A (see below) may help shift the helper/suppressor balance in favour of suppressor cells. We have also found a factor in conditioned media which will increase the relative proportion of Lyt 2 $^+$ T cells in peripheral blood and spleen of mice (Laux, D, Otterness, I et al., unpublished). Whether a factor that increases CD8 levels would be of value for controlling autoimmune disease needs to be tested.

## (h) Inhibition of T cell homing

T lymphocytes have recognition structures for specific homing receptors that regulate their migration from the circulation and lymph into lymphoid organs. For example, Mel-14 is a monoclonal antibody which recognizes a T cell homing structure for lymph node high endothelial venues (HEV) and, when bound to the T cell surface, can block its adherence and entrance into the lymph node[91]. Submitogenic activation of lymphocytes increases the expression of Mel-14[92] and thus the circulation through the lymph node. Mel-14 has been used to prevent lymphadenopathy in MRL/lpr mice. Although Mel-14 prevents homing into the lymph nodes, the aberrant cells accumulate in the spleen instead[93]. These data clearly show the potential to change lymphocyte trafficking and localization patterns. If, as has been suggested, there are specific homing receptors in areas of inflammation, inhibition of such homing receptor activity should keep T cells from circulating through the inflamed area and thereby prevent their continuous recruitment. This is an important area for further research.

## (i) Anti-IL-2 receptor therapy

Resting populations of T cells express little IL-2 receptor (IL-2R) when it is measured by antibody against the low-affinity receptor (p55, also called TAC in man). In cells recently stimulated to proliferate, IL-2R expression is significantly enhanced. Thus targeting removal of IL-2R bearing T cells offers a mechanism for selectively deleting activated T cells. Presumably, during active disease most of the activated T cells would be disease-related. Thus normal, non-activated T cells would be left intact and able to be later recruited to other functions. Administration of monoclonal anti-IL-2R antibody M7/20 was shown to suppress insulitis in autoimmune non-obese spontaneous diabetic (NOD) mice[94]. In NZB/W lupus mice, the anti-IL-2R antibody protected from renal injury as measured by a decreased incidence of pathologic proteinurea. Moreover, deposition of both gp70 and immunoglobulin complexes in the kidney was inhibited. Studies of the mechanism of inhibition suggest that both complement and inhibition of IL-2 binding to the receptor appeared to be required. Anti-IL-2R antibody was ineffective in blocking delayed hypersensitivity in C5-deficient strains of mice, as was a second monoclonal anti-IL-2R antibody (7D4) which failed to block IL-2 binding[95]. Interestingly, *in vitro* 7D4 blocks T cell proliferation by preventing IL-2R internalization[96].

IL-2 itself has been made into a chimeric fusion protein with toxin[97]. Similar substances have been made by chemical linking of toxin with antibodies[98]. As such it has been shown to block delayed hypersensitivity reactions[99]. Presumably it will also be effective in treatment of autoimmune disease. It is targeted, just as is anti-IL-2R antibody, by its binding to the IL-2R, whereupon it can destroy the activated T cells.

In a comparison made at the time of immunization, anti-IL-2R antibodies were as effective as anti-L3T4 antibodies in abrogating delayed hypersensitivity[100]. This suggests that the use of IL-2R antibodies possesses a large advantage in that it eliminates only the responding T cell clones and leaves T cells of other specificities intact and fully capable of responding to infectious insult.

### (j) Inhibition of MHC class II antigen expression

The linkage of the majority of the autoimmune diseases with a particular MHC antigen suggests that the presentation of antigen by IA to T cells is an integral part of the disease[101]. γ-Interferon plays a major role in enhancing the expression of IA[102] in the mouse and DR[103] in man. This facilitates the presentation of antigens to T cells. For example, presentation of myelin basic protein by astrocytes in EAE is γ-interferon-dependent[104,105]. In some autoimmune diseases, such as diabetes in the NOD mice[9], lupus in the NZB/W mouse[106], and experimental thyroiditis[107], it has been shown that disease induction is accelerated by γ-interferon. Moreover, in EAE recovery is associated with the suppression of γ-interferon production by T cells[10]. In NZB/W mice, treatment with γ-interferon exacerbates disease and treatment with anti-γ-interferon antibodies improves disease survival[106]. These data suggest that therapy targeted to removal of γ-interferon in order to decrease antigen presentation might be a useful therapy in man.

Contrary data do however exist. Thus γ-interferon has been shown to have a direct anti-inflammatory effect *in vivo* when applied systemically[108]. This appears also to be the case for EAE where treatment with γ-interferon improves survival, and treatment with anti-γ-interferon causes more severe disease[109]. Moreover, in cases where the autoimmune disease might have an infectious aetiology, γ-interferon might have a therapeutic benefit in its own right.

## (3)  Drug therapy, animal studies

The traditional method of treating disease has been by the use of drugs, that is, small organic chemicals targeted to specific mechanisms. Non-specific immunosuppressive agents exist that have little T cell selectivity[110], but to date, few drugs have been found that are specifically directed at the T cell. Cyclosporin A (CsA) is the best-known T cell-directed drug, and its primary use has been in human transplantation (see below). CP-17,193 was also found to be selective for the T cell limb of the immune response[111,112], and did not act through the cyclosporin binding protein cyclophilin (Handschumacher, unpublished). Unfortunately, in species other than the mouse, hepatoxicity was found to limit its utility[113]. FK-506 is a new immunosuppressive[114] and has been reported to be a T cell-selective agent.

### (a)  Cyclosporin A

Cyclosporin A (CsA) has been shown on the basis of *in vitro* studies to be a drug largely selective for the inhibition of T cell function. It inhibits the synthesis of the T cell lymphokines IL-2[115,116], IL-4[117,118], IL-5[117] and $\gamma$-interferon[119,120]. Although several authors have claimed that IL-2R expression on T cells is inhibited by CsA[121-123], other groups have reported that CsA does not prevent IL-2R expression[124-126]. This difference may be explained by data which show that low- but not high-affinity IL-2R expression on human lymphocytes is inhibited by CsA[127]. Numerous explanations have been marshalled to explain the inhibition of T cell activation by CsA. While it has been suggested that CsA interferes with the binding of $Ca^{2+}$ by calmodulin[128], by displacement of prolactin from the T cell surface[129,130], by inhibiting an enzyme in the activation of ornithine decarboxylase[131] or by blocking of $Ca^{2+}$ influx-dependent $Na^+/H^+$ exchange[132], the evidence presented for CsA acting through cyclophilin[133], a novel cyclosporin binding protein, appears the most compelling.

CsA has been shown to suppress or modulate both spontaneous and induced autoimmune disease in animal models in which T cells play an important role[134]. For example, CsA prevented lymphadenopathy and expansion of T cell subsets without altering autoantibody production in the MRL/1pr mouse[135]. Likewise in the NZB/W lupus mouse model, CsA inhibits the spontaneous renal disease, prevents immune complex deposition[136] but fails to reduce circulating immune complexes[137]. CsA also prevents the early rise of autoantibody titres and causes a fall in the high titres of autoantibody in old NZB/W mice[138]. It also prevents the spontaneous onset of diabetes in the BB rat[139].

Early treatment with CsA also prevents development of disease in several animal models of induced autoimmune disease. Adjuvant arthritis[140,141], streptococcal cell wall arthritis[142], experimental autoimmune uveitis[143], EAE[144,145], and collagen II arthritis[146,147] are all suppressed by

CsA treatment around the time of immunization. By contrast, if treatment is begun after the disease is established, the therapeutic effect may be minimal or, in the case of rat collagen arthritis, disease exacerbation has been reported.

These results suggest CsA is most effective in blocking *de novo* immunization, a finding that suggests CsA acts most efficiently at the time of antigenic triggering of lymphocytes[148]. In some systems it appears to be partially selective for the activation of helper/inducer T lymphocytes and may spare the suppressor T lymphocyte population[149,150].

## (b)  FK506

With the success of CsA, a fungal metabolite, in suppressing the development of immunity to organ grafts in man, fermentation broths have been screened as a source for better-tolerated immunosuppressant compounds for transplantation. A strain of *Streptomyces tsukubaensis* yielded FK506 as a novel immunosuppressant[114]. This substance, a neutral macrolide, demonstrated good immunosuppressive effects in *in vitro* immune systems. It suppressed the mixed lymphocyte reaction[114,151], T cell proliferation, generation of cytotoxic T cells, production of T cell-derived soluble mediators such as IL-2, IL-3 and $\gamma$-IFN, and IL-2 receptor expression[114]. The $IC_{50}$ values of FK506 in these *in vitro* immune systems were approximately 100-fold lower than CsA.

The *in vivo* immunosuppressive properties of FK506 were shown in experimental transplantation. FK506 was found to prolong skin graft survival in rats[152], indefinitely prolong survival of cardiac allografts in rats[153], and prolong the life of canine kidney transplants[154].

FK506 has been tested in the rat collagen arthritis model and was shown to suppress arthritis, but only when administered during the induction phase of the disease[155]. Anti-type II collagen antibody formation and skin responses to type II collagen were also suppressed. The effect of FK506 in this model was similar to that of CsA, except that FK506 did not exacerbate the disease when started during the immediate preclinical phase.

As with CsA, FK506 apparently affects the early stage of T cell activation; data suggest that FK506 affects the biochemical actions post-Ti/T3 complex triggering[156]. Whether the immunosuppressive activity of FK506 will be of value for human transplantation or for treatment of autoimmune disease remains to be determined.

## (4)  Regulation of T cell function in the clinic

### (a)  Inhibition of T cell function

So far, the only major use of T cell-specific antibodies for disease therapy has been in transplantation. Suppression of T cell function is necessary for prolonged graft survival. Anti-thymocyte globulin was used as an immunosuppressive agent and as an acute suppressant during rejection crises[157,158]. Anti-thymocyte globulin has now been largely replaced by monoclonal anti-CD3 antibody for reversal of acute graft rejection crises[159]. It was found effective in reversing the rate of rejection, reducing the rate of retransplantation, and lowering patient mortality[160-162]. It could also be used for sparing of the use of cyclosporin in patients with poor renal function.

Treatment with anti-CD3 leads to the disappearance of detectable levels of T cells in the blood within 1-2 minutes of administration of as little as 1-2 mg of antibody. Virtually all patients experienced a febrile response. Whether this is due to a release of lymphokines triggered by the anti-CD3-CD3 interaction is not known. However, after a single 7-10-day course of antibodies an immune response develops to the idiotypic determinants on the antibody molecule[163,164]. Because of the spectre of serum sickness and the possibility of anaphylactic reaction, the administration of a second course of antibody is unattractive. Moreover, the immune response to the antibody would limit its effectiveness. However, anti-thymocyte globulin or a different isotype or idiotype anti-CD3 antibody can be used after the primary anti-CD3 treatment.

Both the effectiveness of graft prolongation and the number and severity of infectious episodes appear to be related to the number of circulating T cells and the CD4/CD8 ratios[159]. A high CD4/CD8 ratio is associated with a higher incidence of graft rejection. Conversely, viral complications are associated with a lower CD4/CD8 ratio including a possible virally-based renal dysfunction. Anti-CD4 therapy may also be effective in transplantation based upon studies in monkeys[165]. However, human studies, including autoimmune disease, are only now being carried out, and results are not yet published. The results with anti-CD3 antibodies suggest there is no bar to acute therapeutic use of monoclonal antibodies in human disease.

Other more general T cell depletion techniques, such as thoracic duct drainage[166], have been used in arthritis. Thoracic duct drainage was shown to be effective; however, the technique was not practical for more than experimental use. Similarly to anti-CD3 treatment in transplantation[167], as the T cells return in number after depletion by thoracic duct drainage[168], the CD8 cells come back first followed by the CD4 T cells. The observation that disease improved in thoracic duct T-depleted individuals suggests that the disease is at least partially T cell-dependent, and that the disease does not have an active viral component kept in check by T cells.

## (b)  Gamma-interferon

Gamma-interferon ($\gamma$-IFN) may find a role in the treatment of autoimmune disease if the right disease target and the right treatment regimens can be established. In a phase I study in rheumatoid arthritis (RA) patients, a favourable response was reported with low-dose γ-IFN[169]. In a 28-day study, γ-IFN was safe and well-tolerated with fever being the most prominent side-effect[170]. Significant improvement was noted on joint swelling and pain. However, it was not a double-blind placebo-controlled trial. In other open phase II clinical trials[171,172], relatively good short-term efficacy and toleration was indicated. Resting and motion pain, and articular pain, along with general mobility, were improved. Side-effects included fever which was the most prominent, and were reversible upon dosage reduction. A placebo-controlled, double-blind randomized phase III trial with 91 patients for 28 days showed a 30% reduction in the Ritchie or Lansbury index in responding patients, with a reduction in ESR[173]. Preliminary studies of 111 RA patients treated for 12 months suggest a favourable effect in some patients without untoward side-effects.

The mechanism of γ-IFN in arthritis is unclear. Epstein-Barr virus (EBV) has been implicated as a possible aetiological agent in RA[174]. In contrast to normal individuals, the proliferation of EBV-infected B cells from RA patients is not prevented by autologous T cells[175], in large part due to the failure of lymphokine production, including γ-IFN, by rheumatoid T cells. Alternatively, the effect of γ-IFN on IA expression may result in untoward consequences. In man, exacerbation of multiple sclerosis has been associated with γ-IFN therapy[176]. Increased IA expression caused by γ-IFN has been suggested as an explanation for disease exacerbation. Yet, increased IA expression also enhances cytotoxic responses to pathogens. This could be beneficial if a pathogen is involved in the aetiology of RA.

Gamma-IFN appears to be well-tolerated and relatively safe in rheumatoid arthritis. Whether the long-term effect is sufficiently robust to be meaningful remains to be determined by long-term studies and comparisons with other anti-arthritic agents.

## (e) Established therapy

Cyclosporin A (CsA) has been shown to be a selective immunosuppressant agent that appears to act on T cells by inhibiting functional activation and clonal expansion. It influences the early phase of the immune response by blocking the production of IL-2 from T helper cells[116,125,126]. This explains the observation that CsA inhibits T cell-dependent B cell activation[177,178] and unprimed helper and cytotoxic T cell subsets[115,179]. The drug apparently achieves its suppressive effect by interfering with lymphocyte activation and consequently altering the balance of effector and regulatory cells in the earliest phase of the immune response. It is particularly effective in organ transplantation where it can be given prior to antigen exposure[180]. However, in autoimmune diseases such as rheumatoid arthritis and systemic lupus erythematosus, where the immune response has been established prior to initiation of treatment, it may be less effective. There is, nonetheless, a range of autoimmune diseases which have been reported to respond to CsA. Numerous examples exist of its therapeutic use in animal models, and these studies are being extended to man.

Successful treatment of experimental uveitis in rats[143] led to the examination of CsA in patients with Behçet's disease. This ocular disease has an immune complex component[181] and, in some patients, T cells demonstrate responsiveness to S-antigen[182], produce γ-interferon[183], and demonstrate abnormal suppressor cell activity and MLR responses[184]. CsA was effective in reducing or preventing ocular attacks in Behçet's disease.

CsA has also been used to treat type I-diabetes mellitus based upon studies in the BB rat[139]. This disease is associated with both humoral[185,186] and cell-mediated[187] autoimmune components. In a human study of 12 patients with type I diabetes of recent onset, CsA treatment produced remissions[188] or at least reduced insulin dosage[188,189].

There are other individual case reports of successful CsA treatment of other autoimmune diseases, i.e. Crohn's disease[190,191], ulcerative colitis[192], and bullous pemphigoid and pemphigus[193].

Systemic lupus erythematosus is characterized by kidney deposition of immune complexes from the circulation and by the formation of immune complexes by binding of antibody to fixed tissue antigen. By decreasing T cell help, antibody synthesis and thereby immune complex formation might be reduced. After treatment with CsA, some patients showed improvements in arthralgia[194,195], arthritis[195,196] and nephritis[195,196]; however, most experienced at least a transient nephrotoxicity with rises in serum creatinine. At a higher dose, more severe nephrotoxicity forced withdrawal of drug[194].

Rheumatoid arthritis (RA) shows evidence of both T and B cell involvement in the disease. Thus non-specific immunosuppressant drugs such as azathioprine, cyclophosphamide and methotrexate have been found therapeutically useful. Studies of CsA in animal models suggested that it might also be beneficial in treatment of RA. In a number of small studies, patients with definite or classic RA who were refractive to second-line drug therapy showed disease improvement as measured by pain, swollen joints, global assessment and Ritchie articular index[197-200]. No significant changes in T cell subsets were seen after CsA treatment[198]. This is not surprising, as immunosuppressants have been shown to change cell function without changing subset proportions[201]. In each of these studies, nephrotoxicity was a major adverse effect. Nephrotoxicity with CsA in renal transplant patients is largely reversible[202]. Renal function in CsA-treated patients was found to normalize within 2 months after drug withdrawal except for older patients ( > 50 years) and those with RA[203]. It was calculated that CsA administration for not more than 6 months, and at a maximum dosage of 10 mg/kg for 2 months, leads to an irreversible loss of more than 10% of renal function in RA patients[204]. Although renal function parameters were found to gradually normalize, urinary beta2-microglobulin, which is a marker of renal interstitial disease[205], was still increased after 9 months, indicating renal tubular damage[206]. In patients treated only with NSAID, drug-induced renal disturban-ces[207-209] are generally reversible upon discontinuing NSAID therapy[208]. This suggests that it is the combination of CsA and NSAID which leads to the irreversible dysfunction[204]. The near-universal use of NSAID for the treatment of RA effectively precludes the general use of CsA in RA.

While CsA is apparently clinically effective in RA, its utility is limited by its side effects. The search for more specific and less toxic CsA derivatives continues. A derivative (Nva[2])-CsA, has very similar properties to CsA but lacks nephrotoxic and hypertensive side-effects[210]. Another, (Val[2])dihydro-CsA, has a different spectrum of activities; it does not suppress humoral im-munity and allograft rejection as effectively but still suppresses some types of cell-mediated immune responses which may be involved in autoimmune disease. The clinical utility of these new analogues remains to be determined. Clearly, better compounds in terms of therapeutic ratio must be obtained if CsA-like activity is to become a generally useful treatment of autoimmune disease.

## (5) Conclusions

The bulk of the data summarized herein is consistent with the hypothesis that T cells are required for the establishment and maintenance of autoimmune disease. This suggests that the T cell should be a primary therapeutic target. The T cell-specific pharmacological agents developed to date favour inhibi-tion of T cells during the activation process. Thus, based largely on the work in autoimmune disease in animal models, it appears that the immunosup-pressive activities of T cell subset-selective antibodies and drugs are less ef-fective in reversing established autoimmune disease than they are in inhibiting autoimmune disease induction. This is understandable from the viewpoint that an established immune response consists of multiple mech-anisms, only some of which are dependent on concurrent T cell function. Moreover, many effects may be maintained in memory cells and in immature precursor cells which can be called upon to fill a need if the function of ma-ture effector cells is inhibited. Thus, while a single course of antibody ther-apy could be used to destroy certain classes of T cells, the broad utility of such therapy is limited by the host immune response to the heterologous antibody. Cyclosporin A acts to prevent T cell activation, but appears to lose much of its therapeutic effectiveness when T cells have already been primed. Thus cy-closporin A has found a useful therapeutic niche in transplantation, but only limited use in autoimmune disease.

By contrast, targeting therapy to the specifically-activated T cell popu-lation that is involved in the disease process may be effective in established autoimmune disease. Thus destruction of the small population of IL-2 recep-tor-bearing T cells by either anti-IL-2R therapy or by using an IL-2-toxin fu-sion protein appears able to remove acutely responding cells. This provides a method for selectively deleting the T cell circuit activated in disease. By limiting therapy to times of disease exacerbation, deletion therapy would be carried out at times when the activated T cell population was enriched with disease-related T cells. Alternatively, if a limited T cell antigen receptor repertoire is shown, idiotypic therapy against TcAR would be expected to be effective because it would again eliminate the relevant T cell circuit while leaving the rest of the immune system intact. Here the difficulty lies in identifying the appropriate TcAR clones for deletion. With both of these approaches the problem of how to administer an antibody or immunotoxin fusion protein without eliciting a neutralizing antibody response or allergic reaction would have to be resolved. Methods of tolerization exist in animals, but they have not been adequately developed or tested in man.

Under these circumstances, drugs with new characteristics need to be developed for autoimmune disease. In particular, drugs that would convert an activation signal into a tolerogenic signal would be very useful. Additionally, a drug that is selectively toxic for activated T cells but leaves normal T cells intact would be a significant advance. Such a drug would have to be more selectively targeted than current agents which largely just block cell proliferation. Many of the activated T cells secrete factors, serve as non-dividing effector cells or as precursor cells that are not touched by such therapy. New methods and understanding would need to be developed to discover such agents. As our understanding of the T cell limb of the immune response has grown almost exponentially in the past few years, the many new insights into cellular activation and co-operation cannot but leave one optimistic that solutions will be found to the development of selective therapy for autoimmune disease.

## References

1. Meuer, SC, Acuto, O et al. (1984). The human T-cell receptor. Annu Rev Immunol, 2, 23-50
2. Brenner, MB, McLean, J, Dialynas, DP et al. (1986). Identification of a putative second T-cell receptor. Nature, 322, 145-9
3. Koning, F, Kruisbeek, AM, Maloy, WL et al. (1988). T Cell receptor gamma/delta chain diversity. J Exp Med, 167, 676-81
4. Babbitt, BP, Allen, PM, Matsueda, G et al. (1985). Binding of immunogenic peptides to Ia histocompatibility molecules. Nature, 317, 359-61
5. Buus, S, Sette, A, Colon, SM et al. (1987). The relationship between major histocompatibility complex (MHC) restriction and the capacity of Ia to bind immunogenic peptides. Science, 235, 1353-8
6. Gregerson, PK, Silver, J and Winchester, RJ (1987). The shared epitope hypothesis: An approach to understanding the molecular genetics of susceptibility to rheumatoid arthritis. Arthritis Rheum, 30, 1205-13
7. Christadoss, P, Lindstrom, JM, Melvoid, R and Talal, N (1985). Mutation at I-A beta chain prevents experimental autoimmune myasthenia gravis. Immunogenetics, 21, 33-8
8. Rivas, A, Takada, S, Koide, J et al. (1988). CD4 molecules are associated with the antigen receptor complex on activated but not resting T cells. J Immunol, 140, 2912-18

9.    Campbell, IL, Oxbrow, L, Koulmanda, M and Harrison, LC (1988).IFN-γ induces islet cell MHC antigens and enhances autoimmune, streptozotocin-induced diabetes in the mouse. *J Immunol*, **140**, 1111-16

10.   McDonald, AH and Swanborg, RH (1988). Antigen-specific inhibition of immune interferon production by suppressor cells of autoimmune encephalomyelitis. *J Immunol*, **140**, 1132-18

11.   Mosmann, TR and Coffman, RL (1987). Two types of mouse helper T-cell clones. Implications for immune regulation. *Immunol Today*, **8**, 223-7

12.   Janeway, CA, Jr, Carding, S, Jones, B *et al.* (1987). CD4⁺ T cells: specificity and function. *Immunol Rev*, **101**, 39-80

13.   Arthur, RP and Mason, D (1986). T cells that help B cell response to soluble antigen are distinguishable from those producing interleukin 2 on mitogenic or allogeneic stimulation. *J Exp Med*, **163**, 774-86

14.   Reinherz, EL, Morimoto, C *et al.* (1982). Heterogeneity of human T4⁺ inducer T cells defined by a monoclonal antibody that delineates two functional subpopulations. *J Immunol*, **128**, 463-8

15.   Greenbaum, LA, Horowitz, JB, Wood, A *et al.* (1988). Autocrine growth of CD4⁺ T cells. Differential effects of IL-1 on helper and inflammatory T cells. *J Immunol*, **140**, 1555-60

16.   Trenn, G, Takayama, H, Hu-Li, J *et al.* (1988). B cell stimulatory factor 1 (IL-4) enhances the development of cytotoxic T cells from Lyt-2⁺ resting murine T lymphocytes. *J Immunol*, **140**, 1101-6

17.   Duke, O, Panayi, GS, Janossy, G and Poulter, LW (1982). An immunohistological analysis of lymphocyte subpopulations and their microenvironment in the synovial membranes of patients with rheumatoid arthritis using monoclonal antibodies. *Clin Exp Immunol*, **49**, 22-30

18.   Klareskog, L, Forsum, U, Wigren, A and Wigzell, H (1982). Relationships between HLA-DR-expressing cells and T lymphocytes of different subsets in rheumatoid synovial tissue. *Scand J Immunol*, **15**, 501-7

19.   Young, CL, Adamson, III, TC, Vaughan, JH and Fox, RI (1984). Immunohistologic characterization of synovial membrane lymphocytes in rheumatoid arthritis. *Arthritis Rheum*, **27**, 32-9

20.   Rose, LM, Ginsberg, AH, Rothstein, TL *et al.* (1985). Selective loss of a subset of T helper cells in active multiple sclerosis. *Proc Natl Acad Sci USA*, **82**, 7389-93

21.   Sato, K, Miyasaka, N, Yamaoka, K *et al.* (1987). Quantitative defect of CD4+2H4+ cells in systemic lupus erythematosus and Sjögren's syndrome. *Arthritis Rheum*, **30**, 1407-11

22.   Morimoto, C, Reinherz, EL, Borel, Y *et al.* (1981). Autoantibody to an immunoregulatory inducer population in patients with juvenile rheumatoid arthritis. *J Clin Invest*, **67**, 753-61

23.   Emery, P, Gentry, KC, MacKay, IR *et al.* (1987). Deficiency of the suppressor inducer subset of T lymphocytes in rheumatoid arthritis. *Arthritis Rheum*, **30**, 849-56

24.   Lasky, HP, Bauer, K and Pope, RM (1988). Increased helper inducer and decreased suppressor inducer phenotypes in the rheumatoid joint. *Arthritis Rheum*, **31**, 52-9

25.   Greiner, DL, Handler, ES, Nakano, K *et al.* (1986). Absence of the RT-6 T cell subset in diabetes-prone BB/W rats. *J Immunol*, **136**, 148-51

26.   Greiner, DL, Mordes, JP, Handler, ES *et al.* (1987). Depletion of RT6.1⁺ T lymphocytes induces diabetes in resistant biobreeding/Worcester (BB/W) rats. *J Exp Med*, **166**, 461-75

27.   Holmdahl, R, Jonsson, R, Larsson, P and Klareskog, L (1988). Early appearance of activated CD4⁺ T lymphocytes and class II antigen-expressing cells in joints of DBA/1 mice immunized with type II collagen. *Lab Invest*, **58**, 53-60

28.  Holmdahl, R, Rubin, K, Klareskog, L et al. (1985). Appearance of different lymphoid cells in synovial tissue and peripheral blood during the course of collagen II-induced arthritis in rats. Scand J Immunol, 21, 197-204

29.  Klareskog, L, Holmdahl, R, Larsson, E and Wigzell, H (1983). Role of T lymphocytes in collagen II induced arthritis in rats. Clin Exp Immunol, 51, 117-25

30.  Sriram, S, Solomon, D, Rouse, RV and Steinman, L (1982). Identification of T cell subsets and B lymphocytes in EAE lesions. J Immunol, 129, 1649-51

31.  Whittum, J, Goldschneider, I, Greiner, D and Zurier, R (1985). Developmental abnormalities of terminal deoxynucleotidyl transferase positive bone marrow cells and thymocytes in New Zealand mice: Effects of prostaglandin E1. J Immunol, 135, 272-80

32.  Ridge, SC, Zabriske, JB, Oronsky, AL and Kerwar, SS (1985). Streptococcal cell wall arthritis: studies with nude (athymic) inbred Lewis rats. Cell Immunol, 96, 231-4

33.  Allen, JB, Malone, DG, Wahl, SM et al. (1985). Role of the thymus in streptococcal cell wall-induced arthritis and hepatic granuloma formation: comparative studies of pathology and cell wall distribution in athymic and euthymic rats. J Clin Invest, 76, 1042-56

34.  Yocum, DE, Allen, JB, Wahl, SM et al. (1986). Inhibition by cyclosporin A of streptococcal cell wall-induced arthritis and hepatic granulomas in rats. Arthritis Rheum, 29, 262-73

35.  Holoshitz, J, Naparstek, Y, Ben Nun, A and Cohen, IR (1983). Lines of T lymphocytes induce or vaccinate against autoimmune arthritis. Science, 219, 56-8

36.  van Eden, W, Holoshitz, J, Nevo, Z et al. (1985). Arthritis induced by a T-lymphocyte clone that responds to Mycobacterium tuberculosis and to cartilage proteoglycans. Proc Natl Acad Sci USA, 82, 5117-20

37.  Trentham, DE, Dynesius, RA and David, JR (1978). Passive transfer by cells of type II collagen-induced arthritis in rats. J Clin Invest, 62, 359-66

38.  Holmdahl, R, Klareskog, L, Rubin, K et al. (1985). T lymphocytes in collagen type II arthritis in mice. Characterization of arthritogenic collagen II-specific T-cell lines and clones. Scand J Immunol, 22, 295-306

39.  Seki, N, Sudo, Y, Yoshioka, T et al. (1988). Type II collagen-induced murine arthritis. I. Induction and perpetuation of arthritis require synergy between humoral and cell-mediated immunity. J Immunol, 140, 1477-84

40.  Romball, CG and Weigle, WO (1987). Transfer of experimental autoimmune thyroiditis with T cell clones. J Immunol, 138, 1092-8

41.  Pettinelli, CE and McFarlin, DE (1981). Adoptive transfer of experimental allergic encephalomyelitis in SJL/J mice after in vivo activation of lymph node cells by myelin basic protein: requirement for Lyt 1+2- T lymphocytes. J Immunol, 127, 1420-3

42.  Ben-Nun, A, Wekerle, H and Cohen, IR (1981). The rapid isolation of clonable antigen specific T lymphocyte lines capable of mediating autoimmune encephalomyelitis. Eur J Immunol, 11, 195-9

43.  Zamvil, S, Nelson, P, Trotter, J et al. (1985). T cell clones specific for myelin basic protein induce chronic relapsing paralysis and demyelination. Nature, 317, 355-8

44.  Pelletier, L, Pasquier, R, Rossert, J et al. (1988). Autoreactive T cells in mercury-induced autoimmunity. Ability to induce the autoimmune disease. J Immunol, 140, 750-4

45.  Helfgott, SM, Kieval, RI, Breedveld, FC et al. (1988). Detection of arthritogenic factor in adjuvant arthritis. J Immunol, 140, 1838-43

46.  Watanabe, R, Wege, H and ter Meulen, V (1983). Adoptive transfer of EAE-like lesions from rats with coronavirus-induced demyelinating encephalomyelitis. Nature, 305, 150-3

47.  Neu, N, Rose, NR, Beisel, KW et al. (1987). Cardiac myosin induced myocarditis in genetically predisposed mice. J Immunol, 139, 3630-6

48. Schluesener, HJ, Sobel, RA, Linington, C and Weiner, HL (1987). A monoclonal antibody against a myelin oligodendrocyte glycoprotein induces relapses and demyelination in central nervous system autoimmune disease. *J Immunol*, **139**, 4016-21

49. Wofsy, D, Ledbetter, JA, Hendler, PL and Seaman, WE (1985). Treatment of murine lupus with monoclonal anti-T cell antibody. *J Immunol*, **134**, 852-7

50. Wofsy, D (1986). Administration of monoclonal anti-T cell antibodies retards murine lupus in BXSB mice. *J Immunol*, **136**, 4554-60

51. Ranges, GE, Sriram, S and Cooper, SM (1985). Prevention of type II collagen arthritis by *in vivo* treatment with anti-L3T4. *J Exp Med*, **162**, 1105-10

52. Brostoff, SW and Mason, DW (1984). Experimental allergic encephalomyelitis: successful treatment *in vivo* with a monoclonal antibody that recognizes T helper cells. *J Immunol*, **133**, 1938-42

53. Waldor, MW, Sririam, S, Hardy, R *et al.* (1985). Reversal of experimental allergic encephalomyelitis with a monoclonal antibody to a T cell subset marker. *Science*, **227**, 415-17

54. Sriram, S and Roberts, CA (1986). Treatment of established chronic relapsing experimental allergic encephalitis with anti-L3T4 antibodies. *J Immunol*, **136**, 4464-9

55. Christadoss, P and Dauphinee, MJ (1986). Immunotherapy for myasthenia gravis: a murine model. *J Immunol*, **136**, 2437-40

56. Wang, Y, Hao, L, Gill, RG and Lafferty, KJ (1987). Autoimmune diabetes in NOD mouse is L3T4 T-lymphocyte dependent. *Diabetes*, **36**, 535-8

57. Wofsy, D and Seaman, WE (1985). Successful treatment of autoimmunity in NZB/NZW $F_1$ mice with monoclonal antibody to L3T4. *J Exp Med*, **161**, 378-91

58. Bank, I and Chess, L (1985). Perturbations of the T4 molecule transmits a negative signal to T cells. *J Exp Med*, **162**, 1294-1303

59. Tite, JP, Sloan, A and Janeway, Jr, CA (1986). The role of L3T4 in T cell activation: L3T4 may be both an Ia-binding protein and a receptor that transduces a negative signal. *J Mol Cell Immunol*, **2**, 179-90

60. Seaman, WE and Wofsy, D (1988). Selective manipulation of the immune response *in vivo* by monoclonal antibodies. *Annu Rev Med*, **39**, 231-41

61. Waldor, MK, Mitchell, D, Kipps, TJ *et al.* (1987). Importance of immunoglobulin isotype in therapy of experimental autoimmune encephalomyelitis with monoclonal anti-CD4 antibody. *J Immunol*, **139**, 3660-4

62. Brostoff, SW and White, TM (1986). Treatment of clinical experimental allergic encephalitis in the rat with monoclonal antibody. *J Neuroimmunol*, **13**, 233-40

63. Carteron, NL, Wofsy, D and Seaman, WE (1988). Induction of immune tolerance during administration of monoclonal antibody to L3T4 does not depend on depletion of L3T4$^+$ cells. *J Immunol*, **140**, 713-16

64. Rodriguez, M and Sriram, S (1988). Successful therapy of Theiler's virus-induced demyelination (DA strain) with monoclonal anti-Lyt-2 antibody. *J Immunol*, **140**, 2950-5

65. Steinman, L, Rosenbaum, JT, Sriram, S and McDevitt, HO (1981). *In vivo* effects of antibodies to immune response gene products: prevention of experimental allergic encephalitis. *Proc Natl Acad Sci USA*, **78**, 7111-14

66. Sriram, S and Steinman, L (1983). Anti I-A antibody suppresses active encephalomyelitis: treatment model for diseases linked to IR genes. *J Exp Med*, **158**, 1362-9

67. Perry, LL and Green MI (1982). Conversion of immunity to suppression by *in vivo* administration of I-A subregion-specific antibodies. *J Exp Med*, **156**, 480-91

68. Steinman, L, Solomon, D, Lim, M *et al.* (1983). Prevention of experimental allergic encephalitis with *in vivo* administration of anti I-A antibody: decreased accumulation of radiolabelled lymph node cells in the central nervous system. *J Neuroimmunol*, **5**, 91-7

69.  Sriram, S, Topham, DJ and Carroll, L (1987). Haplotype-specific suppression of experimental allergic encephalomyelitis with anti-IA antibodies. *J Immunol*, **139**, 1485-9

70.  Adelman, NE, Watling, D and McDevitt, HO (1983). Treatment of NZB/W F1 disease with anti-I-A monoclonal antibodies. *J Exp Med*, **158**, 1350-5

71.  Rosenbaum, JT, Adelman, NE and McDevitt, HO (1981). *In vivo* effects of antibodies to immune response gene products. I. Haplotype specific suppression of humoral immune responses with a monoclonal anti-I-A. *J Exp Med*, **154**, 1694-1702

72.  Vladutiu, AO and Steinman, L (1987). Inhibition of autoimmune thyroiditis in mice by anti-I-A antibodies. *Cell Immunol*, **109**, 169-80

73.  Wooley, PH, Luthra, HS, Lafuse, WP *et al.* (1985). Type II collagen-induced arthritis in mice. III. Suppression of arthritis by using monoclonal and polyclonal anti-Ia antisera. *J Immunol*, **134**, 2366-74

74.  Waldor, MK, Sriram, S, McDevitt, HO and Steinman, L (1983). *In vivo* therapy with monoclonal anti-I-A antibody suppresses immune responses to acetylcholine receptor. *Proc Natl Acad Sci USA*, **80**, 2713-17

75.  Ben-Nun, A, Wekerle, H and Cohen, IR (1981). Vaccination against autoimmune encephalomyelitis with T lymphocyte line cells reactive against myelin basic protein. *Nature*, **292**, 60-3

76.  Ellerman, KE, Powers, JM and Brostoff, SW (1988). A suppressor T-lymphocyte cell line for autoimmune encephalomyelitis. *Nature*, **331**, 265-7

77.  Maron, R, Zerubavel, R, Friedman, A and Cohen, IR (1983). T lymphocyte line specific for thyroglobulin produces or vaccinates against autoimmune thyroiditis in mice. *J Immunol*, **131**, 2316-22

78.  Brahn, E and Trentham, DE (1987). Attenuation of collagen arthritis and modulation of delayed-type hypersensitivity by type II collagen reactive T-cell lines. *Cell Immunol*, **109**, 139-47

79.  Kakimoto, K, Katsuki, M, Hirofuji, T *et al.* (1988). Isolation of T cell line capable of protecting mice against collagen-induced arthritis. *J Immunol*, **140**, 78-83

80.  Sano, S, Suda, T, Qian, J-H *et al.* (1987). Abrogation of the capacity of delayed-type hypersensitivity responses to alloantigens by intravenous injection of neuraminidase-treated allogeneic cells. *J Immunol*, **139**, 3652-9

81.  Hahn, BH and Ebling, FM (1984). Suppression of murine lupus nephritis by administration of an anti-idiotypic antibody to anti-DNA. *J Immunol*, **132**, 187-90

82.  Fritz, RB and Desjardins, AE (1982). Idiotypes of Lewis rat antibodies to encephalitogenic peptides of guinea pig myelin basic protein: *in vitro* and *in vivo* studies. *J Immunol*, **128**, 247-50

83.  Lennon, VA and Lambert, EHJ (1981). Monoclonal autoantibodies to acetyl choline receptors: evidence for a dominant idiotype and requirement of complement for pathogenicity. *Ann NY Acad Sci*, **377**, 77-96

84.  Hahn, BH and Ebling, FM (1983). Suppression of NZB/NZW murine nephritis by administration of a syngeneic monoclonal antibody to DNA: Possible role of anti-idiotypic antibodies. *J Clin Invest*, **71**, 1728-36

85.  Christadoss, P, Lennon, VA and David, C (1979). Genetic control of experimental autoimmune myasthenia gravis in mice: I. Lymphocyte proliferative response to acetylcholine receptor is under H-2-linked Ir gene control. *J Immunol*, **123**, 2540-3

86.  De Baets, MC, Einarson, B, Lindstrom, JM and Weigle, WO (1982). Lymphocyte activation in experimental autoimmune myasthenia gravis. *J Immunol*, **128**, 2228-35

87.  Krolick, KA and Urso, OE (1986). Influence of T cell specificity on the antibody response to the acetylcholine receptor. *J Neuroimmunol*, **13**, 75-87

88.  Neilson, EG and Phillips, SM (1982). Suppression of interstitial nephritis by auto-anti-idiotypic immunity. *J Exp Med*, **155**, 179-89

89.  Neilson, EG, McCafferty, E, Phillips, SM *et al.* (1984). Antiidiotypic immunity in interstitial nephritis. II. Rats developing anti-tubular basement membrane disease fail

to make an antiidiotypic regulatory response: the modulatory role of an RT7.1[+], OX8[-] suppressor T cell mechanism. *J Exp Med*, **159**, 1009-26

90. Stamenkovic, I, Stegagno, M, Wright, KA *et al*. (1988). Clonal dominance among T lymphocyte infiltrates in arthritis. *Proc Natl Acad Sci USA*, **85**, 1179-83

91. Butcher, EC (1986). The regulation of lymphocyte traffic. *Curr Top Microbiol Immunol*, **128**, 85-122

92. Hamann, A, Jablonski-Westrich, D, Scholz, K-U *et al*. (1988). Regulation of lymphocyte homing. I. Alterations in homing receptor expression and organ-specific high endothelial venule binding of lymphocytes upon activation. *J Immunol*, **140**, 737-43

93. Mountz, JD, Gause, WC, Finkelman, FD and Steinberg, AD (1988). Prevention of lymphadenopathy in MRL/lpr/lpr mice by blocking peripheral lymph node homing with Mel-14 *in vivo*. *J Immunol*, **140**, 2943-9

94. Kelley, VE, Gaulton, GN, Hattori, M *et al*. (1988). Anti-interleukin 2 receptor antibody suppresses murine diabetic insulitis and lupus nephritis. *J Immunol*, **140**, 59-61

95. Kelley, VE, Gaulton, and Strom, TB (1987). Inhibitory effects of anti-interleukin 2 receptor and anti-L3T4 antibodies on delayed type hypersensitivity: the role of complement and epitope. *J Immunol*, **138**, 2771-5

96. Kumar, A, Moreau, J-L, Gibert, M and Thèze, J (1987). Internalization of interleukin 2 (IL-2) by high affinity IL-2 receptors is required for the growth of IL-2-dependent T cell lines. *J Immunol*, **139**, 3680-4

97. Murphy, JR, Bishai, W, Borowski, M *et al* (1986). Genetic construction expression and melanoma selective cytotoxicity of a diptheria toxin-related α-melanocyte-stimulating hormone fusion protein. *Proc Natl Acad Sci USA*, **83**, 8258-62

98. Vitetta, ES and Uhr, JW (1985). Immunotoxins. *Ann Rev Immunol*, **3**, 197-212

99. Kelley, VE, Bacha, P, Pankewycz, O *et al*. (1988). Interleukin-2 toxin fusion protein abolishes cell mediated immunity *in vivo*. *Proc Natl Acad Sci USA*, **85**, 3980-4

100. Kelley, VE, Naor, D, Tarcic, N *et al*. (1986). Anti-interleukin 2 receptor antibody suppresses delayed-type hypersensitivity to foreign and syngeneic antigens. *J Immunol*, **137**, 2122-4

101 Nepom, GT, Hansen, JA and Nepom, BS (1987). The molecular basis for HLA class II associations with rheumatoid arthritis. *J Clin Immunol*, **7**, 1-7

102. Warren, MK and Vogel, SN (1985). Opposing effects of glucocorticoids on interferon-γ-induced murine macrophage Fc receptor and Ia antigen expression. *J Immunol*, **134**, 2462-9

103. Collins, T, Korman, AJ, Wake, CT *et al*. (1984). Immune interferon activates multiple class II major histocompatibility complex genes and the associated invariant chain gene in human endothelial cells and dermal fibroblasts. *Proc Natl Acad Sci USA*, **81**, 4917-21

104. Fontana, A, Fierz, W and Wekerle, H (1984). Astrocytes present myelin basic protein to encephalitogenic T-cell lines. *Nature*, **307**, 273-6

105. Fierz, W, Endler, B, Reske, K *et al*. (1985). Astrocytes as antigen-presenting cells. I. Induction of Ia antigen expression on astrocytes by T cells via immune interferon and its effect on antigen presentation. *J Immunol*, **134**, 3785-93

106. Jacob, CO, van der Meide, PH and McDevitt, HO (1987). *In vivo* treatment of (NZB x NZW)F[1] lupus-like nephritis with monoclonal antibody to γ-interferon. *J Exp Med*, **166**, 798-803

107. Remy, J-J, Salamero, J, Michel-Bechet, M and Charreire, J (1987). Experimental autoimmune thyroiditis induced by recombinant interferon-γ. *Immunol Today*, **8**, 73

108. Heremans, H, Dijkmans, R, Sobis, H *et al*. (1987). Regulation by interferons of the local inflammatory response to bacterial lipopolysaccharide. *J Immunol*, **138**, 4175-9

109. Billiau, A, Heremans, H, Vandekerckhove, F *et al*. (1988). Enhancement of experimental allergic encephalomyelitis in mice by antibodies against IFN-γ. *J Immunol*, **140**, 1506-10

110.   Otterness, IG and Chang, Y-H (1976). Comparative study of cyclophosphamide, 6-mercaptopurine, azathiaprine and methotrexate. Relative effects on the humoral and cellular immune response in the mouse. *Clin Exp Immunol*, **26**, 346-54

111.   Lombardino, JG and Otterness, IG (1981). Novel immunosuppressive agents. Potent immunological activity of some benzothiopyrano[4,3-c]pyrazol-3-ones. *J Med Chem*, **24**, 830-4

112.   Otterness, IG (1981). Comparative activity of CP-17,193 and five established immunosuppressives towards the antigens SRBC and EL4. *Clin Exp Immunol*, **46**, 332-9

113.   Otterness, IG and Bliven, ML (1984). Pharmacologic modulation of immune function: some considerations for design of drug therapy. *Adv Inflam Res*, **7**, 185-99

114.   Kino, T, Hatanaka, H, Hashimoto, N *et al*. (1987). FK-506, a novel immunosuppressant isolated from a *Streptomyces*. I. Fermentation, isolation, and physico-chemical and biological characteristics. *J Antibiot*, **40**, 1249-55

115.   Hess, AD and Tutschka, PJ (1980). Effect of CsA on human lymphocyte responses *in vitro*. I. CsA allows for the expression of alloantigen-activated suppressor cells while preferentially inhibiting the induction of cytolytic effector lymphocytes in MLR. *J Immunol*, **124**, 2601-8

116.   Andrus, L and Lafferty, KJ (1982). Inhibition of T cell activity by cyclosporin A. *Scand J Immunol*, **15**, 449-58

117.   Krusemeier, M and Snow, EC (1988). Induction of lymphokine responsiveness of hapten-specific B lymphocytes promoted through an antigen-mediated T helper lymphocyte intereaction. *J Immunol*, **140**, 367-75

118.   Sideras, P, Funa, K, Zalcberg-Quintana, I *et al*. (1988). Analysis by *in situ* hybridization of cells expressing mRNA for interleukin 4 in the developing thymus and in peripheral lymphocytes from mice. *Proc Natl Acad Sci USA*, **85**, 218-21

119.   Reem, GH, Cook, LA and Vilcek, J (1983). Gamma interferon synthesis by human thymocytes and T lymphocytes inhibited by CsA. *Science*, **221**, 63-5

120.   Herold, KC, Lancki, DW, Moldwin, RL and Fitch, FW (1986). Immunosuppressive effects of cyclosporin A on cloned T cells. *J Immunol*, **136**, 1315-21

121.   Palacios, R (1982). Mechanism of T cell activation: role and functional relationship of HLA-DR antigens and interleukins. *Immunol Rev*, **63**, 73-110

122.   Lillehoj, HS, Malek, TR and Shevach, EM (1984). Differential effects of cyclosporin A on the expression of T and B lymphocyte activation antigens. *J Immunol*, **133**, 244-50

123.   Prince, HE and John, JK (1986). Cyclosporin inhibits the expression of receptors for interleukin 2 and transferrin on mitogen-activated human T lymphocytes. *Immunol Invest*, **15**, 463-72

124.   Larsson, E-L (1980) Cyclosporin A and dexamethasone suppress T cell responses by selectively acting at distinct sites of the triggering process. *J Immunol*, **124**, 2828-33

125.   Miyawaki, T, Yachie, A, Ohzeki, S *et al*. (1983). Cyclosporin A does not prevent expression of the Tac antigen, a probable TCGF receptor molecule on mitogen-stimulated T cells. *J Immunol*, **130**, 2737-42

126.   Dos Reiss, GA and Shevach, EM (1982). Effect of cyclosporin A on T cell function *in vitro*: the mechanism of suppression of T cell proliferation depends on the nature of the T cell stimulus as well as the differentiation state of the responding T cell. *J Immunol*, **129**, 2360-7

127.   Ryffel, B, Muller, S and Foxwell, BC (1987). Cyclosporin-A allows the expression of high-affinity interleukin-2 binding sites on anti-T-cell antibody activated human T lymphocytes. *Trans Proc*, **19**, 1199-1201

128.   Colombani, PM, Robb, A and Hess, AD (1985). Cyclosporin A binding to calmodulin: a possible site of action on T lymphocytes. *Science*, **228**, 337-9

129. Russell, DH, Kibler, DH, Matrisian, L, Larson, DF, Poulos, B and Magun, BE (1985). Prolactin receptors on human T and B lymphocytes: antagonism or prolactin binding of cyclosporine. *J Immunol*, **134**, 3027-31

130. Larson, DF (1986). Mechanism of action: antagonism of the prolactin receptor. *Prog Allergy*, **38**, 222-38

131. Fidelus, RK, Laughter, AH, Twomey, JJ *et al*. (1984). The effect of cylosporine on ornithine decarboxylase induction with mitogens, antigens and lymphokines. *Transplantation*, **37**, 383-7

132. Rosoff, PM and Terres, G (1986). Cyclosporin A inhibits $CA^{2+}$ dependent stimulation of the $Na^+/H^+$ antiport in human T cells. *J Cell Biol*, **103**, 457-63

133. Handschumacher, RE, Harding, MW, Rice, J *et al*. (1984). Cyclophilin: a specific cytosolic binding protein for cyclosporin A. *Science*, **226**, 544-7

134. Borel, JF and Gunn, HC (1986). Cyclosporine as a new approach to therapy of autoimmune diseases. *Ann NY Acad Sci*, **475**, 307-9

135. Mountz, JD, Smith, HR, Wilder, RL *et al*. (1988). Cs-A therapy in MRL-lpr/lpr mice: amerlioration of immunopathology despite autoantibody production. *J Immunol*, **138**, 157-63

136. Gunn, HC and Ryffel, B (1986). Successful treatment of autoimmunity in (NZB x NZW)F$_1$ mice with cyclosporin and (Nva$^2$)-cyclosporin: II. reduction of glomerulonephritis. *Clin Exp Immunol*, **64**, 234-42

137. Jones, MG and Harris, G (1985). Prolongation of life in female NZB/NZW (F$_1$) hybrid mice by cyclosporin A. *Clin Exp Immunol*, **59**, 1-9

138. Gunn, HC (1986). Successful treatment of autoimmunity in (NZB x NZW)F$_1$ mice with cyclosporin and (Nva$^2$)-cyclosporin: I. reduction of autoantibodies. *Clin Exp Immunol*, **64**, 225-33

139. Laupacis, N, Gardell, C, Dupre, J *et al*. (1983). Cyclosporin prevents diabetes in BB Wistar rats. *Lancet*, **i**, 10-12

140. Borel, JF, Feurer, C, Gubler, HU and Stahelin, H (1976). Biological effects of cyclosporin A: a new antilymphocytic agent. *Agents Actions*, **6**, 468-75

141. Kaibara, N, Hotokebuchi, T, Takagishi, K *et al*. (1984). Pathogenetic difference between collagen arthritis and adjuvant arthritis. *J Expt Med*, **159**, 1388-96

142. Yocum, DE, Allen, JB, Wahl, SM *et al*. (1986). Inhibition by cyclosporin A of streptococcal cell wall-induced arthritis and hepatic granulomas in rats. *Arthitis Rheum*, **29**, 262-73

143. Nussenblatt, RB, Rodrigues, MM, Salinas-Carmona, MC *et al*. (1982). Modulation of experimental autoimmune uveitis with cyclosporin A. *Arch Ophthal*, **100**, 1146-9

144. Bolton, C, Borel, JF, Cuzner, ML *et al*. (1982). Immunosuppression by cyclosporin A of experimental allergic encephalomyelitis. *J Neurol Sci*, **56**, 147-53

145. Schuller-Levis, GB, Kozlowski, PB and Wisniewski, HM (1986). Cyclosporin A treatment of an induced attack in a chronic relapsing model of experimental allergic encephalomyelitis. *Clin Immunol Immunopathol*, **40**, 244-52

146. Takagishi, K, Kaibara, N, Hotokebuchi, T *et al*. (1986). Effects of cyclosporin on collagen induced arthritis in mice. *Ann Rheum Dis*, **45**, 339-44

147. Kaibara, N, Hotokebuchi, T, Takagishi, K and Katsuki, I (1983). Paradoxical effects of cyclosporin A on collagen arthritis in rats. *J Exp Med*, **158**, 2007-15

148. Wiesinger, D and Borel, JF (1980). Studies on the mechanism of action of cyclosporin A. *Immunobiology*, **156**, 454-63

149. Leapman, SB, Filo, RS, Smith, EJ and Smith, PG (1980). *In vitro* effects of cyclosporin A on lymphocyte subpopulations. I. Suppressor cell sparing by cyclosporin A. *Transplantation*, **30**, 404-8

150. Kupiec-Weglinski, JW, Filho, MA, Strom, TB and Tilney, NL (1984). Sparing of suppressor cells: a critical action of cyclosporine. *Transplantation*, **38**, 97-101

151. Kino, T, Hatanaka, H, Miyata, S et al. (1987). FK-506, a novel immunosuppressant isolated from a *Streptomyces*. II. Immunosuppressive effect of FK-506 *in vitro*. *J Antibiot*, 40, 1256-65

152. Inamura, N, Nakahara, K, Kino, T et al. (1988). Prolongation of skin allograft survival in rats by a novel immunosuppressive agent, FK-506. *Transplantation*, 45, 206-9

153. Ochiai, T, Nakajima, K, Nagata, M et al. (1987). Studies of the induction and maintenance of long-term graft acceptance by treatment with FK-506 in heterotropic cardiac allotransplantation in rats. *Transplantation*, 44, 734-33

154. Ochiai, T, Nagata, M, Nakajima, K et al. (1987). Studies of the effects of FK-506 on renal allografting in the beagle dog. *Transplantation*, 44, 729-33

155. Inamura, N, Hashimoto, M, Nakahara, K et al. (1988). Immunosuppressive effect of FK506 on collagen-induced arthritis in rats. *Clin Immunol Immunopathol*, 46, 82-90

156. Sawada, S, Suzuki, G, Kawase, Y and Takaku, F (1987). Novel immunosuppressive agent, FK-506. *In vitro* effects on the cloned T cell activation. *J Immunol*, 139, 1797-1803

157. Cosimi, AB (1983). The clinical usefulness of antilymphocyte antibodies. *Transplant Proc*, 15, 583-9

158. Glass, NR, Miller, DT, Sollinger, HW and Belzer, FO (1983). A comparative study of steroids and heterologous antiserum in the treatment of renal allograft rejection. *Transplant Proc*, 15, 617-21

159. Russell, PS, Colvin, RB and Cosimi, AB (1984). Monoclonal antibodies for the diagnosis and treatment of transplant rejection. *Annu Rev Med*, 35, 63-79

160. Ortho Multicenter Transplant Study Group (1985). A randomized clinical trial of OKT3 monoclonal antibody for acute rejection of cadaveric renal transplants. *N Engl J Med*, 313, 337-42

161. Gordon, RD, Starzl, TE, Fung, JJ et al. (1987). Monoclonal antibody therapy with ciclosporin and steroids in nonmatched cadaveric renal transplants. *Nephron*, 46, suppl. I, 56-9

162. Gordon, RD, Tzakis, AG, Iwatsuki, S et al. (1988). Experience with Orthoclone OKT3 monoclonal antibody in liver transplantation. *Am J Kid Dis*, 11, 141-4

163. Chatenoud, L, Jonker, M, Villemain, F et al. (1986). The human response to the OKT3 monoclonal antibody is oligoclonal. *Science*, 232, 1406-8

164. Shield, CF, Norman, DJ, Marlett, P et al. (1987). Comparison of antimouse and antihorse antibody production during the treatment of allograft rejection with OKT3 or antithymocyte globulin. *Nephron*, 46, Suppl. 1, 48-51

165. Cosimi, AB, Burton, RC and Kung, PC (1981). Evaluation in primate renal allograft recipients of monoclonal antibody to human T-cell subclasses. *Transplant Proc*, 13, 499

166. Wegelius, O, Laine, V, Lindstrom, B and Klockars, M (1970). Fistula of the thoracic duct as immunosuppressive treatment in rheumatoid arthritis. *Acta Med Scand*, 187, 539-44

167. Cosimi, AB, Colvin, RB, Burton, RC et al. (1981). Use of monoclonal antibodies to T-cell subsets for immunological monitoring and treatment in recipients of renal allografts. *N Engl J Med*, 305, 308-14

168. Bell, JD, Marshall, GD, Shaw, BA et al. (1983). Alterations in human thoracic duct lymphocytes during thoracic duct drainage. *Transplant Proc*, 15, 677-80

169. Obert, HJ and Hofschneider, PH (1985). Interferon bei chronischer Polyarthritis. *Dtsch Med Wochenschr*, 100, 1766-9

170. Schindler, J, Kennedy, SM and Wolfe, F (1988). Potential of gamma interferon in rheumatoid arthritis. In: *Advances in Inflammation Research*, Vol. 12, ed A Lewis, N Ackerman and I Otterness (New York: Raven Press), pp. 305-11

171. Seitz, M, Manz, G and Franke, M (1986). Einsatz von rekombinatem Human-Interferon Gamma bei Patienten mit rheumatoider Arthritis. *Z Rheumatol*, 45, 93-9

172. Lemmel, EM, Franke, M, Gaus, W et al. (1987). Results of a phase-II clinical trial on treatment of rheumatoid arthritis with recombinant interferon-gamma. *Rheumatol Int*, **7**, 127-32

173. Lemmel, E-M, Obert, HJ and Hofschneider, PH (1988). Low-dose gamma interferon in treatment of rheumatoid arthritis. *Lancet*, **i**, 598

174. Tosato, G, Steinberg, A and Blaese, RM (1981). Defective EBV-specific suppressor T-cell function in rheumatoid arthritis. *N Engl J Med*, **305**, 1238-43

175. Lotz, M, Tsoukas, CD, Fong, S et al. (1985). Regulation of Epstein-Barr virus infection by recombinant interferon. Selected sensitivity to IFN-gamma. *Eur J Immunol*, **15**, 520-5

176. Panitch, HS, Haley, AS, Hirsch, RL and Johnson, KP (1986). A trial of gamma interferon in multiple sclerosis: clinical results. *Neurology*, **36**, Suppl. 1, 285

177. Shidani, B, Colle, JH, Motta, I and Truffa-Bachi, P (1983). Effect of cyclosporin A on the induction and activation of B memory cells by thymus-independent antigens in mice. *Eur J Immunol*, **13**, 359-63

178. Tosato, G, Pike, SE, Koski, IR and Blaese, RM (1982). Selective inhibition of immunoregulatory cell function by cyclosporin A. *J Immunol*, **128**, 1986-91

179. Wang, BS, Heacock, EH, Collins, KH et al. (1981). Suppressive effects of cyclosporin A on the induction of alloreactivity *in vitro* and *in vivo*. *J Immunol*, **127**, 89-93

180. Weil, C (1984). Cyclosporin A: review of results in organ and bone-marrow transplantation in man. *Med Res Rev*, **4**, 221-65

181. O'Connor, GR (1982). Epidemiology and pathogenesis of the ocular and cerebral forms of Behçet's disease. *Behçet's Disease*, ed. G Inaba (Tokyo: University of Tokyo Press), pp. 115-26

182. Nussenblatt, RB, Gery, I, Ballintine, EJ and Wacker, WB (1980). Cellular responsiveness of uveitis patients to retinal S-antigen. *Am J Ophthalmol*, **89**, 173-9

183. Ohno, S (1981). Voght-Koyanagi, and Harada's diseases. *Trans Ophthalmol Soc UK*, **101**, 335-41

184. Sakane, T, Kotani, H, Takada, S and Tsunematsu, T (1982). Functional aberration of T cell subsets in patients with Behçet's disease. *Arthritis Rheum*, **25**, 1343-51

185. Bottazzo, GF, Florin-Christensen, A and Doniach, D (1974). Islet-cell antibodies in diabetes mellitus with autoimmune polyendocrine deficiencies. *Lancet*, **ii**, 1279-83

186. MacCuish, AC and Irvine, WJ (1975). Autoimmunological aspects of diabetes mellitus. *Clin Endocrinol*, **4**, 435-71

187. Nerup, J, Andersen, OO, Bendixen, G et al. (1974). Cell-mediated immunity in diabetes mellitus. *Proc R Soc Med*, **67**, 506-13

188. Assan, R, Debray-Sachs, M, Laborie, C et al. (1985). Metabolic and immunological effects of cyclosporin in recently diagnosed type I diabetes mellitus. *Lancet*, **i**, 67-71

189. Stiller, CR, Dupré, J, Gent, M et al. (1984). Effects of cyclosporine immunosuppression in insulin-dependent diabetes mellitus of recent onset. *Science*, **223**, 1362-7

190. Allison, MC and Pounder, RE (1984). Cyclosporin for Crohn's disease. *Lancet*, **i**, 902-3

191. Bianchi, PA, Mondelli, M, Quatro di Palo, F and Ranzi, T (1984). Cyclosporin for Chrohn's disease. *Lancet*, **i**, 1242

192. Gupta, S, Keshavarzian, A and Hodgson, HJF (1984). Cyclosporin in ulcerative colitis. *Lancet*, **ii**, 1277-8

193. Thivolet, J, Barthelemy, H, Rigot-Muller, G and Bendelac, A (1985). Effects of cyclosporin on bullous pemphigoid and pemphigus. *Lancet*, **i**, 334-5

194. Isenberg, DA, Snaith, ML, Morrow, WJW et al. (1981). Cyclosporin A for the treatment of systemic lupus erythematosus. *Int J Immunopharmacol*, **3**, 163-9

195. Miescher, PA and Miescher, A (1985). Combined ciclosporin steroid treatment of systemic lupus erythematosus. In *Ciclosporin in Autoimmune Diseases*, ed. R Schindler, (Berlin: Springer Verlag), pp. 337-45

196. Feutren, G, Querin, S, Chatenoud, L, Noel, LH *et al.* (1985). The effects of ciclosporin in twelve patients with severe systemic lupus. In *Ciclosporin in Autoimmune Diseases*, ed. R Schindler, (Berlin: Springer Verlag), pp. 366-72

197. van Rijthoven, AWAM, Dijkmans, BAC, Goei The, HS *et al.* (1986). Cyclosporin treatment for rheumatoid arthritis: a placebo controlled, double blind, multicentre study. *Ann Rheum Dis*, **45**, 726-31

198. Forre, O, Bjerkhoel, F, Salvesen, CF *et al.* (1987). An open, controlled, randomized comparison of cyclosporin and azathioprine in the treatment of rheumatoid arthritis: a preliminary report. *Arthritis Rheum*, **30**, 88-92

199. Weinblatt, ME, Coblyn, JS, Fraser, PA *et al.* (1987). Cyclosporin A treatment of refractory rheumatoid arthritis. *Arthritis Rheum*, **30**, 11-17

200. Dougados, M and Amor, B (1987). Cyclosporin A in rheumatoid arthritis: preliminary clinical results of an open trial. *Arthritis Rheum*, **30**, 83-7

201. Bliven, ML, Cunningham, AC and Otterness, IG (1988). A pharmacological study of the relationship between lymphocyte function and surface antigen expression. *Agents Actions*, **25**

202. Chapman, JR, Griffiths, D, Harding, NGL and Morris, PJ (1985). Reversibility of cyclosporin nephrotoxicity after three months' treatment. *Lancet*, **i**, 128-9

203. von Graffenried, B and Harrison, WB (1985). Renal function in patients with autoimmune diseases treated with cyclosporine. *Transplant Proc*, **17**, Suppl. 1, 215-31

204. Dijkmans, BAC, van Rijthoven, AWAM, Goei The, HS *et al.* (1987). Effects of cyclosporin on serum creatinine in patients with rheumatoid arthritis. *Eur J Clin Pharmacol*, **31**, 541-5

205. Bird, HA, Yu, H and Cooper, EH (1984). Renal proximal dysfunction in rheumatic diseases. *Br Med J*, **288**, 1044-5

206. Berg, KJ, Forre, O, Bjerkhoel, F *et al.* (1986). Side effects of cyclosporin A treatment in patients with rheumatoid arthritis. *Kidney Int*, **29**, 1180-7

207. Breedveld, FC, Valentijn, RM, Westedt, ML and Weening, J (1985). Rapidly progressive glomerulonephritis with glomerular crescent formation in rheumatoid arthritis. *Clin Rheumatol*, **4**, 353-9

208. Kimberly, RP, Bowden, RE, Keiser, HR and Plotz, PH (1978). Reduction of renal function by newer nonsteroidal anti-inflammatory drugs. *Am J Med*, **64**, 804-7

209. Wegmueller, E (1985). Nicht-steroidale Antirheumatika und Nephrotoxizitat. *Dtsch Med Wochenschr*, **110**, 469-72

210. Hiestand, PC, Gunn, HC, Gale, JM *et al.* (1985). Comparison of the pharmacological profiles of cyclosporine, $(Nva^2)$-cyclosporine and $(Val^2)$dihydro-cyclosporine. *Immunology*, **55**, 249-55

# 12
# Superoxide dismutase modifications for anti-inflammatory therapy

**F.M. Veronese,* A. Conforti** and G.P. Velo****
*Dipartimento di Scienze Farmaceutiche, Centro di Chimica del Farmaco e dei Prodotti Biologicamente Attivi del CNR, Università di Padova, Padova, Italy; and **Istituto di Farmacologia, Università di Verona, Verona, Italy

## I. INTRODUCTION

In the early 1960s a metalloprotein with anti-inflammatory properties in man and animals was isolated from bovine liver[1], which was, some years later identified as superoxide dismutase (SOD). This is a copper–zinc protein which has subsequently been purified and characterized by McCord and Fridovich[2].

Extensive investigations in animals showed soon the therapeutic values of SOD, in various models of inflammation as carrageenan food oedema, abscess, pleurisy and adjuvant-induced polyarthritis in rats and mice, reversed Arthus reaction in rats and guinea pigs, autoimmune glomerulonephritis in mice and dogs as well as zinc-chloride induced toe abscess in dogs[3].

SOD was also demonstrated able to ameliorate or prevent toxic adverse reaction caused *in vivo* by radiation therapy in various cancer animal models (Walker adenocarcinoma of rats, XHT sarcoma of mice) without influencing the efficacy of the high-intensity radiation[4]. Recently anti-inflammatory effects of SOD were observed in rats with nephritis induced by injection of nephrotoxic serum[5]. The ability of SOD to protect the cardiac ischaemia and re-perfusion injury *in vitro* and *in vivo* was also evaluated[6].

All of these therapeutic effects of SOD were based on the rationale of lowering the abnormally high levels of the very reactive superoxide ion or hydroxyl anion products which appear to have toxic effects *per se*.

In parallel with animal studies, SOD activity was tested and demonstrated also in man and is now marketed in the USA and in five European countries for human use under the trade name "Orgotein", where it is prescribed for treatment of musculoskeletal inflammation.

*New Developments in Antirheumatic Therapy.* Rainsford, KD and Velo, GP (eds), Inflammation and Drug Therapy Series, Volume III.

The efficacy of SOD in osteoarthritis administered intra-articularly into knees and hips was demonstrated in an open clinical study which dates back to 1974[7]. A significant improvement in osteoarthritis determined by parameters of pain, function, use of aids, use of analgesics and doctor's assessment, was also found in a double blind controlled trial *versus* placebo when Orgotein was administered intra-articularly[8].

Trials carried out in different countries demonstrated that the effectiveness of Orgotein in rheumatoid arthritis was comparable to gold and, in some parameters, to D-penicillamine without the serious side-effects of these drugs[3,8]. Other studies suggest that SOD, administered intra-articularly might be more effective than im[9].

A number of clinical trials starting with Marberger (1974) showed the superiority of SOD, give intramurally, over other therapy for the treatment of chronic radiation cystitis, chronic prostatitis, hydrocele, induratio penis plastica both in terms of benefit and outstanding safety[10,11].

Recently however, some authors have raised doubts about the efficacy of SOD as anti-inflammatory agent and have criticized the quality of early experiments[12]. Other investigators have demonstrated the inappropriate use of SOD when given by the oral route of administration[13].

Limits to a more general clinical use seem related to potential immunological responses from the non human source of SOD presently on the market as well as to the short duration of SOD in the circulation. The short half-life which is of the order of minutes following i.v. injection, requires continuous infusion of frequent multiple injections to maintain a therapeutic blood concentration[8]. Immunological reactions and the short duration of action are common problems of many systemic enzyme therapies. The most promising solution seems to modify the enzyme structure so as to mask the protein structure and protect the molecule from degradation, e.g. by enzyme encapsulation.

For surface modification the use of non-toxic, non-immunogenic macromolecules were proposed, both of natural origin as polysaccharides and albumins. Alternatively synthetic molecules were considered, e.g. polyethyleneglycol and acrylic polymers. Among the encapsulating methods the use of liposomes, erythrocytes or artificial cells were proposed and the effects were determined. The results of such enzyme protections appear very promising, so much so that a few derivatized enzymes are already on the market while many are under clinical investigation and several patients have been already presented.

Although derivatized or encapsulated superoxide dismutases are not yet on the market there are many efforts to develop such products in academic and industrial laboratories, so that one may suppose that commercially viable products might appear soon.

Here we briefly report (a) various methods for derivatizing superoxide dismutase, based upon the chemical properties of conjugates described by different authors, (b) the pharmacokinetics of such preparations, and (c) pharmacological properties thereof in various experimental models of inflammation.

## II. POLYSACCHARIDE–SOD CONJUGATES

Early experiments of the effects of modifying the enzyme surface charge on their pharmacokinetic behaviour of enzyme derivatives were performed with *Acinobacter* glutaminase-asparaginase. A lowering of 3.2 pH units in the isoelectric point by glycosylation or succinylation increased up to fifteen fold the clearance time in animals without impairing its enzymatic activity[14].

Positively charged groups at the surface of superoxide dismutase were introduced by coupling N-N-dimethyl-1,3-propanediamine to the existing carboxylic groups with an increase to 8.1 of its isoelectric point. Such positively charged enzyme resulted in increased retention in the joint structure when injected into mouse knee joints, compared with that of the free enzyme. However, the injected enzyme did not suppress the inflammation induced by antigens or zymosan but was instead reduced by catalase and peroxidase. These results were interpreted as an involvement of $H_2O_2$ as promoter of inflammation more than superoxide ions on these models[15,16].

## III. SURFACE PROTEIN CHARGE MODIFICATIONS

Superoxide dismutase was linked to Ficoll, a branched polymeric species with an average molecular weight of 70,000 Da, or to dextran, a linear polysaccharide with similar molecular weight, following cyanogen bromide activation. A dramatic increase in the circulating half time was observed upon modification which was increased from minutes for the native enzyme to 24 and 7 hrs for the Ficoll and dextran derivatives respectively[17,18].

Unfortunately the authors did not report the chemical characteristics of the two SOD derivatives such the degree of substitution, the presence or not of high molecular weight aggregates or the isoelectric point, which might explain the enhanced longevity of the derivatives.

The Ficoll–SOD enzyme intravenously administered was found to possess a significant anti-inflammatory activity on three animal models of inflammation, i.e. the reverse passive Arthus reaction, carrageenan-induced foot oedema in the rat and acute serum sickness glomerulonephritis in mouse. In these models neither Ficoll alone nor the native enzyme, at the same doses (10–24,000 U/kg), showed appreciable activity. The difference was therefore related to the presence in the circulation of the derivatized enzyme with a direct involvement as $O_2^{\cdot -}$ scavenger since catalase, or Ficoll–catalase, or mannitol, quencher of $H_2O_2$ or hydroxyl ions respectively, did not possess any anti-inflammatory activity.

The Ficoll–SOD complex completely suppressed the prostaglandin phase of carrageenan-induced oedema but had no effect on the initial phase of oedema mediated by serotonin, histamine and kinins.

307

Properties of Ficoll–superoxide dismutase conjugates such the sta-bility of the linkage in the body, were not reported. In this regard it is note-worthy that the release of insulin conjugated to Ficoll can occur by nucleophiles present in the circulation[19].

## IV. ALBUMIN–SOD CONJUGATES

Homologous albumin was used as a macromolecule to protect superoxide dismutase from degradation and attack by antibodies. Albumin presents sev-eral advantages as carrier since it may be easily obtained in large amounts as a product of blood processing and, when obtained from the same species, is devoid of antigenicity. However, the potential risk of viral contamination might be evident.

Albumin was covalently linked to superoxide dismutase by the amino groups specific glutaraldehyde reagent, a cross-linking agent extensively em-ployed in enzyme immobilization[20,21]. A limitation of the method is the possibility of forming cross-linked high molecular weight conjugates with variable number of both superoxide and albumin molecules joined together. This was revealed experimentally by the large range of molecular weight ad-ducts separated by gel filtration ranging from $0.7 \times 10^5$ Da to over $3.5 \times 10^5$ Da. As expected, the derivatives with different mass possess large pharma-cokinetic differences. The half life of clearance from circulation of the dis-mutase activity ranged from 2.6 to 15 hrs for the low and high molecular weight materials respectively. In neither case were linear kinetics of clear-ance obtained[22]. However, when the clearance from the circulation was as-sessed by radioactivity using $^{125}I_2$-labelled albumin, non-linear kinetics were obtained which were generally more rapid than that found using enzyme ac-tivity as parameters. The authors suggest that the absence of correlation among the two methods depends upon the fact that by the glutaraldehyde method of coupling results in the formation of albumin–albumin adducts. These are devoid of superoxide activity but are revealed by the presence of radioactively labelled material which may have a different fate in the body as compared to the SOD–albumin adducts. The apparent rapid clearance may also result from $^{125}I_2$ released from the conjugates. The anti-inflammatory potency of the albumin-conjugate SOD, assessed by the inhibition of carra-geenan-induced paw oedema, is superior to that of non-conjugated SOD. The half maximally effective dose appeared to fall between 400–800 U/kg while, to reach a much lower inhibition level, the dose for the free SOD was 3,300 U/kg. For the Ficoll derivative the half maximal inhibition was in contrast observed to be 180 U/kg[17,18].

An increased localization of the derivatives in the inflamed paws was also demonstrated by radioactivity evaluation.

The albumin–SOD did not react with SOD antibodies and presents a reduced immunogenicity in rabbits towards native SOD as assessed by the precipitating method.

## V. PEG–SOD CONJUGATES

Polyethylene glycol, a non toxic, biocompatible polymer has very peculiar properties as a result of the flexibility of its chain and it amphipathic character[23,24]. Once bound to a macromolecule or to other surface[25] the hydrated PEG chains (one-O-CH$_2$-CH$_2$- unit may co-ordinate several water molecules) may act as a screen towards any approaching macromolecule such blood components, antibodies or cells, while the hydrophobic character of PEG itself may facilitate cell interaction (PEG is used in cell fusion) or make a peptide or protein soluble in apolar solvents (PEG-enzymes may be used as biocatalysts in organic solvents)[26].

The use of such polymer to change the pharmacokinetic properties of proteins comes from the reports of Abuchowski *et al.*[27] who described the reduction in antigenicity, increased resistance to proteolytic digestion, reduced clearance from the circulation as well as changes in the properties of some PEG-protein adducts[27,28]. The method of coupling proposed by these authors did not however appear convenient when applied to the formation of SOD-adducts because of the toxicity of the reagent used in the activation and the possibility of cross-linking[29]. Superoxide dismutase was derivatized with PEG using the original method of coupling[29,30], by carbonyldiimidazole[31], trichlorophenyl-chloroformate[32,33] or active esters[34]. PEG derivatization is accompanied by a dramatic increase in half-life which, in contrast to 6 mins for the native enzyme, was prolonged to 15–16 hrs in mice when PEG extensively modified SOD (19 amino grups with linked polymer over the 20 present in the enzyme) was used[30]. In this case, the enzyme which was modified with trichlorotriazine activated PEG, retained 51% of the dismutase activity.

Similar results were reported in rats. The half-life of clearance from circulation is about 30 hrs with the PEG-modified enzyme[29,31,35]. A detailed study of the influence of the derivatization on the time of clearance showed that the clearance is dependent upon the number of linked PEG molecules as well as on the molecular weight of the polymer. Half lives of the polymer derivatives ranged from 1 to 30 hrs for variously modified species[29].

The derivatization reduced the antigenicity of the enzyme, as assessed by the antigen-precipitation test[32], as well as its immunogenicity as verified by the absence of a reduction in clearance time following repeated administration[30]. A detailed study based on the evaluation by ELISA of the antibody titres in mice revealed that the PEG–SOD has a decreased immunogenicity compared to free SOD, since titres of the order of 0.03–0.07% were found. The modified enzyme on the other hand retained the ability to react with preformed antibody to free SOD whereas the antisera raised to PEG–SOD did not react with free form[36].

The anti-inflammatory activity of PEG enzyme, studied using the cotton twine assay on rats showed a slightly improved activity as compared to the native enzyme; the difference in activity among the two samples being observed at high doses[30]. Carrageenan-induced oedema was also used to test the ability of SOD modified with 3 or 18 PEG chains for enzyme molecule. On this model native SOD was almost inactive as an anti-inflammatory agent while both SOD–PEG preparations caused a statistically significant inhibition which was higher for the more extensively modified enzyme. The higher activity of SOD–PEG-18 is parallel with the increase in retention in blood of this derivative[35]. The dose used in this investigation was 5,000 U/kg. The same derivatives were also tested for their anti-inflammatory activity in carrageenan pleurisy in rats at a dose of 3,500 U/kg. Again appreciable anti-inflammatory activity was observed with the long half-life derivative. In parallel with its presence in blood the activity was found to last for more than 24 hrs[34]. The derivatized enzyme diffused into pleural exudate as revealed by the change in time of the exudate/plasma SOD concentration ratio. PEG–SOD used for this study was prepared according to an original and rapid method based on the PEG activation with trichlorophenylchloroformate to give a phenylcarbonate which is reactive towards the protein amino groups. This method of modification allows an extensive enzyme modification with limited activity loss (20–25%).

In another animal model of inflammation, the adjuvant arthritis, SOD–PEG administered i.p. alone or with PEG-catalase, three times a week, did not show significant effects compared with untreated controls[37].

The PEG modified SOD was found to possess limited toxicity when administered at high doses in mice ($50 \times 10^3$ U/kg), or in rats, for five times a week for 3 months, at doses of $10–25 \times 10^3$ U/kg. It was found that the administration did not affect survival rate, appearance, behaviour, and food intake. Only massive doses of PEG–SOD resulted in vacuolation in splenic macrophages in rats[38].

## VI. SOD ENCAPSULATED INTO LIPOSOMES

Encapsulation into liposomes was studied as a method to deliver SOD to lung cells. Liposomes are in fact considered as efficient transmembrane vectors in addition to possess specific organ recognition.

Liposome-entrapped SOD (SOD–LIP) has a circulating half-life of 4 h with respect to the free form[37] which is however much lower than that observed in the enzyme covalently bound to polymers.

SOD concentration in the lung is increased when administered i.v. into liposome but not when administered as free enzyme[40]. Furthermore, only the encapsulated enzyme gives increased survival time in rats exposed to the toxic effects of 100% oxygen. This effect is accompanied by reduction in fluid volume in the pleural cavity and increased lung weight.

Other authors have shown that similar protective effects are obtained by intratracheal administration to rats of liposome encapsulated SOD or catalase separately thus providing a basis for the therapeutic intervention in the hyperoxic lung via inhalation[41].

Some pathological conditions that could benefit by SOD-liposome treatment are detailed by Michelson in a recent review[42]. At the moment most advanced clinical studies are being performed in Japan, where results have been obtained in Behçet as well as Crohn's disease and in rheumatoid arthritis.

LIP–SOD was recently used to treat patients with Kawasaki disease. An improvement in clinical signs was found as compared with conventional aspirin treatment[43].

The method of SOD delivery based on liposomes entrapment has the drawback from the decreased neutrophil bacterial activity both *in vitro* and *in vivo* against *Staphylococcus aureus*[44]. The effect appears related to the liposomes themselves since it also occurs with liposomes devoid of SOD. This result, which suggests a reduction in the defence mechanism of the host, was not observed when PEG was used to improve the activity and delivery of SOD.

## VII. CONCLUSIONS

Limitations for Orgotein therapy such as immunological response or short duration of action, are completely overcome by the chemical modifications to SOD reported here. The large reduction in immunogenicity and antigenicity by PEG conjugation is of particular importance also in relation to the observed immunological reaction still present in homologous proteins obtained by recombinant DNA technologies[45].

The increase in half-life which was observed following polymer conjugation was so dramatic that a reduction of such effect may be considered more desirable. However, as reported above, enzyme species with different circulation time may be obtained by a proper choice of the polymer or of the degree of substitution.

The real problem still existing with SOD derivatives seems to reside on the optimization of the therapeutic doses as well as of the schedule of therapy for the different pathologies. This of course requires a detailed investigation of pharmacokinetics of the conjugates in animals as well in man following various routes of administration. A study of the fate of SOD conjugates in the body may also be of interest.

A reinvestigation of the effectiveness of SOD treatment on some models of inflammation must also be carried out mainly in relation to the criticisms recently reported into literature.

We finally suggest the usefulness of SOD derivatives that, with their different patterns of distribution and pharmacokinetics with respect to the native enzyme, may help in the understanding of the still unresolved question of the anti-inflammatory mechanism of superoxide dismutase.

# References

1.  Huber, W, Schulte, TL, Carson, S, Goldhammer, RE and Vogin, EE (1968). Some chemical and pharmacological properties of a novel anti-inflammatory protein. *Toxicol Appl Pharmacol*, **12**, 308
2.  McCord, JM and Fridovich, I (1969). Superoxide dismutase, an enzymatic function for erythrocuprein. *J Biol Chem*, **244**, 6049–55
3.  Huber, W, Nenander-Huber, KB, Saifer, MGP and Dang, PHC (1977). Studies on the clinical and laboratory pharmacology of drug formulations of bovine Cu-Zn superoxide dismutases (orgotein). In: Willoughby, DA, Giroud, JP and Velo GP (Eds), *Perspectives in Inflammation*, pp. 527–44. (Lancaster: MTP Press)
4.  Edsmyr, F, Huber, W and Nenander-Huber, KB (1976). Orgotein efficacy in ameliorating side effects due to radiation therapy: I double-blind, placebo-controlled trial in patients with bladder tumors. *Curr Ther Res*, **19(2)**, 198–211
5.  Tetsuo, A, Makamoto, F, Yoshimasa, I, Kazuyuki, H, Mamoru, S and Katsuhito, S (1966). Effect of superoxide dismutase on glomerual nephritis. *Biochem Pharmacol*, **35(2)**, 341–5
6.  Huhn-Edholm, M, Ostling, E and Fellenius, E (1986). Superoxide dismutase enhances recovery following myocardial ischemia/reperfusion *in vivo* and *in vitro*. In: Rotilio, G (ed), *Superoxide and Superoxide Dismutase in Chemistry, Biology and Medicine*, pp. 591–3. (Amsterdam, New York, Oxford: Elsevier Science Publisher)
7.  Lund-Olesen, K and Menander, KB (1974). Orgotein: A new anti-inflammatory metalloprotein drug: preliminary evaluation of clinical efficacy and safety in degenerative joint disease. *Curr Ther Res*, **7**, 706–17
8.  Menander-Huber, KB and Huber, W (1980). Orgotein, the drug version of bovine Cu–Zn superoxide dismutase II. A summary account of clinical trials in man and animals. In: Michelson, AM, McCord, JM and Fridovich, I (eds), *Superoxide and Superoxide Dismutase*, pp. 537–549 (London, New York, San Francisco: Academic Press)
9.  Goebel, KM and Storck, V (1983). Effect of intra-articular orgotein versus a corticosteroid on rheumatoid arthritis of the knee. *Am J Med*, **74**, 124–8
10. Marberger, H, Huber, W, Bartsch, G, Schulte, T and Swoboda, P (1974). Orgotein: a new anti-inflammatory metalloprotein drug evaluation of clinical efficacy and safety in inflammatory conditions of the urinary tract. *Int Urol Nephrol*, **6(2)**, 61–74
11. Wilsmann, KM (1986). Ten years of clinical experience with SOD treatment of inflammatory disorders. In: Rotilio, G (ed), *Superoxide and Superoxide Dismutase in Chemistry, Biology and Medicine*, pp. 500–5. (Amsterdam, New York, Oxford: Elsevier Science Publishers)
12. Greenwald, RA (1985). Therapeutic benefits of oxygen radical scavenger treatments remain unproven. *J Free Rad Biol Med*, **1**, 173–7
13. Giri, SN and Misra, HP (1984). Fate of superoxide dismutase in mice following oral route of administration. *Med Biol*, **62**, 285–9
14. Holcenberg, JS, Schmer, G, Teller, DC and Roberts, J (1975). Biologic and physical properties of succinilated and glycosylated Acinetobacter glutaminase-asparaginase. *J Biol Chem*, **250**, 4165–70
15. Van den Berg, WB, Schalkwijk, J, Joosten, LAB and Van de Putte, LBA (1985). Experimental allergic arthritis in mice: effects of local enzyme therapy with native and cationic derivatives. *Agents Actions*, **17**, 350–1
16. Schalkwijk, J, Van den Berg, WB, Van de Putte, LBA, Joosten, LAB and Van den Bersselaar, LJ (1985). Cationization of catalase, peroxidase and superoxide dismutase. *J Clin Invest*, **76**, 198–205
17. McCord, JM, Stokes, SH and Wong, K (1979). Superoxide radical as a phagocyte-produced chemical mediator of inflammation. In: Weissmann, G (ed), *Advances in Inflammation Research*, Vol. 1, pp. 273–80. (New York: Raven Press)

18. McCord, JM and Wong, K (1979). Phagocyte-produced free radicals: roles in cyto-toxicity and inflammation. In: *Oxygen Free Radicals and Tissue Damage, Ciba Foundation Symposium*, Vol. 65, pp. 343–60. (Amsterdam, Oxford, New York: Excerpta Medica)

19. Topper, YJ, Oka, T, Vanderhaar, BK and Wilchek, M (1975). Characterization of super-active insulin, prolactin and placental lactogen. *Biochim Biophis Res Comm*, **66**, 793–8

20. Broun, GB (1976). Chemically aggregated enzymes. *Methods Enzymol*, **44**, 263–80

21. Quiocho, FA (1976). Immobilized proteins in single crystals. *Methods Enzymol*, **44**, 546–58

22. Wong, K, Cleland, LG and Poznanski, MJ (1980). Enhanced anti-inflammatory effects and reduced immunogenicity of bovine liver superoxide dismutase by conjugation with homologous albumin. *Agents Actions*, **10**, 231–9

23. Topchieva, IN (1980). Biochemical applications of poly(ethyleneglycol). *Russian Chem Rev*, **43**, 260–71

24. Ahe, A and Mark, JE (1980). Conformational energies and the random coil dimension and dipole moments of the polyoxides. *J Am Chem Soc*, **98**, 6468–76

25. Nogooka, S, Mori, Y, Takiuchi, H, Yokota, K, Tanzawa, H and Nishiumi, S (1984). Interaction between blood component and hydrogel with poly(oxyethylene) chains. In: Sholoby, SW, Hoffman, AS, Ratner, BD and Horbett, TA (eds), *Polymers as Biomaterials*, pp. 361–74. (New York: Plenum Press)

26. Inada, YI, Takahoshi, K, Yoshimoto, T, Ajima, A, Matsushima, A and Saito, Y (1986). Application of polyethylene glycol-modified enzymes in biotechnological processes: organic solvent soluble enzymes. *Trends Biotech*, **7**, 190–4

27. Abuchowski, A, Van Es, T, Palczuk, NC and Davis, FF (1977). Alteration of immunological properties of bovin serum albumin by covalent attachment of polyethylene glycol. *J Biol Chem*, **252**, 3578–81

28. Abuchowski, A, McCoy, JR, Palczuk, NC, Van Es, T and Davis, FF (1977). Effect of covalent attachment of polyethylene glycol on immunogenicity and circulation life of bovine liver catalase. *J Biol Chem*, **252**, 3582–6

29. Boccù, E, Velo, GP and Veronese, FM (1982). Pharmacokinetic properties of polyethylene glycol derivatized superoxide dismutase. *Pharmacol Res Commun*, **14**, 113–20

30. Pyatak, PS, Abuchowski, A and Davis, FF (1980). Preparation of a polyethylene glycol: superoxide dismutase adduct, and an examination of its blood circulating life and anti-inflammatory activity. *Res Commun Chem Pathol Pharmacol*, **29**, 113–27

31. Beauchamp, CD, Gonias, SL, Menapace, DP and Pizzo, S (1983). A new procedure for the synthesis of polyethylene glycol-protein adducts: effects on function, receptor recognition and clearance of superoxide dismutase, lactoferrin and β-2-macroglobulin. *Anal Biochem*, **131**, 25–33

32. Veronese, FM, Largajolli, R, Boccù, E, Benassi, CA and Schiavon, O (1985). Surface modification of proteins; activation of monomethoxy-polyethylene glycol by phenilchloroformates and modification of ribonuclease and superoxide dismutase. *Appl Biochem Biotechnol*, **11**, 141–52

33. Conforti, A, Marrella, M, Milanino, R, Moretti, U, Velo, GP, Largajolli, R, Veronese, FM, Boccù, E and Schiavon, O (1986). Anti-inflammatory properties of superoxide dismutase derivatives (SOD-PEG-3 and SOD-PEG-18) in carrageenan pleurisy. In: Rotilio, G (ed), *Superoxide and Superoxide Dismutase in Chemistry Biology and Medicine*, pp. 532–4. (Amsterdam, New York, Oxford: Elsevier Sciences Publishers).

34. Conforti, A, Franco, L, Milanino, R, Velo, GP, Boccù, E, Largajolli, R, Schiavon, O and Veronese, FM (1987). PEG superoxide dismutase derivatives: anti-inflammatory activity in carrageenan pleurisy in rats. *Pharmacol Res Commun*, **19**, 187–94

35. Veronese, FM, Boccù, E, Schiavon, O, Velo, GP, Conforti, A, Franco, L and Milanino, R (1983). Anti-inflammatory and pharmacokinetic properties of superoxide dismutase derivatized with polyethylene glycol via active esters. *J Pharm Pharmacol*, **35**, 757–8

36. Nucci, ML, Olejarczyk, J and Abuchowski, A (1986). Immunogenicity of polyethylene glycol-modified superoxide dismutase and catalase. *J Free Rad Biol Med*, **2**, 321–5

37. Greenwald, RA (1986). Treatment of inflammatory arthritis with oxygen radical scavengers. *J Free Rad Biol Med*, **2**, 367–8

38. Viau, AT, Abuchowski, A, Greenspan, S and Davis, FF (1986). Safety evaluation of free radical scavengers PEG-catalase and PEG-superoxide dismutase. *J Free Rad Biol Med*, **2**, 283–8

39. Turrens, JF, Crapo, JD and Freeman, BA (1984). Protection against oxygen toxicity by intravenous injection of liposome-entrapped catalase and superoxide dismutase. *J Clin Invest*, **73**, 87–95

40. Freeman, BA, Turrens, JF, Mirza, Z, Crapo, JD and Young, SL (1985). Modulation of oxidant lung injury by using liposome-entrapped superoxide dismutase and catalase. *Fed Proc*, **44**, 2591–5

41. Pradmanabhan, RV, Gudapaty, R, Liener, IE, Schwartz, BA and Hoidal, JR (1985). Protection against pulmonary oxygen toxicity in rats by the intratracheal administration of liposome-encapsulated superoxide dismutase or catalse. *Am Rev Respir Dis*, **132**, 164–7

42. Michelson, AM, Puget, K and Durosay, P (1985). La superoxyde dismutase et la pathologie des radicaux libres. *CR Soc Biol*, **179**, 429–39

43. Somiya, K, Niwa, K, Shimoda, K, Fukami, S, Puget, K and Michelson, M (1986). Treatment with liposomal superoxide dismutase of patients with Kawasaki disease. In: Rotilio, G (ed), *Superoxide and Superoxide Dismutase in Chemistry Biology and Medicine*, pp. 513–6. (Amsterdam, New York, Oxford: Elsevier Science Publisher)

44. McDonald, RJ, Berger, EM, White, CW, White, JC, Freeman, PA and Resine, JE (1985). Effects of superoxide dismutase encapsulated in liposomes or conjugated with polyethylene glycol on neutrophil bactericidal activity *in vitro* and bacterial clearance *in vivo*. *Am Rev Respir Dis*, **13**, 633–7

45. Thorner, MO, Reschke, J, Chitwood, J, Rogol, AD, Furlanetto, R, Rivier, J, Vale, W and Blizzard, RM (1985). Development of antibody to growth hormone-releasing factor. *N Engl J Med*, **312**, 994

# Index

Note the abbreviations used: NSAIDs (non-steroid anti-inflammatory drugs)

315